Step-Up To USMLE Step 2

Step-Up Series Editors

Samir Mehta, MD
Resident, Department of Orthopaedic Surgery
University of Pennsylvania Health System
Philadelphia, Pennsylvania

Adam J. Mirarchi, MD
Resident, Department of Orthopaedics
Case Western Reserve University
Cleveland, Ohio

Lieutenant Edmund A. Milder, MD
Staff Pediatrician and General Medical Officer
Naval Branch Health Clinic
La Maddalena, Italy

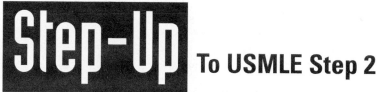

Step-Up To USMLE Step 2

Jonathan P. Van Kleunen, MD

Resident, Department of Orthopaedic Surgery
The Hospital of the University of Pennsylvania
University of Pennsylvania Health System
Philadelphia, PA

LIPPINCOTT WILLIAMS & WILKINS
A **Wolters Kluwer** Company

Philadelphia • Baltimore • New York • London
Buenos Aires • Hong Kong • Sydney • Tokyo

Acquisitions Editor: Donna Balado
Developmental Editor: Nancy Winter and Dvora Konstant
Marketing Manager: Emilie Linkins
Associate Production Manager: Kevin P. Johnson
Designer: Holly McLaughlin
Compositor: TechBooks
Printer: Courier/Kendallville

Printed in the United States of America

Library of Congress Cataloging-in-Publication Data

Van Kleunen, Jonathan P.
  Step-up to USMLE Step 2 / Jonathan P. Van Kleunen.
    p. ; cm.
  Includes bibliographical references and index.
  ISBN 0-7817-5792-4 (alk. paper)
  1. Clinical medicine—Examinations, questions, etc.   2. Physicians—Licenses—
United States—Examinations—Study guides.   I. Title.
  [DNLM: 1. Clinical Medicine—United States—Outlines.   W 18.2 V258s 2006]
RC58.V36   2006
616'.0076—dc22   2005009452

To purchase additional copies of this book, call our customer service department at
(800) 638-3030 or fax orders to **(301) 824-7390**. International customers should call
(301) 714-2324.

Visit Lippincott Williams & Wilkins on the Internet: http://www.LWW.com.
Lippincott Williams & Wilkins customer service representatives are available from
8:30 am to 6:00 pm, EST.

05 06 07 08
1 2 3 4 5 6 7 8 9 10

To my wife, Amy, for her patience, encouragement, and inspiration

To my parents, William and Patricia, and my siblings, Andrew and Nancy, for their support over the years

To all of my teachers, for passing on their knowledge to this generation of physicians

Reviewers

Todd Berland
Medical College of Georgia,
    Class of 2003
Augusta, Georgia

Lisa M. L. Dryer
University of Minnesota Medical School,
    Class of 2003
Minneapolis, Minnesota

Peter F. Kratz
University of Maryland School of Medicine,
    Class of 2004
Baltimore, Maryland

Ajoy Kumar
Ross University School of Medicine,
    Class of 2004
Roseau, Commonwealth of Dominica,
    West Indies

Caren M. Stalburg, MD
Clinical Assistant Professor
Obstetrics and Gynecology
University of Michigan Medical School
Ann Arbor, Michigan

Contents

Preface

In the past several years, the USMLE Step 2 has increased in its importance for measuring clinical acumen during medical school, increasing competitiveness during residency applications, and assessing preparedness for beginning residency. Perception of the role of the USMLE Step 2 in residency applications has changed, and more emphasis is being placed on this exam as a component of the medical student's application. A high Step 2 score can make up for a disappointing Step 1 score, but likewise, a low Step 2 score can reflect negatively on an applicant. Despite this test's increased importance, there is a lack of succinct, efficient, and thorough review texts universally recommended for Step 2 preparation.

Step-Up to USMLE Step 2 builds on the foundation of *Step-Up* and *Step-Up to the Bedside*. The text is designed to present a collection of "high-yield" facts required for the USMLE Step 2 in an easily accessible format. The format is organized according to medical specialties to allow the reader to focus on a particular subject during test preparation. It is designed to utilize a variety of approaches including text, images, tables, and diagrams. Each manner of presentation was selected with the intention of presenting material in a concise yet informative way. By including high-yield information, this book allows the reader to focus on the most relevant facts for test day. The "Quick Hits" found throughout the text are frequently tested facts that deserve particular attention. The "Next Steps" describe steps along the decision-making tree between clinical presentation to diagnosis and treatment and guide the reader through the workup of a patient. This organization was designed to help the reader get the most out of studying in a limited amount of time. Furthermore, the text is to be used as a bridge between the Step 2 examination and the Clinical Skills Assessment.

Please feel free to forward comments to me at *Step-Up@lww.com*. Best of luck in preparing for test day, because you are one step closer to the practice and art of medicine.

Jonathan Van Kleunen

Acknowledgments

I would like to extend thanks to the reviewers whose suggestions helped shape this book. Special thanks go to Samir Mehta for providing direction throughout the writing of this book and to Matt Chansky for his illustrations. I would like to extend a hand of gratitude to Emilie Linkins, Neil Marquardt, and Nancy Winter at Lippincott Williams & Wilkins for their planning and editing of this edition.

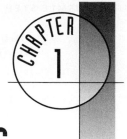

Cardiovascular Disorders

I. Normal cardiac anatomy, physiology, and function

A. **Cardiac and coronary artery anatomy** (see Figure 1-1)

B. **Cardiac cycle** (see Figure 1-2)

C. **Cardiac output (CO)**

1. **Heart rate (HR)**

   a. Beginning of one cardiac cycle to the beginning of the next

   b. If HR is too high (normal = 60–100 bpm), then diastolic filling is decreased

2. **Stroke volume (SV)**

   a. SV is the **change in blood volume** from **before contraction to after**

   b. It is determined by **contractility** (force with which heart contracts), **preload** (amount of myocardial stretch at end of diastole), and **afterload** (resistance ventricles must overcome to empty their contents)

   c. **SV is increased** with catecholamine release, an **increase** in intracellular Ca, a **decrease** in extracellular Na, digoxin use, anxiety, and exercise

   d. **SV is decreased** with β-blockers, heart failure, acidosis, and hypoxia

3. **Fick principle—CO = SV $\times$ HR** = (rate of O_2 use)/(arterial O_2 content – venous O_2 content)

   a. Rate of O_2 use can be determined by comparing O_2 content in expired air to that in inhaled air; arterial and venous O_2 content can be measured directly from the corresponding vasculature

   b. CO increases during exercise, initially by increasing SV and later by increasing HR

4. **Mean arterial pressure** = CO $\times$ total peripheral resistance (TPR) = diastolic arterial pressure + 1/3 pulse pressure

5. **Pulse pressure** = systolic arterial pressure – diastolic arterial pressure

D. **Electrocardiogram (ECG) (see Figure 1-3)**

1. Measures flow of electrical impulses through the heart to provide information regarding **cardiac function**

2. Reviewing an ECG (a consistent order of analysis is useful for picking up abnormalities)

   a. Check calibration on tracing

   b. Rhythm (regular, irregular, pathognomonic signs?)

   c. Rate (normal, tachycardia, bradycardia?)

   d. Intervals (PR, QRS, ST)

   e. QRS axis (normal, deviated?)

   f. P wave (normal, abnormal?)

   g. QRS complex (normal, hypertrophy, widened, infarction?)

   h. ST segment and T wave (normal, depressed, elevated, inverted?)

3. Morphology of action potentials varies with location in the heart (see Figure 1-4)

 The **left anterior descending artery** is the most common site of coronary artery occlusion.

 In 10% of patients, the posterior descending artery derives from the left coronary artery.

 Coronary arteries fill during **diastole**, while systemic arteries fill during **systole**; conditions or drugs that reduce diastolic filling allow less coronary perfusion.

CARDIOVASCULAR DISORDERS

FIGURE 1-1 **A.** Anterior and posterior views of the heart. LA, left atrium; LV, left ventricle; RA, right atrium; RV, right ventricle; SVC, superior vena cava. **B.** Coronary artery hierarchy and regions of the heart supplied by branches. AV, atrioventricular; SA, sinoatrial.

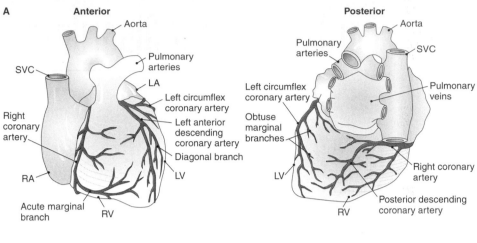

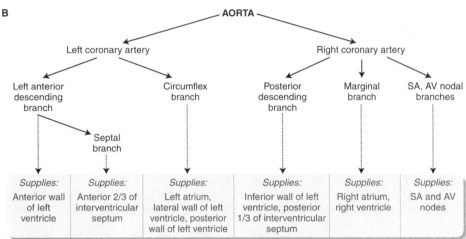

(Modified from Lilly LS. *Pathophysiology of Heart Disease.* 2nd Ed. Baltimore: Williams & Wilkins; 1998. Used with permission of Lippincott Williams & Wilkins.)

II. Ischemic heart disease

A. Brief introduction to ischemic heart disease

1. **Inadequate** supply of O_2 for a given myocardial demand leads to **myocardial hypoxia** and an accumulation of waste products

2. The vast majority of cases of ischemic heart disease arise from **atherosclerosis of the coronary arteries (coronary artery disease, or CAD)**

B. **Atherosclerosis**

1. Gradual narrowing of arteries due to formation of plaques (which consist of lipids and smooth muscle)

2. Plaques may calcify, rupture and thrombose leading to further narrowing of arteries and progressive occlusion of blood flow

3. **History and Physical (H/P)** = asymptomatic for most of disease progression; later sequelae include angina, claudication, progressive hypertension (HTN), retinal changes, extra heart sounds, myocardial infarction (MI), and stroke

4. **Labs** = stress testing, echocardiography, nuclear studies, or angiography may be used to detect ischemic heart disease

FIGURE 1-2 **A.** Pressure relationships between left-sided heart chambers, and timing with normal heart sounds and the electrocardiogram for one full cardiac cycle. **B.** Normal left ventricular pressure-volume loop for one full cardiac cycle. AV, aortic valve; ECG, electrocardiogram; LA, left atrium; LV, left ventricle; MV, mitral valve.

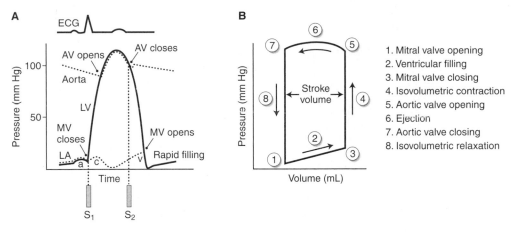

(Modified from Lilly LS. *Pathophysiology of Heart Disease.* 2nd Ed. Baltimore: Williams & Wilkins; 1998. Used with permission of Lippincott Williams & Wilkins.)

a. Exercise stress test—patient exercises on an aerobic fitness machine at increasingly strenuous workloads; heart rate and ECG are constantly monitored; test is continued until patient develops angina or signs of ischemia are seen on ECG; ischemic heart disease is diagnosed with signs of **reproducible angina** or obvious signs of **ischemia at low workloads**

b. Nuclear exercise test—thallium-201 or technetium-99m-sestamibi is injected during exercise testing, and scintigraphy is performed to assess myocardial perfusion; used in cases of suspected ischemic heart disease in which results of regular exercise stress testing is equivocal

c. Exercise stress test with echocardiography—exercise stress testing performed in conjunction with echocardiography to increase sensitivity of detecting myocardial ischemia

d. Pharmacologic stress testing—administration of cardiac inotropes in place of exercise to increase myocardial demand; performed in patients for whom comorbidities interfere with ability to perform exercise

FIGURE 1-3 General structure of the electrocardiogram tracing and significance of specific regions. AV, atrioventricular.

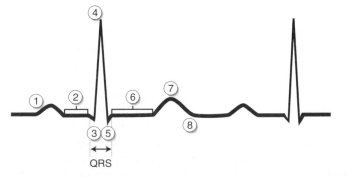

1. P wave–atrial depolarization
2. PR interval–conduction through AV node (< 0.2 sec)
3. Q wave ⎤ QRS complex–
4. R wave ⎬ ventricular depolarization;
5. S wave ⎦ < 0.12 sec
6. ST segment–isoelectric ventricular contraction
7. T wave–ventricular repolarization
8. U wave–relative hypokalemia

(Modified from Lilly LS. *Pathophysiology of Heart Disease.* 2nd Ed. Baltimore: Williams & Wilkins; 1998. Used with permission of Lippincott Williams & Wilkins.)

FIGURE 1-4 Morphology of action potentials at different locations along the conduction pathways of the heart and their relation to the electrocardiogram. AV, atrioventricular; SA, sinoatrial.

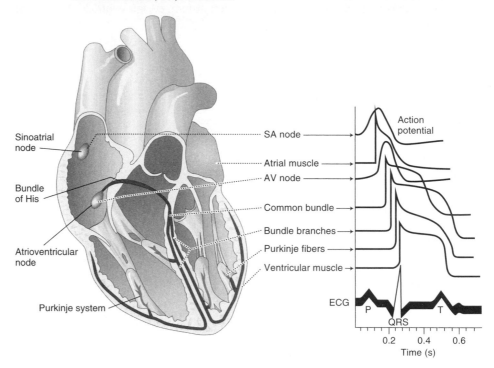

e. Coronary angiography—gold standard for identifying CAD, but more invasive than other techniques

5. **Treatment** = management is primarily intended to minimize risk factors (including tobacco use, HTN, hyperglycemia, hypercholesterolemia); diet low in fats and cholesterol and high in antioxidants (vitamins E and C and β-carotene) is helpful in preventing disease

C. **Hypercholesterolemia**

1. Abnormal serum cholesterol levels (**high** low-density lipoprotein [**LDL**] and/or **low** high-density lipoprotein [**HDL**]) associated with increased risk of ischemic heart disease

2. May be due to congenital disorder or acquired condition

3. **Normal cholesterol physiology**
   a. Cholesterols and triglycerides are carried by lipoproteins
   b. Increased LDL leads to increased CAD risk; increased HDL is protective
   c. Increased LDL and decreased HDL result from diet high in fatty foods, tobacco use, obesity, alcohol use, diabetes mellitus (DM), and certain medications (oral contraceptive pills [OCPs], diuretics)

4. **H/P** = usually asymptomatic; extremely high triglycerides and LDL lead to xanthomas (lipid deposits in tendons), xanthelasmas (lipid deposits in eyelids), and cholesterol emboli in retina (visible on fundoscopic examination); symptoms are more severe and appear earlier in life in primary disorders compared to acquired conditions

5. **Labs** = increased total cholesterol and LDL; possible decreased HDL; total cholesterol may be > 300–600 mg/dL in primary disorders; screening for hyperlipidemia is performed in men > 35 yr old and women > 45 yr old (earlier ages if family history of congenital condition)

6. **Treatment** = focuses on **prevention** of cardiovascular disease and includes tobacco cessation, exercise, and dietary restrictions (such as low

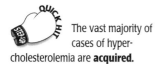
The vast majority of cases of hyper-cholesterolemia are **acquired.**

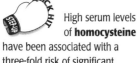
High serum levels of **homocysteine** have been associated with a three-fold risk of significant atherosclerosis.

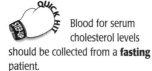
Blood for serum cholesterol levels should be collected from a **fasting** patient.

FIGURE 1-5 Decision tree for screening for hypercholesterolemia. CAD, coronary artery disease; DM, diabetes mellitus; HDL, high-density lipoprotein; HTN, hypertension; LDL, low-density lipoprotein.

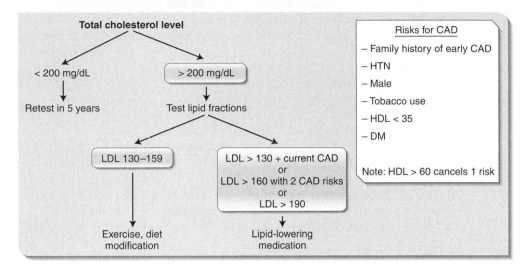

fat and low cholesterol); cholesterol-lowering medications are used in patients with increased cardiac risk

D. **Angina pectoris**
1. **Etiology**
   a. **Temporary myocardial ischemia** during exertion that causes chest pain
   b. Most commonly due to **CAD;** also occurs secondary to arterial vasospasm (Prinzmetal's angina) and valvular disease
   c. Gastroesophageal reflux disease (GERD) and esophageal spasm may mimic symptoms
2. **H/P — substernal chest pain** that may radiate to left shoulder, arm, jaw, or back

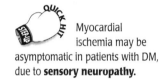 Myocardial ischemia may be asymptomatic in patients with DM, due to **sensory neuropathy.**

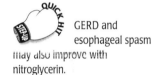 GERD and esophageal spasm may also improve with nitroglycerin.

TABLE 1-1 Lipid-Lowering Agents

Drug	Site of Action	Effect on LDL	Effect on HDL	Effect on Triglycerides	Side Effects
Fibric acids (gemfibrozil, fenofibrate)	Blood (all stimulate lipoprotein lipase)	↓	↑	↓↓↓	Myositis, increased LFTs (must monitor)
Bile acid sequestrants (cholestyramine, colestipol, colesevelam)	GI tract	↓↓	—	—/↑	Bad taste, GI upset
Niacin	Liver	↓↓	↑↑	↓	Facial flushing
HMG-CoA reductase inhibitors (e.g., lovastatin, pravastatin, simvastatin)	Liver	↓↓↓	↑	↓	Myositis, increased LFTs (must monitor)

GI, gastrointestinal; HDL, high-density lipoprotein; LDL, low-density lipoprotein; LFTs, liver function tests; ↑ = Increased; ↑↑ = More increased; ↑↑↑ = Most increased;—/↑ = Normal or increased.

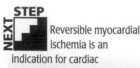

NEXT STEP
Reversible myocardial ischemia is an indication for cardiac catheterization to assess need for PTCA or CABG.

3. **Labs** = stress testing or nuclear studies used for diagnosis
   a. Important in assessment of chest pain
   b. Seeks to increase cardiac workload to assess myocardial ischemia
   c. Accomplished either through exercise or pharmacologic testing
4. **Treatment = sublingual nitroglycerin** and rest; full work-up (including stress testing or nuclear studies) for cause is needed to define long-term treatment

E. **Unstable angina**
   1. **Worsening angina** that occurs at rest
   2. Frequently due to **plaque rupture,** hemorrhage, or thrombosis in coronary arteries
   3. 1/3 of patients have an MI within three years
   4. **H/P** = angina with worse pain and increased frequency than in past; **symptoms occur at rest;** less responsive to prior treatment regimens
   5. **ECG = ST depression,** T wave flattening or inversion
   6. Any patient suspected of having an MI must be worked up in a hospital setting with an ECG and serial cardiac enzymes
   7. **Treatment** = seeks to relieve cause of ischemia and decrease myocardial O_2 demand
      a. **Pharmacotherapy** = aspirin (ASA), O_2, nitroglycerin, and β-blockers initially; calcium-channel blockers and angiotensin converting enzyme inhibitors (ACE-I) are additional useful medications
      b. **Percutaneous transluminal coronary angioplasty (PTCA)**
         (1) Suggested in cases that are nonresponsive to medications
         (2) Catheter inserted through femoral or brachial artery and maneuvered through heart to stenotic vessel
         (3) Balloon on catheter inflated to dilate stenosis
         (4) Catheters may also be used for arthrectomy (plaque is shaved by burr on catheter) or stent placement (intravascular support structure)
      c. **Coronary artery bypass grafting (CABG)**
         (1) Considered for left main stenosis > 50%, 3-vessel disease, or history of CAD and DM
         (2) Donor vessel grafted to coronary artery to bypass obstruction
         (3) Saphenous vein and internal mammary artery are most commonly used

F. **Myocardial infarction (MI)**
   1. **Tissue death** resulting from ischemia caused by **occlusion of coronary vessels** or **vasospasm;** often secondary to thrombus formation following plaque rupture
   2. **Risk factors** = increased age, HTN, hypercholesterolemia, family history of CAD, DM, and tobacco use; males > females; postmenopausal females > pre-menopausal females
   3. **H/P** = chest pain ("elephant on chest") in distribution similar to episodes of angina; possible shortness of breath, diaphoresis, nausea and vomiting; exam may include tachycardia, decreased blood pressure, pulmonary rales, new S_4, and new systolic murmur
   4. **ECG = ST elevation** and T wave changes; possible new arrhythmia, left bundle branch block (LBBB), or Q wave changes
   5. **Labs** = serial cardiac enzymes
      a. Changes in enzymes in the initial **24 hr** after MI are helpful for making a diagnosis of acute infarction, so enzymes are measured every 8 hr in the first 24 hr after presentation (three sets total)
      b. Creatine phosphokinase myocardial fraction (CPK-MB) increases 2–12 hr post-MI, peaks in 12–40 hr, and decreases in 24–72 hr
      c. Lactase dehydrogenase (LDH) increases in 6–24 hr and peaks in 3–6 days (rarely used for diagnosis)

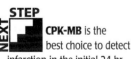

NEXT STEP
CPK-MB is the best choice to detect infarction in the initial 24 hr post-MI, but troponin I is considered sensitive up to 7 days post-MI.

QUICK HIT
Because general CPK will be increased with significant muscular trauma or degradation, CPK-MB is a better indicator of cardiac muscle damage.

FIGURE 1-6 Acute myocardial infarction shown on electrocardiogram. Note the pathological Q waves and ST elevation in leads II, III, and aVF suggesting an inferior-wall infarct, and tall R waves in V_1 and V_2 suggesting posterior-wall involvement.

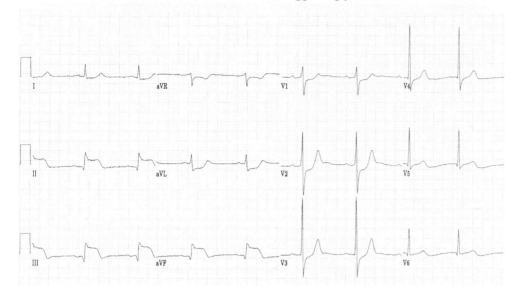

(Taken from Lilly LS. *Pathophysiology of Heart Disease.* 2nd Ed. Baltimore: Williams & Wilkins; 1998. Used with permission of Lippincott Williams & Wilkins.)

    d. Troponin-I increases in 3 hr, peaks in 6 hr, and gradually decreases over 7 days

6. **Treatment**

    a. Acutely, give O_2, ASA, β-blockers, nitroglycerin, morphine (pain control may improve cardiac demand); consider thrombolysis (t-PA, urokinase) or angioplasty if patient presents in initial 12 hr after start of MI; if patient is hypotensive stop nitroglycerin and give intravenous (IV) fluids; in hospital, continue monitoring, ASA, β-blockers, heparin, ACE-I, give antiarrhythmics for frequent premature ventricular contractions (PVCs) or ventricular tachycardia (Vtach)

    b. Perform stress test or nuclear study after 5-days post-MI to assess future risk; if test is suggestive of increased risk for repeat MI, perform cardiac catheterization to measure vessel patency and consider possible PTCA or CABG if significant occlusion is found (Color Figure 1-1)

    c. Long-term treatment = **low dose ASA, β-blockers, ACE-I**, exercise, dietary modifications, possible lipid-lowering agent

NEXT STEP
Treatment for MI:
BeMOAN =
Beta-blocker, **M**orphine, **O**$_2$,
ASA, **N**itroglycerin.

TABLE 1-2	Relation of ECG Changes to Location of Infarct	
ECG Leads with Changes	**Area of Infarct**	**Coronary Artery Branch**
V_2, V_3, V_4	Anterior	Left anterior descending
V_1, V_2, V_3	Septal	Left anterior descending
II, III, aVF	Inferior	Posterior descending or marginal branch
I, aVL, V_4, V_5, V_6	Lateral	Left anterior descending or circumflex
V_1, V_2 (frequent comorbid inferior MI)	Posterior	Posterior descending
ECG, electrocardiogram; MI, myocardial infarction.		

CARDIOVASCULAR DISORDERS

TABLE 1-3   Common Medications Used in Ischemic Disease

Drug	Indications	Cardiovascular	Contraindications
ASA	MI prevention; during and after MI	Decreases thrombosis risk	High risk of GI bleeding
Nitroglycerin	During angina and MI	Decreases venous pressure causing decrease in preload and end-diastolic volume; as a result, blood pressure, ejection time, and O_2 consumption decrease while contractility and heart rate increase	Significant hypotension
β-Blocker	MI prevention; during angina; during and post-MI	Decreases blood pressure, contractility, heart rate, and O_2 consumption; increases end-diastolic volume and ejection time; **decreases mortality** following MI	Long-term use with PVD, asthma, COPD, DM (may mask hypoglycemia), and depression (may worsen symptoms)
ACE-I	Post-MI	Decreases afterload leading to decreased O_2 consumption and blood pressure; **decreases mortality** following MI; particularly helpful with comorbid CHF or DM	Pregnancy
Heparin	Immediately post-MI, inpatient setting	Decreases risk of thrombus formation	Active hemorrhage
Warfarin	Post-MI	Decreases risk of thrombus formation	Pregnancy, active hemorrhage
Morphine	During and immediately post-MI	No direct cardiac benefit, but decreases pain during MI leading to decreased heart rate, blood pressure, and O_2 consumption	Respiratory distress
Thrombolytics (t-PA, urokinase)	Immediately post-MI, inpatient setting	Breaks up thrombus; **decreases mortality** if used within 12 hr post-MI	High bleeding risk

ACE-I, angiotensin converting enzyme inhibitors; ASA, acetylsalicylic acid; CHF, congestive heart failure; COPD, chronic obstructive pulmonary disease; DM, diabetes mellitus; ECG, electrocardiogram; GI, gastrointestinal; MI, myocardial infarction; PVD, peripheral vascular disease.

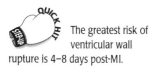

The greatest risk of sudden cardiac death from arrhythmias is in the first few hours post-MI, due to **Vtach, Vfib,** or **cardiogenic shock.**

The greatest risk of ventricular wall rupture is 4–8 days post-MI.

7. **Complications** = infarct extension, arrhythmias, myocardial dysfunction, papillary muscle necrosis, wall rupture, aneurysm, mural thrombus, pericarditis, **Dressler's syndrome** (fever, pericarditis, and increased erythrocyte sedimentation rate [ESR] 2–4 weeks post-MI)

III. Arrhythmias

   A. **Heart block**

      1. Impaired myocardial conduction that occurs when electrical impulses encounter tissue that is electronically unexcitable, resulting in an arrhythmia

      2. First degree

         a. **Cause** is increased vagal tone

         b. **H/P** = asymptomatic

         c. **ECG** = PR > 0.2 sec (see Figure 1-7A)

         d. **Treatment** = none necessary

      3. Second degree—Mobitz I (Wenckebach)

         a. **Caused** by **intranodal** conduction defect, drug effects (β-blockers, digoxin, calcium-channel blockers), or increased vagal tone

FIGURE

1-7 **A.** Primary heart block: regular PR prolongation without skipped QRS.
B. Secondary-Mobitz I heart block: progressive lengthening of PR until QRS is skipped. **C.** Secondary-Mobitz II heart block: regular PR with random skipped QRS. **D.** Tertiary heart block: no relationship between P and QRS.

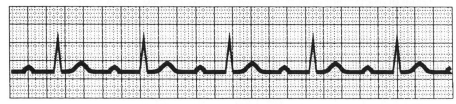

A

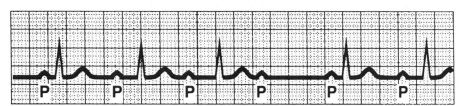

B

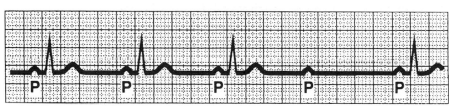

C

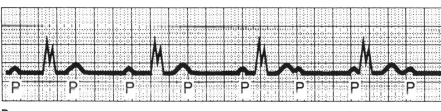

D

(Taken from Lilly LS. *Pathophysiology of Heart Disease*. 2nd Ed. Baltimore: Williams & Wilkins; 1998. Used with permission of Lippincott Williams & Wilkins.)

       b. **H/P** = asymptomatic
       c. **ECG** = **progressive PR lengthening** until skipped QRS; PR
          progression then resets and begins again (see Figure 1-7B)
       d. **Treatment** = adjust medications; treatment usually not necessary
    4. Second degree—Mobitz II
       a. **Cause** is **infranodal** conduction problem (bundle of His, Purkinje
          fibers)
       b. **H/P** = usually asymptomatic
       c. **ECG** = **randomly skipped QRS** without changes in PR interval
          (see Figure 1-7C)
       d. **Treatment** = ventricular pacemaker
       e. **Complications** = may progress to third-degree heart block
    5. Complete or third-degree heart block
       a. **Cause** is absence of conduction between atria and ventricles
       b. **H/P** = syncope, dizziness, hypotension
       c. **ECG** = no relationship between P waves and QRS (see Figure 1-7D)
       d. **Treatment** = ventricular pacemaker

FIGURE 1-8 Mechanism of atrioventricular nodal reentry tachycardia. **A.** Action potential reaches division in conduction pathway with both fast and slow fibers. **B.** Conduction proceeds quickly down fast pathway to reach distal fibers and also proceeds up slow pathway in retrograde fashion. **C.** Impulse returns to original division point after fibers have repolarized, allowing a reentry conduction loop and resultant tachycardia. AV, atrioventricular.

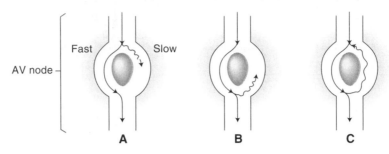

B. **Paroxysmal supraventricular tachycardia (PSVT)**
   1. Tachycardia (HR > 100 bpm) arising in atria or atrioventircular (AV) junction
   2. Occurs mostly in **young patients** with **healthy hearts**
   3. Cause frequently is **reentry** anomaly
      a. **AV nodal reentry**—presence of both slow and fast conduction pathways in AV node; conduction proceeds quickly through fast pathway and progresses up slow pathway in retrograde fashion; conduction loop is created resulting in reentrant tachycardia
      b. **AV reentry** as found in **Wolff-Parkinson-White (WPW) syndrome**—similar to AV nodal reentry, but instead of fast and slow pathways existing in the AV node, a separate accessory conduction pathway exists between the atria and ventricles that returns a conduction impulse to the AV node to set up a reentry loop; ECG shows a delta wave and slurred upstroke of the QRS
   4. **H/P** = sudden tachycardia; possible chest pain, shortness of breath, palpitations, syncope
   5. **ECG** = P waves hidden in T waves; 150–250 bpm HR; normal QRS
   6. **Treatment** = carotid massage or Valsalva maneuver may halt an acute arrhythmia, but pharmacologic therapy or catheter ablation of accessory conduction pathways is usually used for long-term control
C. **Multifocal atrial tachycardia (MAT)**
   1. **Caused** by several ectopic foci in the atria that discharge automatic impulses (multiple pacemakers), resulting in tachycardia

QUICK HIT

Antiarrhythmics other than class IA or IC are contraindicated for Wolff-Parkinson-White syndrome because they may speed up conduction through the accessory pathway.

FIGURE 1-9 Wolff-Parkinson-White syndrome on electrocardiogram. The arrow indicates the presence of a delta wave, a slurred upstroke of the QRS that is characteristic of the condition.

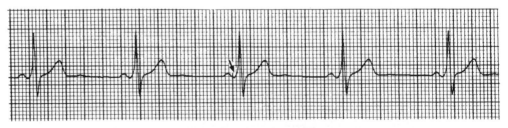

(Courtesy of Dr. Eric Isselbacher, Massachusetts General Hospital, Boston, Massachusetts. From Lilly LS. *Pathophysiology of Heart Disease.* 2nd Ed. Baltimore: Williams & Wilkins; 1998. Used with permission of Lippincott Williams & Wilkins.)

FIGURE 1-10 Multifocal atrial tachycardia (MAT). The arrows indicate P waves of variable morphology.

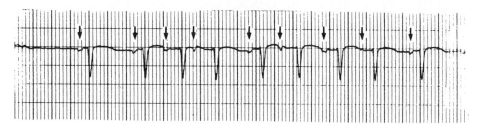

(Courtesy of Dr. Eric Isselbacher, Massachusetts General Hospital, Boston, Massachusetts. From Lilly LS. *Pathophysiology of Heart Disease.* 2nd Ed. Baltimore: Williams & Wilkins; 1998. Used with permission of Lippincott Williams & Wilkins.)

2. **H/P** = usually asymptomatic
3. **ECG** = **variable morphology of P waves;** HR > 100 bpm
4. **Treatment** = calcium-channel blockers; catheter ablation or surgery to eliminate abnormal pacemakers

D. **Bradycardia**
1. HR < 50 bpm
2. Caused by increased vagal tone or nodal disease
3. **Risk factors** = elderly, history of CAD
4. **H/P** = frequently asymptomatic; possible weakness, syncope
5. Predisposition to development of ectopic beats
6. **Treatment** = pacemaker if severe

E. **Atrial fibrillation (Afib)**
1. Sporadic ventricular contractions
2. Cause is rapid, disorderly firing from a second atrial focus
3. **Risk factors** = pulmonary disease, CAD, HTN, anemia, valvular disease, pericarditis, hyperthyroidism, rheumatic heart disease (RHD), sepsis, alcohol use
4. **H/P** = possibly asymptomatic; shortness of breath, chest pain, palpitations, **irregularly irregular pulse**
5. **ECG** = **no discernible P waves,** irregular QRS rate
6. **Treatment** = **anticoagulation; rate control** via calcium-channel blockers, β-blockers, or digoxin; electric or chemical (class IA, IC, or III antiarrhythmics) cardioversion if presenting within initial two days; if presenting after two days or if thrombus is seen on echocardiogram then wait three to four weeks before cardioversion
7. **Complications** = increased risk of MI, heart failure; poor atrial contraction causes blood stasis which leads to mural thrombi formation and a risk of embolization

 Common risk factors for Afib: **PIRATES** — **P**ulmonary disease, **I**schemia (CAD), **R**heumatic heart disease, **A**nemia, hyper**T**hyroid, **E**thanol, and **S**epsis.

 STEP In a patient with Afib, echocardiogram should be performed **before** cardioversion to rule out mural thrombus formation.

FIGURE 1-11 Atrial fibrillation—irregular QRS rate and no discernable P waves.

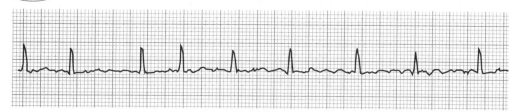

(Taken from Lilly LS. *Pathophysiology of Heart Disease.* 2nd Ed. Baltimore: Williams & Wilkins; 1998. Used with permission of Lippincott Williams & Wilkins.)

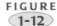

FIGURE 1-12 Atrial flutter—rapid sawtooth P waves (*arrows*) preceding QRS.

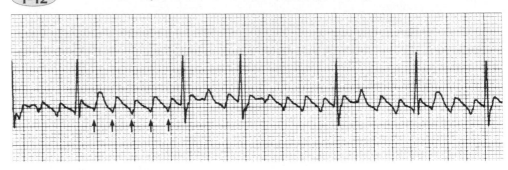

(Taken from Lilly LS. *Pathophysiology of Heart Disease.* 2nd Ed. Baltimore: Williams & Wilkins; 1998. Used with permission of Lippincott Williams & Wilkins.)

F. **Atrial flutter (Aflutter)**
1. Cause is rapid firing of an ectopic focus in the atria
2. **Risk factors** = CAD, congestive heart failure (CHF), chronic obstructive pulmonary disease (COPD), valvular disease, pericarditis
3. **H/P** = possibly asymptomatic; palpitations, syncope
4. **ECG** = regular tachycardia > 150 bpm with occasionally set ratio of P waves to QRS; **sawtooth pattern of P waves**
5. **Treatment** = **rate control** with calcium-channel blockers, β-blockers; electrical or chemical (class IA, IC, or III antiarrhythmics) cardioversion if unable to be controlled with medication; catheter ablation to remove atopic focus may be possible in some cases
6. **Complications** = may degenerate into Afib
G. **Premature ventricular contraction (PVC)**
1. Caused by ectopic beats from a ventricular origin
2. Common, frequently benign; may be caused by hypoxia, abnormal serum electrolyte levels, hyperthyroidism, caffeine use
3. **H/P** = usually asymptomatic; possible palpitations, syncope
4. **ECG** = early and wide QRS without preceding P wave followed by brief pause in conduction
5. **Treatment** = none if patient is healthy; β-blockers in patients with CAD
6. **Complications** = associated with increased risk of sudden death in patients with CAD
H. **Ventricular tachycardia (Vtach)**
1. Series of **3+ PVCs** with HR 160–240 bpm
2. **Risk factors** = CAD, history of MI
3. **H/P** = possibly asymptomatic if brief; palpitations, syncope, hypotension

FIGURE 1-13 Ventricular tachycardia—wide, rapid QRS with no discernable P waves.

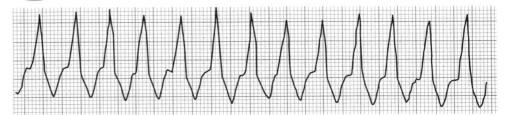

(Taken from Lilly LS. *Pathophysiology of Heart Disease.* 2nd Ed. Baltimore: Williams & Wilkins; 1998. Used with permission of Lippincott Williams & Wilkins.)

TABLE 1-4   Classes of Antiarrhythmic Medications

Class	General Mechanism of Action	Examples	Potential Uses
IA	Na-channel blockers (prolong action potential)	Quinidine, procainamide	PSVT, Afib, Aflutter, Vtach
IB	Na-channel blockers (shorten action potential)	Lidocaine, tocainide	Vtach
IC	Na-channel blockers (no effect on action potential)	Flecainide, propafenone	PSVT, Afib, Aflutter, PSVT
II	β-Blockers	Propanolol, esmolol, metoprolol	PVC, PSVT, Afib, Aflutter, Vtach
III	K-channel blockers	Amiodarone, sotalol, bretylium	Afib, Aflutter, Vtach (not bretylium)
IV	Calcium-channel blockers	Verapamil, diltiazem	PSVT, MAT, Afib, Aflutter
Other	K-channel activation, decrease in intracellular cAMP	Adenosine	PSVT

Afib, atrial fibrillation; Aflutter, atrial flutter; MAT, multifocal atrial tachycardia; PSVT, paroxysmal supraventricular tachycardia; PVC, premature ventricular contraction; Vtach, ventricular tachycardia.

4. **ECG** = series of regular, wide QRS complexes independent of P waves
5. **Treatment** = electrical cardioversion followed by antiarrhythmic medications; role of antiarrhythmic drugs for asymptomatic Vtach uncertain; for recurrent Vtach, internal defibrillator may be necessary (senses ventricular arrhythmia and automatically releases electric pulse to restore normal rhythm)
6. **Complications** = sustained Vtach can quickly deteriorate into Vfib if not corrected

I. **Ventricular fibrillation (Vfib)**
1. Lack of ordered ventricular contraction leads to **no CO** which is rapidly fatal
2. Frequently occurs post-severe MI, post-Vtach
3. **Risk factors** = CAD, MI
4. **H/P** = syncope, hypotension, pulselessness
5. **ECG** = **totally erratic tracing;** no P waves or QRS
6. **Treatment** = CPR, immediate electric (+/− chemical) cardioversion
J. **Antiarrhythmic medications**

IV. Heart failure
A. **Heart physiology**
1. Three important principles
a. Larger diastolic ventricular volume causes increased cardiac muscle fiber stretching; this increased stretching leads to increased contraction force (this is the Frank-Starling relationship, i.e., increased **preload** causes increased ventricular output)
b. Pressure generated by ventricles and end-systolic volume are dependent on load opposing contraction (i.e., **afterload,** approximated at the mean arterial pressure) but independent of stretch on fibers prior to contraction.

 Torsades de pointes is Vtach with a sine wave morphology. It carries a poor prognosis and may rapidly convert to Vfib; Mg may be useful in treatment.

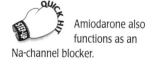 Amiodarone also functions as an Na-channel blocker.

The heart does well in adjusting to changes in blood volume and work demands, but persistently high demands placed on it will cause it to gradually fail.

COPD leads to right-side hypertrophy that ends in right-sided failure (i.e., **cor pulmonale**).

S$_3$ is the most frequent sign of CHF.

STEP NEXT
ACE-I and **spironolactone** have been shown to decrease mortality in CHF; consider incorporating these drugs in the treatment plans, as other medications have not been proven to reduce mortality.

In aortic stenosis, Valsalva will **decrease** the murmur; in hypertrophic obstructive cardiomyopathy (HOCM), Valsalva will **increase** the murmur.

Successful treatment and surgical correction of valvular diseases depend upon diagnosing the disorder before severe symptoms develop.

STEP NEXT
Perform an echocardiogram to diagnose any suspected valvular lesion.

c. Increasing **contractility** (force of contraction independent of preload and afterload) leads to greater tension at isometric contraction for a given preload

2. Ejection fraction (EF) = SV/end-diastolic volume (**normal EF = 55–75%**)

3. Changes in volume-pressure relationship determine compliance of heart

4. Insufficient CO for systemic demand results from progressive heart dysfunction (i.e., CHF)

B. **Systolic dysfunction**
   1. Inadequate CO for systemic demand
   2. Caused by decreased contractility, increased preload, increased afterload, HR abnormalities, or high output conditions (e.g., anemia, hyperthyroidism)

C. **Diastolic dysfunction**
   1. Decreased ventricular compliance leads to decreased ventricular filling, increased diastolic pressure, and decreased CO
   2. Caused by hypertrophy or restrictive cardiomyopathy

D. **Congestive heart failure (CHF)**
   1. Left side of heart
      a. Left ventricle **unable to produce adequate CO**
      b. Blood backs up leading to pulmonary edema that eventually causes pulmonary HTN
      c. Progressive **left ventricular hypertrophy (LVH)** to compensate for poor output causes eventual failure because the heart is unable to keep pace with systemic need for CO
   2. Right side of heart
      a. Increased pulmonary vascular resistance leads to **right ventricular hypertrophy (RVH)** and systemic venous stasis
      b. **Most commonly due to left-sided failure** (Eisenmenger's syndrome); also may be due to unrelated pulmonary HTN, valvular disease, or congenital defects
   3. **Risk factors** = CAD, HTN, valvular disease, cardiomyopathy, drug toxicity, alcohol use
   4. **H/P** = fatigue, dyspnea on exertion, orthopnea, paroxysmal nocturnal dyspnea, nocturia, cough; displaced point of maximum impulse, **S**$_3$, jugular vein distention (JVD) peripheral edema, hepatomegaly
   5. **Radiology** = chest x-ray (CXR) shows cardiac enlargement, **Kerley B lines** (increased marking of lung interlobular septa due to pulmonary edema), **cephalization of pulmonary vessels** (increased marking of superior pulmonary vessels due to congestion and stasis); echocardiogram can assess chamber size and function
   6. **ECG** = possible findings consistent with ischemic disease
   7. **Treatment** = treat underlying conditions that cause dysfunction; salt restricted diet; **diuretics** (decrease preload), **ACE-I** or angiotensin receptor blockers (ARBs) (decrease preload and afterload and increase CO), digoxin (increases contractility), spironolactone (as adjunct to ACE-I) and diuretics (K-sparing diuretic); β-blockers and vasodilators may be helpful in long-standing cases; assistive devices or cardiac transplant may be required in progressive cases

V. **Valvular diseases (see Table 1-5)**

TABLE 1-5 Valvular Diseases

Valvular Disease (Description)	Causes	Symptoms	Exam	Radiology	Treatment
Mitral regurgitation (mitral valve incompetency causes blood backflow to LA)	– Mitral valve prolapse (floppy valve) – **RHD** – Papillary muscle dysfunction – Endocarditis – LV dilation	– Asymptomatic in early/mild cases – Palpitations – Dyspnea on exertion – Orthopnea – Paroxysmal nocturnal dyspnea	– Harsh blowing **holosystolic murmur** radiating from apex to axilla – S_3 – Widely split S_2 – Midsystolic click	– LVH, LA enlargement on CXR – Echo helpful for diagnosis	– Surgical repair in severe or acute cases – Prophylactic antibiotics for increased infection risk
Mitral stenosis (obstructed blood flow to LV causes increased LA volume)	– RHD	– Initially asymptomatic ($\sim$10 yr) – Dyspnea on exertion – Orthopnea – Paroxysmal nocturnal dyspnea – Peripheral edema – Hepatomegaly	– Opening snap after S_2 – Diastolic rumble – Loud S_1	– RVH, LA enlargement, mitral valve calcification on CXR – Echo helpful for diagnosis	– Diuretics (reduce preload) – Antiarrhythmics for Afib secondary to atrial enlargement – Surgical repair prior to symptomatic progression
Aortic regurgitation (aortic valve incompetency causes blood backflow to LV)	– Congenital defect – Endocarditis – RHD – Tertiary syphilis – Aortic-root dilatation (possibly from aortic dissection)	– Initially asymptomatic – Dyspnea on exertion – Chest pain – Orthopnea	– Bounding pulses – Widened pulse pressure – **Diastolic decrescendo murmur** at right 2nd intercostal space – Late diastolic rumble (**Austin-Flint murmur**) – Capillary pulsations in nail bed, more visible when pressure is applied (**Quincke's sign**)	– Dilated aorta, LV enlargement on CXR – Echo helpful for diagnosis	– ACE-I, calcium-channel blockers, or nitrates (decrease afterload) – Valve replacement
Aortic stenosis (narrowing of aortic valve causes obstructed blood flow from LV)	– **Congenital defect** – RHD – Calcification in elderly patients	– Chest pain – Dyspnea on exertion – **Syncope**	– Weak prolonged pulse – **Crescendo-decrescendo systolic murmur** radiating from right upper sternal border to carotids – Weak S_2 – Valsalva decreases murmur	– Calcified aortic valve, dilated aorta on CXR – Echo and cardiac cath. helpful for diagnosis	– β-Blockers – Valvuloplasty – Valve replacement

ACE-I, angiotensin converting enzyme inhibitors; Afib, atrial fibrillation; CXR, chest x-ray; Echo, echocardiogram; LA, left atrium; LV, left ventricle; LVH, left ventricular hypertrophy; RHD, rheumatic heart disease; RVH, right ventricular hypertrophy.

FIGURE
1-14 Renin-angiotensin-aldosterone system and its end effects which contribute to hypertension; ACE-I act to inhibit the conversion of angiotensin I to angiotensin II, and ARBs block angiotensin II activity at the receptor level.

ANGIOTENSINOGEN
(secreted by liver)

↓ *Renin (secreted by kidney)*

ANGIOTENSIN I

↓ *Angiotensin converting enzyme*

ANGIOTENSIN II

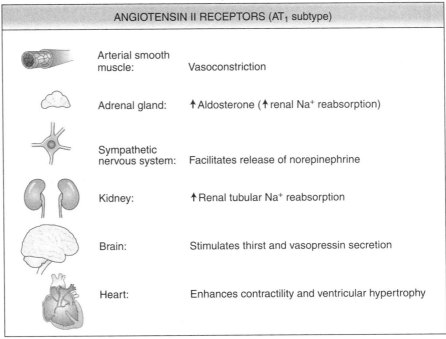

ANGIOTENSIN II RECEPTORS (AT$_1$ subtype)	
Arterial smooth muscle:	Vasoconstriction
Adrenal gland:	↑Aldosterone (↑renal Na$^+$ reabsorption)
Sympathetic nervous system:	Facilitates release of norepinephrine
Kidney:	↑Renal tubular Na$^+$ reabsorption
Brain:	Stimulates thirst and vasopressin secretion
Heart:	Enhances contractility and ventricular hypertrophy

(Modified from Lilly LS. *Pathophysiology of Heart Disease.* 2nd Ed. Baltimore: Williams & Wilkins; 1998. Used with permission of Lippincott Williams & Wilkins.)

FIGURE
1-15 Common murmurs associated with valvular diseases.

Diagram	S$_1$ S$_2$	S$_1$ S$_2$	S$_1$ S$_2$	S$_2$ S$_1$	S$_2$ S$_1$
Murmur Type	Systolic ejection	Pansystolic	Late systolic	Early diastolic	Mid/late diastolic
Examples	Aortic stenosis Pulmonic stenosis	Mitral regurgitation Tricuspid regurgitation	Mitral valve prolapse	Aortic regurgitation Pulmonic regurgitation	Mitral stenosis
Location & Radiation	2nd right interspace→neck (but may radiate widely) 2nd-3rd left interspace	Apex→axilla Left lower sternal border →right lower sternal border	Apex→axilla	Along left side of sternum Upper left side of sternum	Apex

(Modified from Lilly LS. *Pathophysiology of Heart Disease.* 2nd Ed. Baltimore: Williams & Wilkins; 1998. Used with permission of Lippincott Williams & Wilkins.)

TABLE 1-6 **Cardiomyopathies**

Cardiomyopathy (Description)	Causes	Symptoms	Exam	Radiology	Treatment
Hypertrophic obstructive (HOCM) (Ventricular hypertrophy, thickened septum causes decreased filling, LV outflow obstruction, both systolic and diastolic dysfunction)	• Congenital (**autosomal dominant**)	• Syncope • Dyspnea • Palpitations • Chest pain • **Symptoms worse with exertion**	• S_4 • Systolic murmur • Sustained apical impulse • ECG may show arrhythmia, LVH, abnormal Q waves	• Boot-shaped heart on CXR • Echo helpful for diagnosis	• β-Blockers • Calcium-channel blockers • Pacemaker • Partial septal excision
Dilated (Ventricular dilation causes systolic dysfunction)	• **Idiopathic** • Alcohol use • Beriberi • Coxsackie virus B • Cocaine use • Doxorubicin • HIV	• Similar to CHF and bi-valvular regurgitation	• S_3 • **Systolic and diastolic murmurs** • ECG may show ST and T wave changes, weak QRS, tachycardia, LBBB	• Balloon-like heart on CXR • Echo helpful in diagnosis	• Stop alcohol or cocaine use • Diuretics • ACE-I • β-Blockers • Anti-coagulation
Restrictive (Decreased heart compliance causes impaired diastolic filling)	• Sarcoidosis • Amyloidosis	• Similar to CHF with right-sided symptoms worse	• Ascites • JVD • Biopsy is diagnostic	• Often normal	• Treat underlying cause • Palliative treatment for heart failure

ACE-I, angiotensin converting enzyme inhibitors; CHF, congestive heart failure; CXR, chest x-ray; ECG, electrocardiogram; Echo, echo cardiogram; JVD, jugular vein distention; LBBB, left bundle branch block; LV, left ventricle; LVH, left ventricular hypertrophy.

VI. Cardiomyopathies (see Table 1-6)

VII. Pericardial diseases

A. **Acute pericarditis**

1. Acute inflammation of the pericardial sac accompanied by pericardial effusion
2. Caused by **viral infection,** tuberculosis, systemic lupus erythematosus (SLE), uremia, neoplasm, drug toxicity (isoniazid, hydralazine), post-MI inflammation (**Dressler's syndrome**), **radiation, recent heart surgery**
3. H/P = chest pain with breathing (i.e., **pleuritic chest pain**), dyspnea, cough; **pain worsens with leaning forward** or shallow breathing; fever, **friction rub** (best heard when leaning forward); pulsus paradoxus (fall in systolic blood pressure > 10 mm Hg with inspiration) occurs because increased physiologic right ventricle (RV) filling during inspiration combined with pathologic left ventricle (LV) compression by pericardial effusion causes impaired LV filling, decreased stroke volume, and decreased inspiratory systolic blood pressure
4. **ECG = ST elevation,** PR depression
5. **Radiology =** CXR helpful in ruling out other systemic causes; effusion frequently seen on echocardiogram

Squatting relieves symptoms in HOCM.

HOCM is the most common cause of sudden death in **young athletes.**

Dilated cardiomyopathy accounts for 90% of all cardiomyopathies.

ST elevation is seen in acute pericarditis as well as in MI, but acute pericarditis also demonstrates **PR depression** and ST elevation in **most leads** (MI frequently does not show PR depression, and ST elevation is focal).

STEP NEXT If ST elevation is seen on ECG, full work-up is required to rule out MI.

STEP NEXT Pericardial effusions are usually **transudates** (low in proteins, specific gravity < 1.012); if **exudates** (rich in proteins, specific gravity > 1.020) are collected during pericardiocentesis, perform workup for neoplasm or fibrotic disease.

STEP NEXT Differentiate restrictive cardiomyopathy from constrictive pericarditis with CT or MRI.

STEP NEXT If you find **Beck's triad**–hypotension, distant heart sounds, and distended neck veins–perform urgent pericardiocentesis!

QUICK HIT Myocarditis in South and Central America is commonly due to *Trypanosoma cruzi* (**Chagas' disease**), and in these cases may be associated with **achalasia.**

QUICK HIT Several of the drugs that cause myocarditis are used in **cancer** therapy (cyclophosphamide, doxorubicin, daunorubicin).

QUICK HIT RHD only occurs in 3% of untreated streptococcal infections.

6. **Treatment** = treat underlying cause; pericardiocentesis for large effusions; nonsteroidal anti-inflammatory drugs (NSAIDs) for pain, inflammation
7. **Complications** = chronic constrictive pericarditis if untreated

B. **Chronic constrictive pericarditis**
1. Sequelae of chronic untreated pericardial irritation
2. Diffuse thickening of pericardium with possible calcifications leads to decreased diastolic filling and decreased CO
3. Most commonly caused by **radiation** or **heart surgery**
4. **H/P** = symptoms consistent with right-sided heart failure (JVD, dyspnea on exertion, orthopnea, peripheral edema, increasing JVD with inspiration (**Kussmaul's sign**)); Afib common
5. **Labs** = cardiac catheterization shows **equal pressure in all chambers**
6. **Radiology** = possible pericardial calcifications on CXR; echocardiogram, computed tomography (CT), and magnetic resonance imaging (MRI) show pericardial thickening
7. **Treatment** = surgical excision of pericardium (high mortality)

C. **Cardiac tamponade**
1. Large pericardial effusion causes compression of heart and **greatly decreased CO;** may result from progressive **acute pericarditis, chest trauma,** LV rupture following MI, or dissecting aortic aneurysm
2. High mortality
3. **H/P** = dyspnea, tachycardia, tachypnea; JVD, pulsus paradoxus
4. **Radiology** = enlarged heart shadow on CXR; large effusion seen on echocardiogram
5. **ECG** = very weak
6. **Treatment** = **immediate pericardiocentesis**

VIII. **Myocardial infections**
A. **Myocarditis**
1. Inflammatory reaction in heart limited to cardiac muscle involvement
2. Most commonly caused by infection (**Coxsackie virus,** bacteria, rickettsiae, fungi, parasites)
3. Occasionally due to **drug toxicity** (doxorubicin, chloroquine, penicillins, sulfonamides, cocaine, radiation), toxins, or endocrine abnormalities
4. **H/P** = patient may report history of recent upper respiratory infection; pleuritic chest pain or symptoms similar to heart failure
5. **ECG** = ST and T wave changes, conduction abnormalities
6. **Radiology** = possible cardiomegaly on CXR; echocardiogram useful in assessing heart function
7. **Labs** = difficult to diagnose because of variations in lab findings; viral titers and serology may help suggest a particular infectious agent; myocardial biopsy frequently shows myocyte inflammation with primarily monocytes and macrophages, and focal areas of necrosis
8. **Treatment** = treat infection; stop offending medications

B. **Rheumatic heart disease (RHD)**
1. Caused by **untreated group A streptococcus** infection
2. Streptococcus infection may provoke autoantibodies that attack heart valves and joints (mitral valve more commonly affected than aortic valve, which is more commonly involved than right-sided valves)
3. Incidence is low in the United States due to antibiotic treatment
4. **H/P** = migratory arthritis, hot and swollen joints, fever, subcutaneous nodules on extensor surfaces, Sydenham's chorea, erythema marginatum (painless rash)
5. Diagnosis of RHD using JONES mnemonic shown in Figure 1-16
6. **Labs** = increased ESR and white cell count (WBC); 90% of patients have antistreptococcal antibodies

FIGURE 1-16 JONES Criteria mnemonic for diagnosis of rheumatic heart disease (RHD). ESR, erythrocyte sedimentation rate; PR, pulse rate.

JONES CRITERIA— Think J♥NES

J: **J**oints
♥: **H**eart
N: **N**odules
E: **E**rythema marginatum
S: **S**ydenham's chorea

Diagnosis of RHD is made either with 2 JONES criteria or 1 JONES criteria plus 1 of the following: fever, arthralgia, increased PR, increased ESR, recent streptococcal infection, or history of rheumatic fever.

7. **ECG** = increased PR interval
8. **Treatment** = NSAIDs for joint inflammation; use corticosteroids if carditis is severe; β-lactam (penicillin family) antibiotic for infection; if valves have been damaged, patient will need **prophylactic antibiotics** before surgery or dentistry
9. **Complications** = progressive valve damage if untreated

C. **Endocarditis**
1. Bacterial infection of endocardium (inner lining of heart) with or without valve involvement
2. More common in patients with **congenital heart defects, intravenous drug abuse,** or prosthetic valves
3. SLE patients may present in a similar manner with non-infective endocarditis (**Libman-Sacks endocarditis**)
4. Both acute (sudden presentation) and subacute (insidious progression) forms
   a. **Acute endocarditis** is caused by *Staphylococcus aureus, Streptococcus pneumoniae, Staphylococcus pyogenes, Neisseria gonorrhoeae*
   b. **Subacute endocarditis** due to viridans streptococcus, *Enterococcus,* fungi, and *Staphylococcus epidermidis*
5. **H/P** = fever (very high in acute form), chills, night sweats, fatigue, arthralgias; possible new murmur, small tender nodules on finger and toe pads (**Osler's nodes**), peripheral petechiae (**Janeway lesions**), subungual petechiae (**splinter hemorrhages**), retinal hemorrhages (**Roth's spots**)
6. **Labs** = serial blood cultures will grow same pathogen; increased ESR
7. **Radiology** = echocardiogram may show vegetations on valves; CXR may reveal congestion consistent with septic emboli and right-sided heart failure
8. **Treatment** = **long-term (28 days) IV antibiotics** (initially broad-spectrum, then bug-specific); antibiotic prophylaxis before surgery or dental work if valves are damaged; valve replacement may be necessary for severely damaged valves
9. **Complications** = severe damage to endocardium and valves, **septic embolization,** or abscess formation if untreated

IX. **Hypertension (HTN)**
A. **Primary (essential) HTN**
1. Cause is idiopathic
2. Accounts for > 95% all cases of HTN
3. Diagnosed when systolic blood pressure > 140 and/or diastolic blood pressure > 90 as measured in three readings taken at three separate appointments

 Negative-culture endocarditis can result from the HACEK bacteria: *Haemophilus, Actinobacillus, Cardiobacterium, Eikenella,* and *Kingella.*

 Prosthetic valves are particularly susceptible to *Staphylococcus epidermidis* infection.

 The patient should be sitting quietly for five min before blood pressure is measured to minimize **false high readings.**

CARDIOVASCULAR DISORDERS

TABLE 1-7 Common Antihypertensive Agents

Class of Medication	Examples	Mechanism of Action	Prescription Strategy	Side Effects
Diuretics	Thiazides (HCTZ, etc.); K-sparing (spironolactone, etc); loop diuretics too potent for regular anti-HTN use	Reduce circulatory volume to decrease CO and mean arterial pressure	Early; particularly effective in African Americans and salt-sensitive patients	Increased serum glucose, cholesterol, or triglycerides; hypokalemia
α-Blockers	Prazosin, doxazosin, terazosin	Block α-adrenergic receptors (primary controllers of vascular tone) to decrease total peripheral resistance	Adjunct to other medications; less commonly used	Postural hypotension, headache, rebound HTN if stopped
β-Blockers	Nonselective (propranolol, timolol); β_1-selective (metoprolol, atenolol, esmolol)	Decrease HR, contractility, CO, and decrease renin secretion to decrease total peripheral resistance	Early; many important cardiac uses; more effective in Caucasian patients	Sexual dysfunction in males, bronchoconstriction if non-β_1 selective, HDL reduction, increased triglycerides
Calcium-channel blockers	Non-dihydropyridines (diltiazem, verapamil); dihydropyridines (nifedipine, amlodipine)	Reduce influx of calcium during cardiac and vascular smooth muscle contraction to cause vasodilation	Second line; nondihydropyridines mainly effect the myocardium; dihydropyridines mainly effect vascular smooth muscle and are utilized more often for HTN	Hypotension, headache, constipation, increased GI reflux
Vasodilators	Hydralazine, minoxidil	Direct relaxation of vascular smooth muscle	Adjunct to other medications; less commonly used	Reflex tachycardia, possible adverse cardiovascular incidents
ACE-I	Lisinopril, captopril, enalopril	Block conversion of angiotensin I to angiotensin II and increase circulating bradykinin to decrease angiotensin II vasopressor activity and aldosterone secretion, causing decrease in total peripheral resistance	Early or second line; important cardiac and renal uses; more effective in young Caucasian patients	Dry cough, azotemia, hyperkalemia
ARBs	Irbesartan, losartan	Block binding of angiotensin II to receptors to inhibit vasopressor activity and decrease aldosterone secretion	Second line	Few side effects; high cost

ACE-I, angiotensin converting enzyme inhibitors; ARBs, angiotensin receptor blockers; CO, cardiac output; GI, gastrointestinal; HCTZ, hydrochlorothiazide; HDL, high-density lipoprotein; HR, heart rate; HTN, hypertension.

4. **Risk factors** = family history of HTN, high salt diet (especially if salt-sensitive), tobacco use, obesity, increased age; African Americans > Caucasians

5. **H/P** = asymptomatic until progression, then headache may be the only symptom until complications develop; blood pressure > 140/90; arteriovenous nicking (apparent retinal-vein narrowing secondary to arterial-wall thickening), cotton-wool spots, or retinal hemorrhages (**flame hemorrhages**) on eye exam; loud S_2, possible S_4

TABLE 1-8 Recommendations and Contraindications for Antihypertensive Drug Selection

Comorbid Condition	Recommended Antihypertensive	Recommended Reason	Contraindicated Antihypertensive	Contraindicated Reason
DM	ACE-I	Delays renal damage	Thiazide diuretic β-Blocker	Impaired glucose tolerance May mask signs of hypoglycemia
CHF	ACE-I Diuretic	Improves mortality Improves mortality	Calcium-channel blocker	Reduced rate/contractility may exacerbate heart failure
Post-MI	β-Blocker ACE-I	Improves mortality Improves mortality		
Benign prostatic hypertrophy	Selective β₁-blocker	Improves symptoms		
Migraine headache	β-Blocker	May improve symptoms		
Osteoporosis	Thiazide diuretic	Maintains normal/high serum calcium		
Asthma/COPD			Non-selective β-blocker	Exacerbates bronchoconstriction
Pregnancy			Thiazide diuretic	Increased blood volume during pregnancy should be maintained
			ACE-I ARB	Teratogenic Teratogenic
Gout			Diuretic	Increase serum uric acid
Depression			β-Blocker	May worsen symptoms

ACE-I, angiotensin converting enzyme inhibitors; ARB, angiotensin receptor blocker; CHF, congestive heart failure; COPD, chronic obstructive pulmonary disease; DM, diabetes mellitus; MI, myocardial infarction.

6. **Treatment** = do not start medications until three consecutive high readings have been recorded
   a. Initially prescribe weight loss, exercise, salt restriction, and alcohol reduction
   b. Diuretics and β-blockers are good initial medications; ACE-I, ARBs, calcium-channel blockers may be added later
   c. Comorbid conditions may dictate a change in prescription strategy
7. **Complications** = untreated or poorly treated disease increases risk of CAD, stroke, aortic aneurysm, aortic dissection, CHF, kidney disease, and ophthalmologic disease

B. **Secondary HTN**
   1. Due to identifiable cause
   2. Some causes may be reversible while others are progressive
C. **Hypertensive emergency**
   1. Blood pressure >**200/120** (non-pregnant patient)
   2. **H/P** = possibly asymptomatic or mildly symptomatic; signs of renal failure, hematuria, change of mental status, papilledema, retinal vascular changes, unstable angina, MI, pulmonary edema
   3. **Malignant HTN** = progressive renal failure, encephalopathy, papilledema
   4. **Treatment** = for malignant HTN, rapidly reduce diastolic blood pressure to 100 mm Hg using IV nitroprusside, labetalol, nicardipine, or fenoldopam; once blood pressure is controlled, use oral β-blockers and

NEXT STEP If patient has been normotensive in the past and now systolic blood pressure is > 140 or diastolic blood pressure > 90, recheck in two months.

Renal diseases are the most common cause of secondary HTN.

ACE-I drugs are contraindicated in cases of **bilateral renal artery stenosis** since they may accelerate renal failure by impeding sufficient renal perfusion and lowering glomerular filtration rate.

TABLE 1-9 Causes of Secondary HTN

Condition	Common Patient Group	Signs/Symptoms	Diagnosis	Treatment
Renal diseases (various)		Depends on disease identity	Depends on disease identity	ACE-I (delays progression)
Renal artery stenosis	<25 years old (fibromuscular dysplasia) or >50 years old (atherosclerosis)	Renal artery bruit	Arteriography; renal vein renin ratio	Angioplasty; stent placement; ACE-I if one-sided; surgical repair
OCPs (combination pill)	Women >35 years old; obese women; long-term OCP use		History	Stop use; change to progestin-only pill or intramuscular medroxy-progesterone
Pheochromocytoma	Young patients; patients with history of endocrine tumors	Episodic HTN, diaphoresis, headaches; symptoms occur suddenly	Increased 24-hr urinary catecholamines or vanillylmandelic acid; CT, MRI	Surgical removal of tumor with pharmacologic control of HTN up until time of surgery
Primary hyper-aldosteronism (excess aldosterone = Conn's disease; excess glucocorticoids = Cushing's disease)		Central obesity, hirsutism, buffalo hump, striae, and glucose intolerance in Cushing's disease	Decreased serum K, increased urinary K, increased serum/urine aldosterone	Surgical removal of tumor
Coarctation of the aorta	Male > female; Turner's syndrome, aortic valve pathology, PDA	HTN in arm but not in legs, weak femoral pulse	Possible LVH on ECG; echocardiogram can localize defect	Surgical repair

ACE-I, angiotensin converting enzyme inhibitors; CT, computed tomography scan; ECG, electrocardiogram; HTN, hypertension; LVH, left ventricular hypertrophy; MRI, magnetic resonance imaging; OCP, oral contraceptive pill; PDA, patent ductus arteriosus.

ACE-I to gradually reduce mean diastolic pressure to 85–90 mm Hg over two months; use diuretics to reduce pulmonary edema

X. Shock (see Table 1-10)
  A. Circulatory collapse in which blood delivery is inadequate for tissue demands
  B. High mortality without timely treatment

XI. Vascular Diseases
  A. **Aortic conditions**
    1. **Aortic aneurysm**
      a. Localized dilation of aorta
      b. The majority occur in abdomen below renal arteries (abdominal aortic aneurysm (**AAA**))
      c. **Risk factors** = atherosclerosis, HTN, tobacco use, family history, age > 55 years
      d. Marfan's syndrome and syphilis are the most common causes of thoracic aortic aneurysms
      e. **H/P** = AAAs are **frequently asymptomatic** until later progression; possible lower back pain; **pulsating abdominal mass, abdominal bruits;** thoracic aneurysms may cause dysphagia, hoarseness,

TABLE 1-10	Common Types of Shock		
Type of Shock	**Mechanism**	**Cause**	**Treatment**
Cardiogenic	Failure of myocardial pump	MI, arrhythmias, cardiac tamponade, pulmonary embolism	IV fluids, pressor agents, intra-aortic balloon pump, PTCA
Septic	Decreased total peripheral resistance	Gram neg. bacteria, DIC; possibly endotoxin mediated	Treat underlying infection, pressor agents
Hypovolemic	Inadequate blood or plasma volume	Hemorrhage, severe burns, trauma	IV fluids, transfusions, surgery may be required to stop volume loss; specialized dressings, skin grafts may be required with severe burns to prevent ongoing fluid loss
Anaphylactic	Generalized hypersensitivity type I reaction	Massive release of mast cells and basophils in response to allergic reaction	Maintain airway, epinephrine, diphenhydramine, cimetidine, IV fluids
Neurogenic	Widespread peripheral vasodilation	CNS or spinal cord injury	IV fluids, pressor agents

CNS, central nervous system; DIC, disseminated intravascular coagulation; IV, intravenous; MI, myocardial infarction; PTCA, percutaneous transluminal coronary angioplasty.

dyspnea, hemoptysis, upper body edema; hypotension and severe pain occur with any rupture

   f. **Radiology** = ultrasound (US) can detect location and size quickly; CT or MRI are used for more accurate localization and size determination

   g. **Treatment** = monitor with periodic US if <5 cm diameter; surgical repair (open or using endovascular stenting) if symptomatic or >5 cm diameter; thoracic aneurysms are repaired if >6 cm diameter or rapidly enlarging

   h. **Complications** = if untreated, possible MI, rupture, renal insufficiency, ischemic colitis, stroke, or paraplegia

2. **Aortic dissection**

   a. Intimal tear leads to blood entering media causing formation of false lumen

   b. Stanford classification—**Stanford A** aortic dissection involves ascending aorta; **Stanford B** is distal to left subclavian artery

   c. **Risk factors** = HTN, trauma, coarctation of the aorta, syphilis, Ehlers-Danlos syndrome, Marfan's syndrome

   d. **H/P** = acute "**ripping**" chest pain, syncope; decreased peripheral pulses, normal or increased blood pressure

   e. **ECG** = normal or LVH

   f. **Radiology** = widening of aorta and superior mediastinum on CXR; CT with contrast, echocardiogram, MRI, MRA, or angiography good for definite diagnosis

   g. **Treatment** = stabilize blood pressure (nitroprusside, β-blockers) if unstable; Stanford A dissections need emergency surgery; Stanford B dissections may be treated medically unless rupture or occlusion develops

B. **Arterial condition—peripheral vascular disease (PVD)**

   1. Occlusion of peripheral blood supply secondary to atherosclerosis

   2. **Risk factors** = HTN, DM, CAD

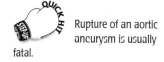

Rupture of an aortic aneurysm is usually fatal.

NEXT STEP If a patient presents with new severe chest pain, an immediate ECG can differentiate an aortic dissection from an acute MI (ECG will be normal or will show mild left ventricular hypertrophy in aortic dissection).

Remember the six Ps to grade PVD severity: **P**ain, **P**allor, **P**oikilothermia, **P**ulselessness, **P**aresthesia, and **P**aralysis.

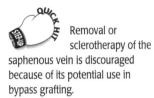

Removal or sclerotherapy of the saphenous vein is discouraged because of its potential use in bypass grafting.

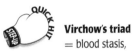

Virchow's triad = blood stasis, hypercoagulability, and vascular damage increase patient's risk of DVT.

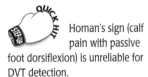

Homan's sign (calf pain with passive foot dorsiflexion) is unreliable for DVT detection.

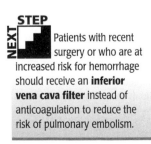

STEP NEXT
Patients with recent surgery or who are at increased risk for hemorrhage should receive an **inferior vena cava filter** instead of anticoagulation to reduce the risk of pulmonary embolism.

3. **H/P** = leg pain with activity that improves with rest (**intermittent claudication**), resting leg pain in severe disease; dry skin, skin ulcers, decreased hair growth in affected area; male impotence with aorto-iliac disease
4. **Labs** = ankle-brachial index (ABI) is ratio of systolic blood pressure at ankle to that at brachial artery; ABI < 1 indicates vascular insufficiency at ankle; ABI < 0.4 indicates severe disease (frequently seen with resting pain)
5. **Radiology** = US is useful for locating stenosis and variations in blood pressure; arteriography will map narrowing in the arterial distribution of interest
6. **Treatment** = exercise (increases collateral circulation), instruction in foot examination (early detection of ulcers from vascular insufficiency), treat underlying diseases; ASA, **pentoxifylline** or **cilostazol** to help to slow occlusion; bypass grafting if incapacitating claudication, resting pain, or necrotic foot lesions develop; prolonged ischemia may require limb amputation

C. **Venous conditions**
   1. **Varicosities**
      a. Incompetent venous valves that cause elongation, dilation, and tortuosity of veins
      b. **H/P** = usually asymptomatic; pain and fatigue that improves with leg elevation; possible visible or palpable veins, increased local pigmentation, edema, or ulceration
      c. **Treatment** = exercise, compression hosiery, leg elevation; surgical removal or injection sclerotherapy for cosmetic improvement or symptomatic varicosities
   2. **Arteriovenous malformations (AVMs)**
      a. Abnormal communications between arteries and veins
      b. May be congenital or acquired
      c. **H/P** = palpable, warm, pulsating masses if superficial; painful if mass compresses adjacent structures
      d. Large AVMs may cause local ischemia and may increase the risk of thrombus formation
      e. **Treatment** = surgical removal or sclerosis if symptomatic or if located in brain or bowel
   3. **Deep vein thrombosis (DVT)**
      a. Development of thrombosis in large vein; most common in lower extremity
      b. Location, in order of decreasing frequency: **calf,** femoral, popliteal, and iliac veins
      c. May cause inflammation of affected vein (**thrombophlebitis**)
      d. **Risk factors** = **prolonged inactivity** (travel, immobilization), heart failure, disorders of coagulation, neoplasm, **pregnancy,** OCP use, **tobacco use,** vascular trauma
      e. **H/P** = possibly asymptomatic; deep leg pain, swelling, warmth
      f. **Radiology** = US and contrast venography are used for detection
      g. **Treatment** = leg elevation; heparin initially, warfarin for long-term management
      h. **Complications** = clot can embolize to lungs (**pulmonary embolus**) with 40% mortality; chronic DVTs can cause chronic venous insufficiency

D. **Vasculitis**
   1. **Polyarteritis nodosa**
      a. Inflammation of small or medium arteries leads to ischemia
      b. Affects kidneys, heart, gastrointestinal (GI) tract, muscles, nerves, joints (anything with a vascular supply)
      c. **Risk factors** = **hepatitis B or C;** young > elderly; men > women

    d. **H/P** = fever, HTN, hematuria, anemia, neuropathy, weight loss, joint pain, palpable purpura or ulcers on skin

    e. **Labs** = increased WBC, decreased hemoglobin (Hgb) and hematocrit, increased ESR, proteinuria, hematuria; **p-ANCA** in 50–80% patients; arterial biopsy may help in diagnosis

    f. **Radiology** = angiography may show numerous aneurysms

    g. **Treatment** = corticosteroids, immunosuppressive agents

2. **Temporal (giant cell) arteritis**

    a. Commonly due to subacute granulomatous inflammation of the external carotid and vertebral arteries

    b. **Risk factors = women** > men, **50 years old and older**

    c. Half of patients also have **polymyalgia rheumatica**

    d. **H/P = new onset of headache** (unilateral or bilateral) with scalp pain, **temporal region tenderness,** jaw claudication, transient or permanent monocular blindness, weight loss, myalgias, arthralgias, fever; fundoscopic exam should be performed to address vision loss (may show thrombosis of ophthalmic or ciliary arteries)

    e. **Labs** = increased ESR; temporal artery biopsy shows inflammation in vessel media and lymphocytes, plasma cells, or giant cells in vessel adventitia

    f. Treatment = prednisone for one to two months followed by taper; ophthalmology follow-up

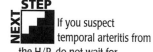

STEP
NEXT If you suspect temporal arteritis from the H/P, do not wait for temporal artery biopsy to start prednisone.

3. **Takayasu's arteritis**

    a. Inflammation of aorta and its branches

    b. **H/P** = fever, malaise, decreased carotid and limb pulses

    c. May cause cerebrovascular and myocardial ischemia

    d. **Labs** = biopsy of affected vessel shows plasma cells and lymphocytes in media and adventitia, giant cells, and vascular fibrosis

    e. **Treatment** = corticosteroids, immunosuppressive agents; bypass grafting of obstructed vessels

4. **Churg-Strauss disease (allergic angiitis)**

    a. Inflammation of small or medium arteries

    b. **H/P = asthmatic symptoms,** fatigue, malaise

    c. **Labs** = increased serum eosinophils; lung biopsy may show eosinophilic granulomas

    d. **Treatment** = corticosteroids, immunosuppressive agents

5. **Henoch-Schönlein purpura**

    a. IgA immune-complex-mediated vasculitis affecting arterioles, capillaries, and venules

    b. More frequently in **children** than adults

    c. **H/P = recent upper respiratory infection;** polyarticular arthritis, fever, hemorrhagic urticaria, palpable purpura, **abdominal pain,** possible GI bleeding

    d. **Labs** = biopsy of purpura demonstrates **IgA deposition;** similar findings in **renal** biopsy

    e. **Treatment** = frequently self-limited; use corticosteroids for severe GI symptoms

6. **Kawasaki's disease**

    a. Necrotizing inflammation of large, medium, and small vessels

    b. Most commonly seen in **young children**

    c. **H/P** = fever, lymphadenopathy, conjunctival lesions, maculopapular rash, edema, eventual desquamation of hands and feet

    d. Coronary vasculitis develops in 25% of patients leading to possible aneurysm, MI, or sudden death

    e. **Labs** = possible autoantibodies to endothelial cells

    f. **Treatment** = ASA, IV gamma globulin; frequently self-limited

FIGURE 1-17 Diagram of fetal circulation—arrows indicate the direction of blood flow; three shunts (ductus venosus, foramen ovale, ductus arteriosus) exist in utero but close shortly after birth.

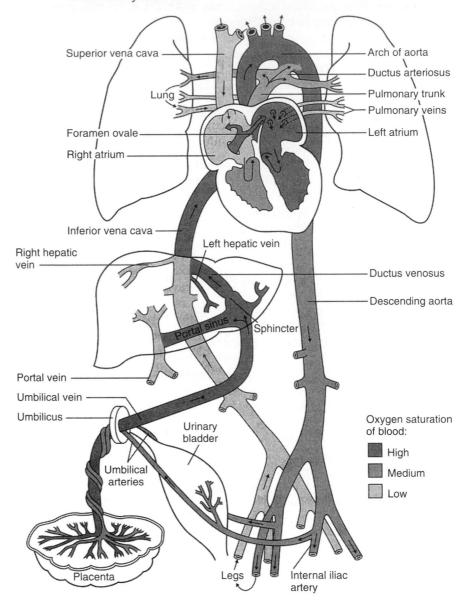

(Taken from Lilly LS. *Pathophysiology of Heart Disease.* 2nd Ed. Baltimore: Williams & Wilkins; 1998. Used with permission of Lippincott Williams & Wilkins.)

XII. Pediatric cardiology

A. **Fetal circulation**

1. Gas exchange occurs in uteroplacental circulation
2. Fetal Hgb has greater O_2 affinity than adult Hgb and pulls O_2 from maternal blood
3. Umbilical arteries carry deoxygenated blood to placenta; umbilical veins carry oxygenated blood from placenta to portal system
4. Changes occurring after birth
   a. Lung expansion causes increased pulmonary blood flow leading to an increase in relative blood oxygenation
   b. A decreasing serum level of prostaglandin E_2 results in **ductus arteriosus closure;** umbilical cord clamping results in end of placental circulation and an increase in systemic vascular resistance

FIGURE
1-18 Ventricular septal defect (VSD)–the arrow depicts shunting of blood from the left to right ventricle. Ao, aorta; IVC, inferior vena cava; LA, left atrium; LV, left ventricle; PA, pulmonary artery; RA, right atrium; RV, right ventricle; SVC, superior vena cava.

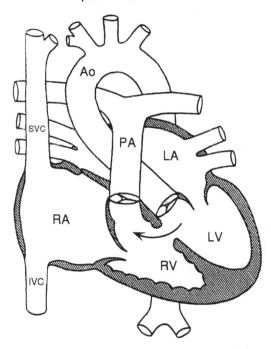

(Taken from Lilly LS. *Pathophysiology of Heart Disease.* 2nd Ed. Baltimore: Williams & Wilkins; 1998. Used with permission of Lippincott Williams & Wilkins.)

    c. This increased vascular resistance, in turn, induces **ductus venosus closure** and umbilical artery and vein constriction

    d. Left atrial pressure increases (due to increased pulmonary blood flow) and umbilical circulation decreases causing decrease in inferior vena cava pressure

    e. Decrease in inferior vena cava and right atrial pressures lead to **foramen ovale closure**

B. **Ventricular septal defect (VSD)**
  1. Opening in ventricular septum allowing shunting of blood
  2. **Most common** congenital heart defect
  3. **H/P** = asymptomatic if small; frequent respiratory infections, failure to thrive, dyspnea, shortness of breath, heart failure symptoms with larger defects; pansystolic murmur at lower left sternal border, loud pulmonic S_2, systolic thrill
  4. **ECG** = left ventricular hypertrophy, right ventricular hypertrophy; frequently normal
  5. **Radiology** = echocardiogram shows shunt
  6. **Treatment** = clinically follow small defects; repair large defects soon (before Eisenmenger's develops)
  7. **Complications** = if untreated, Eisenmenger's syndrome develops (irreversible); increased risk of endocarditis

C. **Atrial septal defect (ASD)**
  1. Opening in atrial septum allowing movement of blood between atria
  2. Initially, blood flow is left-to-right across defect
  3. **H/P** = possibly asymptomatic; large defects may cause cyanosis, heart failure symptoms, dyspnea, fatigue, or failure to thrive; strong impulse at lower left sternal border, **wide fixed split S$_2$,** systolic ejection murmur at upper left sternal border

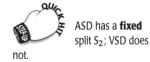

ASD has a **fixed** split S_2; VSD does not.

FIGURE 1-19 Atrial septal defect (ASD)—the arrow depicts shunting of blood from the left to right atrium. Ao, aorta; IVC, inferior vena cava; LA, left atrium; LV, left ventricle; PA, pulmonary artery; RA, right atrium; RV, right ventricle; SVC, superior vena cava.

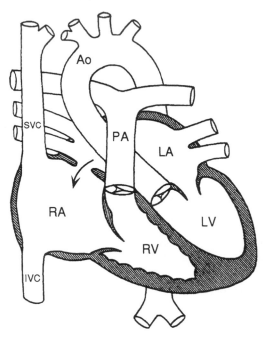

(Taken from Lilly LS. *Pathophysiology of Heart Disease.* 2nd Ed. Baltimore: Williams & Wilkins; 1998. Used with permission of Lippincott Williams & Wilkins.)

    4. **ECG** = right axis deviation
    5. **Radiology** = echocardiogram shows blood flow between atria, dilated RV, and large heart; CXR shows increased pulmonary vascular markings due to pulmonary HTN
    6. **Treatment** = small defects do not need repair but require **antibiotic prophylaxis** prior to surgery or dental work; surgical closure for symptomatic infants or when pulmonary blood flow is twice that of systemic blood flow
    7. **Complications** = untreated ASD leads to right-to-left shunt (**Eisenmenger's syndrome**), RV dysfunction, pulmonary HTN, arrhythmias
  D. **Patent ductus arteriosus (PDA)**
    1. Failure of ductus arteriosus to close after birth
    2. Left-to-right shunt (aorta to pulmonary artery)
    3. **Risk factors** = **prematurity,** high altitude, 1st-trimester maternal rubella, maternal prostaglandin administration; females > males
    4. **H/P** = possibly asymptomatic; heart failure symptoms, dyspnea; wide pulse pressure, continuous "**machinery**" **murmur** at 2nd left intercostal space, loud S_2, bounding pulses
    5. **ECG** = possible LVH
    6. **Radiology** = possible cardiomegaly on CXR; echocardiogram shows large left atrium (LA) and LV; angiography confirms diagnosis
    7. **Treatment** = **indomethacin** induces closure; surgical closure if unresponsive
  E. **Transposition of the great vessels**
    1. Parallel pulmonary and systemic circulations; aorta connected to RV; pulmonary artery connected to LV

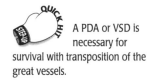

A PDA or VSD is necessary for survival with transposition of the great vessels.

FIGURE 1-20 Patent ductus arteriosus (PDA)—the arrow depicts shunting of blood from the aorta to pulmonary artery. Ao, aorta; IVC, inferior vena cava; LA, left atrium; LV, left ventricle; PA, pulmonary artery; RA, right atrium; RV, right ventricle; SVC, superior vena cava.

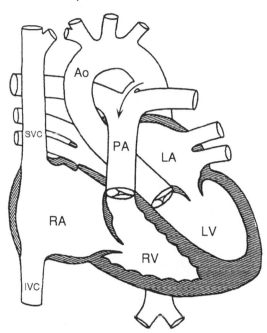

(Taken from Lilly LS. *Pathophysiology of Heart Disease.* 2nd Ed. Baltimore: Williams & Wilkins; 1998. Used with permission of Lippincott Williams & Wilkins.)

FIGURE 1-21 Transposition of the great vessels—the aorta arises from the right ventricle, and the pulmonary artery arises from the left ventricle. Ao, aorta; IVC, inferior vena cava; LA, left atrium; LV, left ventricle; PA, pulmonary artery; RA, right atrium; RV, right ventricle; SVC, superior vena cava.

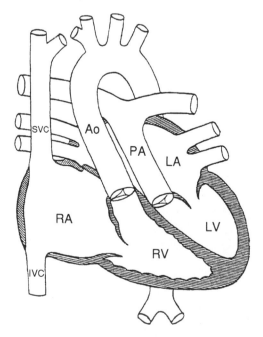

(Taken from Lilly LS. *Pathophysiology of Heart Disease.* 2nd Ed. Baltimore: Williams & Wilkins; 1998. Used with permission of Lippincott Williams & Wilkins.)

2. Cause is poorly understood but is likely linked to cardiac septal development in the truncus arteriosus
3. Incompatible with life (fetus is stillborn) unless comorbid PDA or VSD
4. **Risk factors** = Apert's syndrome, Down's syndrome, cri-du-chat syndrome, trisomy 13 or 18
5. **H/P** = cyanosis after birth; cyanosis worsens as PDA closes; loud S_2
6. **Radiology** = narrow heart base, abnormal pulmonary markings on CXR; echocardiogram used for diagnosis
7. **Treatment = keep PDA open with prostaglandin E;** balloon atrial septostomy to widen VSD; prompt surgical correction

F. **Persistent truncus arteriosus**
1. Failure of aorta and pulmonary artery to separate during development results in a single vessel that supplies systemic and pulmonary circulation
2. **H/P** = cyanosis after birth; dyspnea, fatigue, failure to thrive; heart failure symptoms soon develop; harsh systolic murmur at lower left sternal border, loud S_1 and S_2, bounding pulses
3. **ECG** = likely LVH, RVH
4. **Radiology** = angiography or echocardiogram used for diagnosis; CXR may show boot-shaped heart, no pulmonary artery, large aorta arcing to right side
5. **Treatment** = surgical correction

G. **Endocardial cushion defect**
1. Malformation of atrioventricular valves, atrial septum, and/or ventricular septum during fetal development causes variety of valvular and septal defects

FIGURE
1-22 Tetralogy of Fallot—combination of ventricular septal defect *(hollow arrow indicates right to left shunt),* right ventricular outflow obstruction *(solid arrow),* overriding aorta, and right ventricular hypertrophy. Ao, aorta; IVC, inferior vena cava; LA, left atrium; LV, left ventricle; PA, pulmonary artery; RA, right atrium; RV, right ventricle; SVC, superior vena cava.

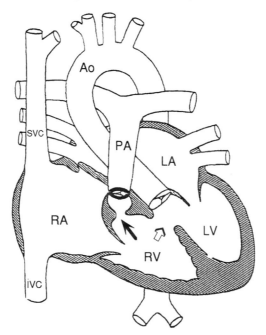

(Taken from Lilly LS. *Pathophysiology of Heart Disease.* 2nd Ed. Baltimore: Williams & Wilkins; 1998. Used with permission of Lippincott Williams & Wilkins.)

2. **Complete defect** has ASD, VSD, and single atrioventricular canal
3. **Incomplete defect** has ASD and minor atrioventricular valve abnormalities
4. Found in **20% of Down's syndrome children**
5. **H/P** = incomplete form resembles presentation for ASD; complete form causes heart failure symptoms, pneumonitis; murmurs consistent with particular defect
6. **ECG** = left axis deviation
7. **Radiology** = echocardiogram or cardiac catheterization used for diagnosis
8. **Treatment** = surgical correction

H. **Tetralogy of Fallot**
   1. VSD, RV outflow obstruction, RVH, and overriding aorta
   2. **Risk factors** = Down's syndrome, cri-du-chat syndrome, trisomy 13 and 18
   3. **H/P** = early cyanosis, dyspnea, fatigue; children squat for relief during hypoxemic episodes; systolic ejection murmur at left sternal border, RV lift, single S_2
   4. **ECG** = right axis deviation
   5. **Radiology** = echocardiogram or cardiac catheterization used for diagnosis; boot-shaped heart seen on CXR
   6. **Treatment** = prostaglandin E to maintain PDA; O_2, propranolol, IV fluids, morphine, knee-to-chest positioning during cyanotic episodes; surgical correction

Pulmonary Disorders

I. Measures of pulmonary function

A. Pulmonary function tests (PFTs)

1. Uses for PFTs
   a. Categorizing various types of lung processes and changes in lung air volumes
   b. Assessing severity of pulmonary disease
   c. Evaluating success of treatment
2. Specific measurements
   a. **Lung volumes (see Figure 2-1)**
   b. **Airflow**
      (1) FEV_1/FVC is ratio of air volume expired in 1 second to functional vital capacity (FEV = forced expiratory volume)
      (2) $FEF_{25\%-75\%}$ is forced expiratory flow rate between 25% and 75% of FVC
   c. **Alveolar membrane permeability**
      (1) Diffusing capacity of lungs, or D_{Lco}, is a relative measurement of lungs' ability to transfer gases from alveoli to pulmonary capillaries
      (2) PFTs usually list D_{Lco} as a percentage of the normal expected value

B. Alveolar-arterial (A-a) gradient (see Table 2-3)

1. This measurement compares the oxygenation status of arterial blood (Pa_{O_2}) to alveoli (PA_{O_2})
2. **Normal A-a gradient = 5–15 mm Hg**
3. Increased A-a gradient is seen in pulmonary embolism (PE), pulmonary edema, and right-to-left vascular shunts
4. False-normal A-a gradient may be seen in cases of hypoventilation or at high altitudes

II. Respiratory infections

A. Upper respiratory infections (URIs)

1. Common cold (viral rhinitis) is the inflammation of upper airways
   a. Most commonly due to rhinovirus, coronavirus, or adenovirus
   b. **History and Physical (H/P)** = nasal and throat irritation, sneezing, **rhinorrhea** (nasal congestion and increased secretions), **non-productive cough;** possible fever, no exudates or productive cough
   c. **Labs** = negative throat culture
   d. **Treatment** = rest, analgesia, treat symptoms; antibiotics are NOT helpful
2. **Pharyngitis**
   a. Pharyngeal infection caused by **group A β-hemolytic streptococci ("strep throat")** or common cold virus

Normal FEV_1/FVC is 80%; <80% suggests obstructive pathology; >110% suggests a restrictive pattern.

Upper respiratory infections are those that occur in the **sinuses** or **pharynx; lower** respiratory infections are those that occur in the **lungs** or **bronchi.**

Prescribing antibiotics for viral rhinitis is a contributing factor to the development of resistant strains of bacteria.

FIGURE
2-1 Healthy lung volumes. ERV, expiratory reserve volume; FRC, functional reserve capacity; FVC, functional vital capacity; IC, inspiratory capacity; IRV, inspiratory reserve volume; RV, residual volume; TLC, total lung capacity; TV, tidal volume.

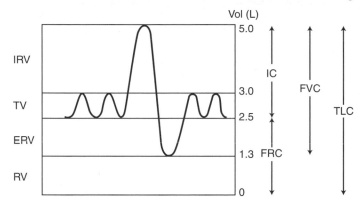

b. **H/P** = **sore throat,** lymphadenopathy, possible nasal congestion; fever, red and swollen pharynx, **tonsillar exudates** (more common with bacterial infection)

c. **Labs** = throat culture grows streptococcal species and rapid streptococcal antigen test is positive for strep throat; negative culture suggests viral etiology

d. **Treatment** = self-limited; β-lactam antibiotics (penicillin, amoxicillin, etc.) reduce infection time

e. **Complications** = untreated infection may cause **rheumatic heart disease** or glomerulonephritis (characterized by a high antistreptolysin O titer)

3. **Tonsillar infections**

a. Spread of streptococcal pharyngitis to palatine tonsils leading to tonsillar inflammation (**tonsillitis**)

 It is important to complete the full prescribed course of an antibiotic to achieve cure and prevent relapse and complications as well as prevent development of **antibiotic-resistant strains.**

TABLE 2-1	Definitions of Lung Volume Terms and Formulas
Lung Volume	**Definition**
Inspiratory reserve volume (IRV)	Air volume beyond normal tidal volume that is filled during maximum inspiration
Tidal volume (TV)	Inspiratory volume during normal respiration
Expiratory reserve volume (ERV)	Air volume beyond tidal volume that can be expired during normal respiration
Residual volume (RV)	Remaining air volume left in lung following maximum expiration
Inspiratory capacity (IC)	Total inspiratory air volume considering both tidal volume and inspiratory reserve volume (IC = TV + IRV)
Functional reserve capacity (FRC)	Air volume remaining in lungs after expiration of tidal volume (FRC = RV + ERV)
Functional vital capacity (FVC)	Maximum air volume that can be inspired and expired (FVC = IC + ERV)
Total lung capacity (TLC)	Total air volume of lungs (TLC = FVC + RV)

ERV, expiratory reserve volume; FRC, functional reserve capacity; FVC, functional vital capacity; IC, inspiratory capacity; IRV, inspiratory reserve volume; RV, residual volume; TLC, total lung capacity; TV, tidal volume.

FIGURE 2-2 Spirometry tracings for normal respiration compared to obstructive and restrictive pulmonary diseases. FEV_1, one-second forced expiratory volume.

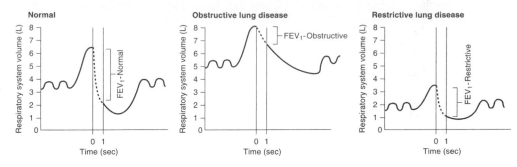

(Modified from Mehta S, Milder EA, Mirachi AJ, Milder E. *Step-Up: A High-Yield, Systems-Based Review for the USMLE Step 1*. 2nd Ed. Philadelphia: Lippincott Williams & Wilkins; 2003.)

> **QUICK HIT**
> **Signs of a peritonsillar abscess** include difficulty opening the mouth, asymmetric tonsils, and displacement of the uvula away from the abscess.

b. **H/P** = similar to streptococcal pharyngitis; ear pain, difficulty swallowing; possible high fever, **tonsillar exudates**

c. **Treatment** = same as streptococcal pharyngitis

d. **Complications** = airway compromise; abscess (require intravenous [IV] antibiotics and surgical incision and drainage followed by tonsillectomy after resolution to prevent recurrence)

4. **Viral influenza**

a. Generalized infection with URI symptoms caused by one of several influenza viruses

b. **H/P** = arthralgias, **myalgias,** sore throat, nasal congestion, non-productive cough, nausea, **vomiting, diarrhea; high fevers** (typically >100° F and may reach up to 106° F)

c. **Labs** = serologic tests are definitive but rarely required for diagnosis

> **QUICK HIT**
> **Mortality from influenza** is greater in the elderly and chronically ill, and these patients should receive annual vaccination.

d. **Treatment** = treat symptoms; **fluid intake important** to replace losses from vomiting and diarrhea; self-limited (several days) but **amantadine** may shorten course of disease; elderly patients, healthcare workers, immunocompromised patients, and patients with lung disease should receive annual vaccine to reduce risk of infection

5. **Sinusitis**

a. Sinus infection associated with allergic rhinitis, barotrauma, viral infection, prolonged nasogastric tube placement, or asthma

b. **Acute sinusitis** is usually due to *Streptococcus pneumoniae, Haemophilus influenzae, Moraxella catarrhalis,* viral infection

TABLE 2-2 Changes in PFTs From Normal Lung to Obstructive and Restrictive Disease States

Measurement	Obstructive	Restrictive
TLC	↑	↓
FVC	↑	↓
RV	↑	↓
FRC	↓↓	↓
FEV_1	↓	↓
FEV_1/FVC	↓	Normal or ↑

FEV_1, one-second forced expiratory volume; FRC, functional reserve capacity; FVC, functional vital capacity; RV, residual volume; TLC, total lung capacity; ↑, increase; ↓, decrease; ↓↓, large decrease.

TABLE 2-3	Calculation of the A-a Gradient	
Variable	**Definition**	**Value**
Pa_{O_2}	Arterial O_2 content	Measured directly from arterial blood gas sample; normal value is ~**90 – 100 mmHg**
PA_{O_2}	Alvcolar O_2 content	(Atmospheric air pressure) × (Fi_{O_2}) – ([$Pa_{CO_2}/0.8$]); for **room air** this becomes (713 mmHg) × (0.21) – ([$Pa_{CO_2}/0.8$]) = **150 mmHg – ([$Pa_{CO_2}/0.8$])**
Pa_{CO_2}	Arterial CO_2 content	Measured directly from arterial blood gas sample; normal value is ~**40 mmHg**
Fi_{O_2}	Fraction of O_2 in inspired air	For room air this fraction is typically **0.21**
A-a gradient	Difference between alveolar and arterial oxygenation status	$PA_{O_2} - Pa_{O_2}$ = (713 mmHg) × (Fi_{O_2}) – [(Pa_{CO_2})/0.8] – Pa_{O_2}; **5–15 mmHg is considered a normal A-a gradient**

c. **Chronic sinusitis** (lasting >3 months) is usually due to sinus obstruction, anaerobic infection; patients with DM predisposed to mucormycosis

d. **H/P = pain over infected sinuses,** purulent nasal discharge, maxillary toothache pain; illumination test (light held close to sinuses) may detect congestion in frontal of maxillary sinuses but is **unreliable**

e. **Radiology** = radiograph shows opacification and fluid levels in affected sinuses; computed tomography (CT) is diagnostic; frequently radiological tests are not needed because of clinical diagnosis

f. **Treatment** = treat symptoms; amoxicillin × two weeks in acute cases and for 6–12 weeks in chronic cases; surgical drainage or correction of anatomical obstruction may be required for full cure

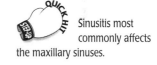

Acute sinusitis may spread to the CNS and cause **meningitis** if untreated.

Sinusitis most commonly affects the maxillary sinuses.

FIGURE 2-3 Diagram of the upper and lower respiratory regions and appropriate sites of infection.

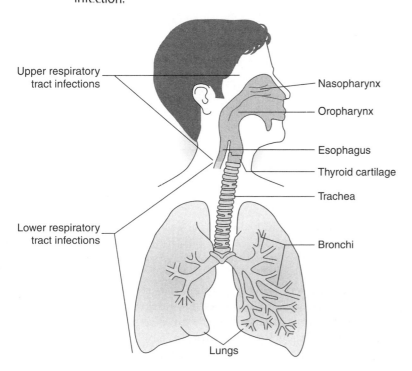

Upper respiratory tract infections

Nasopharynx

Oropharynx

Esophagus

Thyroid cartilage

Trachea

Lower respiratory tract infections

Bronchi

Lungs

TABLE 2-4	Overview of Etiologies of Pneumonia		
Pathogen	**Patients Affected**	**Characteristic Symptoms**	**Treatment**
Viral Pneumonia			
Viral (influenza, parainfluenza, adenovirus, cytomegalovirus, respiratory syncytial virus	**Most common pneumonia in children;** common in adults	Classic symptoms;[a] **non-productive cough**	**Self-limited;** amantidine may be used for influenza A virus
Typical Bacterial Pneumonia			
Streptococcus pneumoniae	**Most common pneumonia in adults;** higher risk of infection in sickle cell patients	Classic symptoms; high fevers, pleuritic pain, **productive cough**	β-Lactams, macrolides
Haemophilus influenzae	COPD patients; higher risk of infection in sickle cell patients	Classic symptoms; **slower onset**	β-Lactams, TMP-SMX
Staphylococcus aureus	Nosocomial pneumonia, immunocompromised patients	Classic symptoms; abscess formation	β-Lactams
Atypical Bacterial Pneumonia			
Klebsiella pneumoniae	Alcoholics, patients with high risk of aspiration, patients staying in the hospital for extended amounts of time, sickle cell patients	**"Currant-jelly"** sputum; classic symptoms	Both cephalosporins and aminoglycosides (gentamicin, tobramycin)
Mycoplasma pneumoniae	**Young adults**	Less severe symptoms; possible rash; **positive cold-agglutinin test**	Macrolides (azithromycin, clarithromycin, erythromycin)
Pseudomonas aeruginosa	Chronically ill and immunocompromised patients, **patients with cystic fibrosis,** nosocomial pneumonia	Classic symptoms; rapid onset	Fluoroquinolones (ciprofloxacin), aminoglycosides, 3rd-generation cephalosporins
Legionella pneumophilia	Associated with **aerosolized water** (air-conditioners)	Slow onset of classic symptoms; nausea, diarrhea, confusion, or ataxia	Macrolides, fluoroquinolones
Fungal Pneumonia			
Fungi	Travelers to **southwest U.S.** (coccidioidomycosis), **caves** (histoplasmosis), or Central America (blastomycosis)	Less severe symptoms; subacute disease for initial history	Antifungal agents (amphotericin B, ketoconazole)
Pneumocystis carinii (fungi-like)	Immunocompromised patients (HIV) (CD4 count <200)	Slow onset of classic symptoms; GI symptoms	TMP-SMX

[a]Classic symptoms = productive or nonproductive cough, dyspnea, chills, night sweats, pleuritic chest pain.
COPD, chronic obstructive pulmonary disease; GI, gastrointestinal; TMP-SMX, trimethoprim-sulfamethoxazole.

Mycoplasma pneumoniae is the most common bacterial cause of acute bronchitis in non-smokers and may be diagnosed by a high cold agglutinin titer; *Streptococcus pneumonia* and *Haemophilus influenzae* are common causes in smokers.

B. **Lower respiratory infections**
1. **Acute bronchitis**
   a. Inflammation of trachea and bronchi caused by spread of URI or exposure to inhaled irritants
   b. **H/P = productive cough,** sore throat; fever, wheezing, tight breath sounds
   c. **Treatment** = self-limited if viral (vast majority of cases); patient groups with an increased risk of bacterial infection (smokers, elderly, patients with other lung disease) may be given antibiotics (fluoroquinolones, tetracycline, or erythromycin)

TABLE 2-5	Most Common Etiologies of Pneumonia by Age Group
Age Group	**Common Etiologies of Pneumonia (in Decreasing Frequency)**
Birth–20 yr of age	Respiratory syncytial virus *Mycoplasma pneumoniae* *Chlamydia pneumoniae* *Streptococcus pneumoniae*
20–40 years of age	*Mycoplasma pneumoniae* *Streptococcus pneumoniae*
40–60 years of age	*Streptococcus pneumoniae* *Mycoplasma pneumoniae* *Haemophilus influenzae*
>60 years of age	*Streptococcus pneumoniae* Anaerobes *Haemophilus influenzae* Respiratory syncytial virus

(Modified from Mehta S, Milder EA, Mirachi AJ, Milder E. *Step-Up: A High-Yield, Systems-Based Review for the USMLE Step 1*. 2nd Ed. Philadelphia: Lippincott Williams & Wilkins; 2003.)

2. **Pneumonia**
    a. Infection of the bronchoalveolar tree—may be due to common nasopharyngeal bacteria (**typical** pneumonia), or bacteria, viruses, or fungi from the surrounding environment (**atypical** pneumonia); common etiologies vary by age group
    b. **H/P** = productive or non-productive cough, dyspnea, chills, night sweats, **pleuritic chest pain; decreased breath sounds,** rales, wheezing, **dullness to percussion,** egophony (change in voice quality heard during auscultation over a consolidated region of lung), tactile fremitus, **tachypnea**
    c. **Labs** = increased white blood cell count (WBC) (slight increase with viral cause, significant increase with bacterial or fungal cause) with left shift (more immature forms); positive sputum culture and possible positive blood culture with bacterial or fungal cause (Color Figure 2-1)
    d. **Radiology** = CXR shows **lobar consolidation,** infiltrates, or general increased density of lung fields
    e. **Treatment** = viral pneumonia is self-limited and only requires supportive care; bacterial and fungal pneumonias require antibiotics (given orally on an outpatient basis for most patients and given IV on an inpatient basis for elderly patients or those with other respiratory conditions)
3. **Tuberculosis (TB)**
    a. Pulmonary infection caused by *Mycobacterium tuberculosis*
    b. Most of the active cases are due to formerly dormant infections that are reactivated
    c. While the number of yearly cases in the U.S. decreased with the advent of pharmacologic treatment in the 1950s, the incidence of cases has slowly **increased** since 1985 (now ~ 10 new cases per 100,000 people each yr), in large part because of the **HIV epidemic**
    d. **Risk factors** = immunosuppression, alcoholism, lung disease, DM, advanced age, homelessness, malnourishment, crowded living conditions, and close proximity to infected patients (e.g., **healthcare**

TABLE 2-6	Criteria Used to Determine Positive PPD for Tuberculosis
Size of Induration[a]	**When Considered Positive**
5 mm	HIV-positive, close contact with TB-infected patient, signs of TB seen on CXR
10 mm	Homeless patients, immigrants from developing nations, IVDA patients, chronically ill patients, healthcare workers, patients with recent incarceration
15 mm	Always considered positive

[a] Induration is considered the firm cutaneous region and not the region of erythema
CXR, chest x-ray; IVDA, intravenous drug abuse; PPD, purified protein derivative tuberculin skin test; TB, tuberculosis.

NEXT STEP Patients should be given an anergy test (subcutaneous *Candida* preparation) in addition to a PPD to check for an appropriate immune response.

NEXT STEP A positive PPD should be followed with a CXR to look for signs of TB.

Recipients of the BCG vaccine (commonly used in other countries) will show a false-positive PPD.

The multi-drug regimen for TB may be remembered as **RIPE** (**R**ifampin, **I**soniazid, **P**yrazinamide, **E**thambutol).

workers); TB is significantly more common in **developing nations** than in the U.S.

e. **H/P** = cough, hemoptysis, dyspnea, weight loss, night sweats, fever
f. **Labs** = positive sputum acid-fast stain, positive culture (may take weeks, so not useful in planning therapy), positive purified protein derivative tuberculin skin test (PPD) (Color Figure 2-2)
g. **Radiology** = chest x-ray (CXR) may show apical fibronodular infiltrates (reactivated disease), lower-lobe infiltrates (primary lesion), and calcified granulomas/lymph nodes (Ghon complexes)
h. **Treatment** = **respiratory isolation;** report all diagnosed cases to local and state health agencies; **multi-drug treatment** initially with isoniazid (INH), rifampin, pyrazinamide, and ethambutol or streptomycin; adjust treatment per susceptibility (INH and rifampin for six months is a common course); give vitamin B_6 with INH to prevent peripheral neuritis (INH competes with vitamin B_6 as a cofactor in neurotransmitter synthesis, so supplemental vitamin B_6 helps offset this competition); give prophylactic INH to patients with an asymptomatic positive PPD who are immunocompromised, have a history of intravenous drug abuse (IVDA), are less than 35 years of age, have a history of close contact with TB-infected people, or are indigent patients (reporting is unnecessary unless TB is diagnosed)
i. **Complications** = meningitis, bone involvement (Pott's disease), widespread dissemination to multiple organs (miliary TB)

III. Acute respiratory distress syndrome (ARDS)

A. Acute respiratory failure due to sepsis, trauma, aspiration, near drowning, drug overdose, shock, or lung infection that is characterized by **refractory hypoxemia,** decreased lung compliance, and pulmonary edema, and carries a **high mortality**
B. **H/P** = acute dyspnea, cyanosis; tachypnea (begins within 48 hours of initial insult), wheezing, rales, rhonchi
C. **Labs** = arterial blood gas (ABG) shows respiratory alkalosis, decreased O_2 (due to impairment of O_2 transfer to pulmonary capillaries by pulmonary edema), decreased CO_2 (due to hyperventilation)
D. **Radiology** = bilateral pulmonary edema and infiltrates
E. **Treatment** = treatment in **intensive care** usually necessary; treat underlying condition; mechanical ventilation with positive end-expiratory pressure (PEEP), increased inspiratory times, and Fio_2 adjusted to maintain O_2 saturation (Sao_2) >90%; keep fluid volumes low to prevent pulmonary edema; use of extracorporeal membrane oxygenation (ECMO) may improve outcome

IV. Obstructive airway diseases

A. Asthma

1. **Reversible** airway obstruction secondary to bronchial hyperactivity, acute airway inflammation, mucous plugging, and smooth muscle hypertrophy

2. **Exacerbations** (sudden bronchoconstriction and airway inflammation) are triggered by allergens (dust, smoke, pollen, fumes), URIs, exercise, stress, β-antagonist drugs, aspirin (rare) and sulfites (rare)

3. While the prevalence of asthma in the U.S. has increased in the past 20 years, the reasons for this trend are poorly understood

4. **Risk factors** = family history of asthma, allergies, atopic dermatitis, low socioeconomic status

5. Disease may be worse in childhood; improves with age

6. **H/P** = cough, dyspnea, wheezing, chest tightness; tachypnea, tachycardia, **prolonged expiratory duration** (extended time required to expire smaller inspiratory capacity; refer to Figure 2-2), decreased breath sounds, wheezing, **accessory muscle use,** possible pulsus paradoxus; cyanosis, decreased arterial O_2 saturation (SaO_2) on pulse oximetry, or difficulty talking in severe attacks

7. **Labs** = ABG may show mild hypoxia and respiratory alkalosis; **PFTs show decreased FEV_1**

8. **Radiology** = CXR shows hyperinflation

9. **Treatment** =

   a. Acute exacerbations—**inhaled rapid-acting β_2-agonists** (albuterol, pirbuterol, bitolterol) are the cornerstone of therapy; inhaled corticosteroids, cromolyn, inhaled leukotriene inhibitors, or inhaled anticholinergics may be used for refractory exacerbations

NEXT STEP Status asthmaticus is a prolonged, non-responsive asthma attack that can be fatal and should be treated with **aggressive** bronchodilator therapy, corticosteroids, O_2, and possible intubation.

NEXT STEP A normal CO_2 during an exacerbation signals impending respiratory failure and requires additional β_2-agonists, supplemental O_2, and possible ventilation.

FIGURE 2-4 Medication protocols for treatment of chronic asthma.

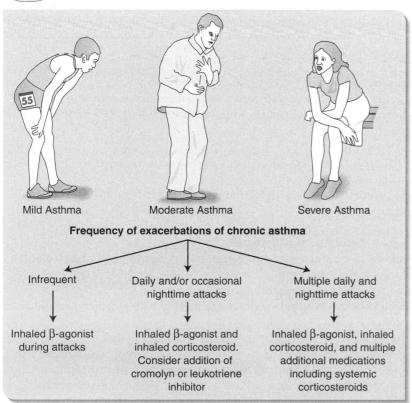

Mild Asthma   Moderate Asthma   Severe Asthma

Frequency of exacerbations of chronic asthma

Infrequent	Daily and/or occasional nighttime attacks	Multiple daily and nighttime attacks
Inhaled β-agonist during attacks	Inhaled β-agonist and inhaled corticosteroid. Consider addition of cromolyn or leukotriene inhibitor	Inhaled β-agonist, inhaled corticosteroid, and multiple additional medications including systemic corticosteroids

TABLE 2-7	Commonly Used Medications for Treatment of Asthma	
Medication	**Mechanism of Action**	**Role**
Rapid-acting β_2-agonists (albuterol, pirbuterol, bitolterol)	Bronchodilators that relax airway smooth muscle; have rapid onset of action	First-line therapy in acute exacerbations
Long-acting β_2-agonists (salmeterol, formoterol, sustained-release albuterol)	Bronchodilators that relax airway smooth muscle; have gradual onset and sustained activity	Regular use in patients with moderate chronic asthma
Inhaled corticosteroids (beclomethasone, flunisolide)	Decrease number and activity of cells involved with airway inflammation	Moderate-to-severe asthma; frequently combined with β_2-agonist use
Leukotriene inhibitors (zafirlukast, zileuton)	Block activity or production of leukotrienes that are involved in inflammation and bronchospasm	Oral agents; adjunctive therapy in moderate-to-severe cases
Cromolyn	Stabilizes mast cells; anti-inflammatory prophylaxis	Not useful acutely; anti-inflammatory prophylaxis in moderate-to-severe cases
Theophylline	Bronchodilator	Former first-line therapy but now replaced by β_2-agonists because of side effects and interactions with other drugs; may be useful in acute attacks but no longer commonly used
Anticholinergic agents (ipratropium)	Blocks vagal-mediated smooth muscle contraction	Adjunctive therapy in moderate-to-severe cases
Systemic steroids (methylprednisolone, prednisone)	Similar action to inhaled steroids; stronger effect than inhaled preparation	Adjunctive therapy in severe, refractory cases

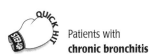

Patients with **chronic bronchitis** are "**blue bloaters**" because secondary development of cor pulmonale causes cyanosis and peripheral edema; patients with **emphysema** are "**pink puffers**" because of their pursed-lip breathing, dyspnea, and barrel-chests.

b. Long-term therapy—avoidance of exacerbating factors and regular use of **long-acting β_2-agonists** (salmeterol, formoterol, sustained-release albuterol), **inhaled corticosteroids,** cromolyn, and/or oral leukotriene inhibitors

B. **Chronic bronchitis**
  1. Chronic bronchial inflammation **associated with tobacco use** (common) or chronic asthma (uncommon)
  2. **H/P** = productive cough, recurrent respiratory infections, dyspnea; wheezing
  3. Diagnosis made with history of **productive cough for three months of the year for more than two years**
  4. **Treatment = tobacco cessation,** antibiotics given for URI due to greater incidence of bacterial etiology; bronchodilators and inhaled corticosteroids during exacerbations
  5. **Complications** = emphysema may frequently result without smoking cessation

C. **Emphysema** (chronic obstructive pulmonay disease [COPD])
  1. Long-term tobacco use leads to chronic bronchoalveolar inflammation associated with release of proteolytic enzymes by neutrophils and macrophages; **destruction of alveoli and bronchioles** results with panacinar airspace enlargement and a decreased capillary bed

2. Less common form (appears at younger age) caused by α_1-antitrypsin deficiency
3. **H/P = dyspnea,** barrel-chested; **pursed-lip breathing,** prolonged expiratory duration, decreased heart sounds, decreased breath sounds, rhonchi, accessory muscle use, jugular venous distension (JVD); exacerbations present with worsening symptoms
4. **Labs** = PFTs show decreased FEV_1, **decreased FEV_1/FVC,** increased total lung capacity (TLC); ABG during acute exacerbations shows decreased O_2, increased CO_2 (beyond a baseline increase already seen in these patients)
5. **Radiology** = CXR shows **flat diaphragm, hyperinflated lungs,** subpleural blebs and bullae (small fluid-filled sacs), and decreased vascular markings
6. **Treatment** = smoking cessation; O_2, inhaled β_2-agonists, inhaled anticholinergics, inhaled steroids; antibiotics given for respiratory infections; pneumococcal and influenza vaccines; enzyme replacement may have a role in α_1-antitrypsin deficiency therapy; lung transplant may be an option in late severe disease
7. **Complications** = chronic respiratory decompensation, cor pulmonale, frequent respiratory infections, frequent comorbid lung cancer

D. **Bronchiectasis**
1. **Permanent dilation** of small and medium bronchi due to destruction of bronchial elastic components
2. Occurs secondary to TB, fungal infections, severe pneumonia, or cystic fibrosis
3. **H/P** = persistent productive cough, hemoptysis, frequent respiratory infections; **copious sputum,** wheezing, crackles, and hypoxemia
4. **Radiology** = multiple cysts and bronchial crowding seen on CXR; CT shows dilation of bronchi and bronchial wall thickening
5. **Treatment** = bronchodilators, chest physical therapy, antibiotics given when sputum production increases
6. **Complications** = cor pulmonale, massive hemoptysis, abscess formation

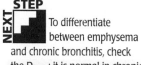
The common form of emphysema has a centrilobular distribution while the form associated with α_1-antitrypsin deficiency has a panlobular distribution.

NEXT STEP To differentiate between emphysema and chronic bronchitis, check the D_{LCO}; it is normal in chronic bronchitis but decreased in emphysema.

FIGURE 2-5 Chest x-ray demonstrating a solitary pulmonary nodule (*arrows*); in this patient the finding was determined to be a loculated pleural effusion.

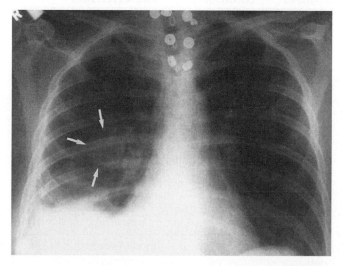

(Taken from Daffner RH. *Clinical Radiology: The Essentials.* 2nd Ed. Philadelphia: Lippincott Williams & Wilkins; 1999.)

FIGURE 2-6 Workup of the solitary pulmonary nodule.

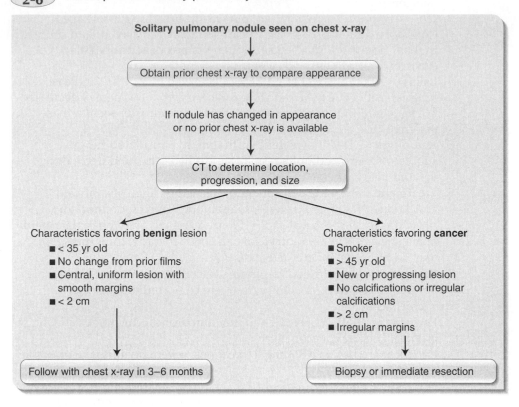

V. Respiratory neoplasms

  A. **Solitary pulmonary nodule**

   1. A lung nodule <5 cm diameter may be discovered incidentally on CXR or CT

   2. May be granuloma, hamartoma, cancer (primary or metastasis), carcinoid tumor, pneumonia

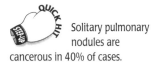

Solitary pulmonary nodules are cancerous in 40% of cases.

TABLE 2-8 Common Types of Primary Lung Cancer

Primary Lung Cancer Type	% of Primary Malignancies	Location	Characteristics
Squamous cell carcinoma	25–35%	Central	Cavitary lesions; direct extension to hilar lymph nodes
Adenocarcinoma	25–35%	Peripheral	Wide metastases; may be caused by asbestos; pleural effusions show increased hyaluronidase levels; bronchiolar cancer is subtype that is low grade and occurs in single nodules
Small cell carcinoma	20–25%	Central	Rapidly growing; early distant metastases; several paraneoplastic syndromes
Large cell carcinoma	5–15%	Peripheral	Late distant metastases, early cavitation

TABLE 2-9	Common Paraneoplastic Syndromes Associated with Primary Lung Cancers
Primary Lung Cancer Type	**Associated Paraneoplastic Syndromes**
Squamous cell	Hypercalcemia Dermatomyositis
Adenocarcinoma	Disseminated intravascular coagulation (DIC) Thrombophlebitis Microangiopathic hemolytic anemia Dermatomyositis
Small cell	Cushing's syndrome Syndrome of inappropriate ADH secretion (SIADH) Ectopic growth hormone and ACTH secretion Peripheral neuropathy Subacute cerebellar degeneration Eaton-Lambert syndrome (similar presentation to myasthenia gravis) Subacute sensory neuropathy Limbic encephalitis Dermatomyositis
Large cell	Gynecomastia Dermatomyositis

ACTH, adrenocorticotropic hormone; ADH, antidiuretic hormone.

B. **Lung cancer**
1. Most frequently **associated with tobacco use** (approximately 90% of cases). Also may be due to occupational exposures (e.g., smoke, asbestos)
2. Four types of primary lung cancer are described in Table 2-7
3. **H/P** = possibly asymptomatic; hemoptysis, cough, dyspnea, pleuritic chest pain, fatigue, weight loss, frequent pulmonary infections; additional symptoms may accompany paraneoplastic syndromes; local extension of tumors may result in:
    a. **Horner's syndrome** (miosis, ptosis, and anhidrosis due to invasion of cervical ganglia)
    b. **Pancoast's syndrome** (Horner's syndrome plus brachial plexus involvement)
    c. **Superior vena cava syndrome** (obstruction of venous drainage through superior vena cava and associated head swelling and [CNS] symptoms)
4. **Radiology** = initially seen on CXR or CT as pulmonary nodule; bronchoscopy with biopsy and brushings or fine needle aspiration of lesion are diagnostic
5. **Treatment**
    a. Squamous cell carcinoma, adenocarcinoma, and large cell carcinoma are treated with surgical resection (lobectomy), radiation, and chemotherapy; unresectable lesions treated with radiation and chemotherapy
    b. Small cell carcinoma treated with radiation and chemotherapy (usually unresectable, so surgery is not an option); mass effect of substantial tumors may be palliated with radiation; additional palliative treatment is used for metastases
6. **Complications = poor prognosis** (~10% five-yr survival); recurrence common for primary tumors

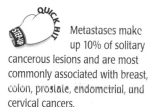

Metastases make up 10% of solitary cancerous lesions and are most commonly associated with breast, colon, prostate, endometrial, and cervical cancers.

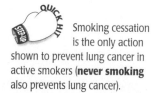

Smoking cessation is the only action shown to prevent lung cancer in active smokers (**never smoking** also prevents lung cancer).

C. Laryngeal cancer
   1. Squamous cell cancer of the larynx **associated with tobacco and alcohol use**
   2. **H/P = hoarseness that worsens with time** (over several weeks), dysphagia
   3. **Labs** = biopsy is diagnostic
   4. **Radiology** = laryngoscopy may detect lesion; magnetic resonance imaging (MRI) or CT with contrast detects soft tissue mass
   5. **Treatment** = radiation to shrink tumor; surgery to remove mass; advanced cases may require total laryngectomy

VI. **Interstitial lung diseases and other lung diseases**
   A. **Idiopathic pulmonary fibrosis (IPF)**
      1. Inflammatory lung disease causing lung fibrosis; it is of unknown etiology and generally affects patients >50 years of age
      2. **H/P** = progressive exercise intolerance, dyspnea; dry crackles, JVD, tachypnea, and possible digital clubbing
      3. **Labs** = PFTs will show **restrictive lung disease** characteristics (FEV_1/FVC normal, decreased FVC, decreased TLC, decreased compliance); bronchioalveolar lavage shows increased polymorphonuclear cells (PMNs)
      4. **Radiology** = CXR shows reticulonodular pattern and "**honeycomb**" lung; CT will show lung fields with "**ground glass**" appearance
      5. **Treatment** = corticosteroids are helpful in some patients (follow PFTs to evaluate effectiveness)
      6. **Complications** = progressive lung fibrosis with frequent mortality within five years
   B. **Sarcoidosis**
      1. Systemic disease characterized by **noncaseating granulomas;** unknown etiology
      2. **Risk factors** = African Americans >Caucasians; females >males; most frequently occurs between 30 and 40 years of age
      3. **H/P** = cough, malaise, weight loss, dyspnea, arthritis (knees, ankles); fever, erythema nodosum (tender red nodules on shins and arms), lymphadenopathy, vision loss, cranial nerve palsies
      4. **Labs** = increased serum angiotensin converting enzyme (ACE), increased calcium, hypercalciuria, increased alkaline phosphatase, decreased WBC, increased erythrocyte sedimentation rate (ESR); PFTs show decreased FVC, decreased D_{LCO}
      5. **Radiology** = CXR shows bilateral hilar lymphadenopathy, pulmonary infiltrates (ground glass appearance)
      6. **Treatment** = occasionally self-resolving; corticosteroids in chronic cases
   C. **Pneumoconioses**
      1. Interstitial lung diseases that result from long-term **occupational exposure** to substances that cause pulmonary inflammation
      2. **H/P** = symptoms begin when significant pulmonary fibrosis has occurred; cough, dyspnea on exertion, heavy sputum production; rales and wheezing are heard on auscultation
      3. **Labs** = PFTs show a restrictive pattern
      4. **Radiology** = CT shows signs of pulmonary fibrosis
      5. **Treatment** = there are usually no successful treatments for these conditions; **prevention** (proper air filters, following safe-handling recommendations) **is vital to avoiding disease**
   D. **Goodpasture's syndrome**
      1. Progressive autoimmune disease of lungs and kidneys characterized by intra-alveolar hemorrhage and glomerulonephritis

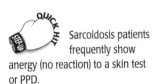

Sarcoidosis patients frequently show anergy (no reaction) to a skin test or PPD.

TABLE 2-10 Common Pneumoconioses and How to Diagnose Them

Disease	Exposure	Labs	Radiology	Complications
Asbestosis	Working with insulation, construction, demolition, building maintenance, automobiles	Asbestos fibers seen in **pleural biopsy**	Linear opacities at base of lungs; thickened pleura	Increased risk of **malignant mesothelioma** and lung cancer; synergistic effect with tobacco
Silicosis	Mining, pottery making, sandblasting, cutting granite	PFTs show restrictive pattern	Small apical nodular opacities; hilar adenopathy	**Increase risk of TB infection;** progressive fibrosis
Coal worker's disease	**Coal mining**	PFTs show restrictive pattern	Small apical nodular opacities	Progressive fibrosis
Berylliosis	**Electronics,** ceramics, tool, die manufacturing	Pulmonary edema, diffuse granuloma formation	Diffuse infiltrates; hilar adenopathy	Increased risk of lung cancer; may need chronic corticosteroid treatment to maintain respiratory function

PFTs, pulmonary function tests; TB, tuberculosis.

2. **H/P** = hemoptysis, dyspnea, recent respiratory infection
3. **Labs** = positive **anti-GBM antibodies;** PFTs show restrictive pattern
4. **Radiology** = bilateral alveolar infiltration
5. **Treatment** = plasmapheresis to remove auto-antibodies; corticosteroids and immunosuppressive agents

E. **Wegener's granulomatosis**
1. Rare disease with granulomatous inflammation and necrosis of lung and other organ systems
2. Due to systemic vasculitis that mainly affects lung and kidney causing formation of noncaseating granulomas and destruction of lung parenchyma
3. **H/P** = hemoptysis, dyspnea, myalgias, chronic sinusitis; ulcerations of nasopharynx, fever; additional symptoms from renal, CNS, ophthalmologic, and cardiac involvement
4. **Labs** = **positive c-ANCA;** biopsy shows **noncaseating granulomas;** renal workup should aid in diagnosis
5. **Treatment** = cytotoxic therapy, corticosteroids
6. **Complications** = rapidly fatal if untreated

VII. Vascular and thromboembolic pulmonary conditions
A. **Pulmonary embolism (PE)**
1. Occlusion of pulmonary vasculature by a dislodged thrombus
2. Increasing pulmonary artery pressure due to occlusion leads to right-sided heart failure, hypoxia, and pulmonary infarction
3. **Risk factors** = **immobilization, cancer,** prolonged travel, recent surgery, pregnancy, oral contraceptive use, hypercoagulability, obesity, bone fracture, prior deep vein thrombosis (DVT), or severe burns
4. **H/P** = **sudden dyspnea,** pleuritic chest pain, cough, syncope, hemoptysis, cyanosis; fever, tachypnea, tachycardia, loud S_2
5. **Labs** = ABG shows increased CO_2, decreased O_2 (<80), **increased A-a gradient;** ventilation-perfusion scan (**V/Q scan**) may show areas of mismatch
6. **Electrocardiogram (ECG)** = tachycardia, may show S wave in lead I and T-wave inversion in lead V_3

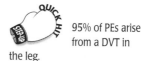

95% of PEs arise from a DVT in the leg.

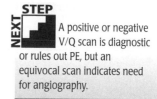

A positive or negative V/Q scan is diagnostic or rules out PE, but an equivocal scan indicates need for angiography.

Low-molecular-weight heparin (LMWH) is an acceptable alternative to heparin and does not require PTT monitoring (but may be assessed by measuring anti-factor Xa levels).

7. **Radiology** = CXR may be normal or may show pleural effusion or wedge-shaped infarct; pulmonary angiography is diagnostic; spiral CT may detect proximal PE
8. **Treatment** = administer heparin until prothrombin time (PTT) is 1.5–2.5 times normal; warfarin given 3–6 months with an international normalized ratio (INR) between 2–3; inferior vena cava filter may be placed if anticoagulation is contraindicated; thrombolysis or embolectomy are only performed for massive PE

B. **Pulmonary hypertension**
   1. Increased pulmonary artery pressure due to **PE, valvular disease,** left-to-right shunts, COPD, or idiopathic causes
   2. Idiopathic pulmonary hypertension has a high mortality rate within a few years of diagnosis
   3. **H/P** = dyspnea, fatigue, deep chest pain, cough, syncope, cyanosis; digital clubbing, **loud S_2,** JVD, hepatomegaly
   4. **Labs** = increased RBC and WBC
   5. **ECG** = right ventricular hypertrophy
   6. **Radiology** = CXR shows large pulmonary artery and large right ventricle; echocardiogram and angiography are helpful in making diagnosis
   7. **Treatment** = treat underlying condition; supplemental O_2 helps maintain blood oxygenation; vasodilators decrease pulmonary vascular resistance; anticoagulants decrease risk of pulmonary thrombus formation

C. **Pulmonary edema**
   1. Increased fluid in lungs caused by increased pulmonary venous pressure
   2. Due to **left-sided heart failure,** MI, **valvular disease,** arrhythmias, ARDS
   3. **H/P** = dyspnea, **orthopnea, paroxysmal nocturnal dyspnea;** tachycardia, frothy sputum, wheezing, rhonchi, rales, dullness to percussion, peripheral edema
   4. **Radiology** = CXR shows fluid throughout lungs, cephalization of vessels (increased vascular markings in upper lung fields), Kerley B lines (prominent horizontal interstitial markings in lower lung fields)
   5. **Treatment** = treat underlying condition; diuretics, salt restriction, O_2, morphine, vasodilators

VIII. Pleural diseases
A. **Pleural effusion**
   1. Serous or lymphatic fluid collection in pleural space classified according to protein and lactate dehydrogenase (LDH) content and due to **changes in hydrostatic and oncotic pressure** (transudative), **inflammation** (exudative), or lymphatic duct rupture (lymphatic)
   2. **H/P** = possibly asymptomatic; dyspnea, pleuritic chest pain, weakness; decreased breath sounds, dullness to percussion, decreased tactile fremitus, egophony

TABLE 2-11 **Distinctive Characteristics and Causes of Types of Pleural Effusions**

Effusion	Pleural:Serum Protein Ratio	Pleural:Serum LDH Ratio	Total Pleural Protein	Causes
Transudate	<0.5	<0.6	<3 g/dL	CHF, cirrhosis, kidney diseases (nephrotic syndrome)
Exudate	>0.5	>0.6	>3 g/dL	Infection, cancer, vasculitis

CHF, congestive heart failure; LDH, lactate dehydrogenase.

TABLE 2-12	Types of Pneumothorax and Their Causes	
Type of Pneumothorax	**Mechanism**	**Causes**
Closed	Internal rupture of respiratory system; chest wall intact	Spontaneous, COPD, TB
Open	Passage of air through opening in chest wall	Trauma, iatrogenic (central line placement, thoracocentesis, biopsy)
Tension	Open pneumothorax; "ball-valve" condition allows air to enter but not leave pleural space	Trauma

COPD, chronic obstructive pulmonary disease; TB, tuberculosis.

3. **Labs** = pleural fluid analysis utilized for protein and LDH levels, CBC, gram stain, and cytology
4. **Radiology** = CXR shows blunting of costophrenic angles; decubitus CXR can demonstrate whether fluid is loculated or free flowing
5. **Treatment** = treat underlying condition; relieve pressure on lung with thoracocentesis and chest tube placement; for cases with empyema (effusion of pus due to infection) a chest tube is required; if recurrent malignant effusion occurs, use pleurodesis (talc or other irritant) to scar the pleural layers together

B. **Pneumothorax**
1. Collection of air in pleural space that predisposes patient to pulmonary collapse
2. **H/P = unilateral chest pain,** dyspnea; **decreased chest wall movement,** decreased breath sounds, increased resonance to percussion, decreased tactile fremitus; respiratory distress, decreased Sao$_2$, hypotension, JVD, or tracheal deviation suggest tension pneumothorax
3. **Radiology** = CXR shows lung retraction and mediastinal shift away from affected side (See Figure 2-7)
4. **Treatment**
   a. Small pneumothorax may self-resolve
   b. Large pneumothorax requires **chest tube placement**
   c. Tension pneumothorax requires **immediate needle decompression** and chest tube placement (4th or 5th intercostal space at the maxillary line)
   d. Recurrent pneumothorax may require pleurodesis

C. **Hemothorax**
1. Collection of blood in pleural space due to trauma, malignancy, TB, or pulmonary infarction
2. **H/P** = dyspnea, pleuritic chest pain, weakness; decreased breath sounds, dullness to percussion, decreased tactile fremitus, egophony
3. **Labs** = thoracocentesis shows bloody effusion
4. **Radiology** = CXR resembles that for pleural effusion (i.e., lung retraction, mediastinal shift from affected side)
5. **Treatment** = chest tube placement; treat underlying cause
6. **Complications** = thrombi formation, fibrosis may occur if blood is not drained from pleural space

D. **Malignant mesothelioma**
1. Uncommon tumor occurring on visceral pleura with very poor prognosis
2. **Increased incidence with asbestos exposure** (occurs 20 years after exposure)

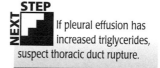
If pleural effusion has increased triglycerides, suspect thoracic duct rupture.

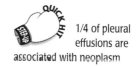
1/4 of pleural effusions are associated with neoplasm

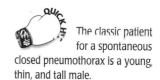
The classic patient for a spontaneous closed pneumothorax is a young, thin, and tall male.

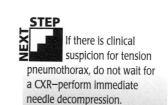
If there is clinical suspicion for tension pneumothorax, do not wait for a CXR—perform immediate needle decompression.

FIGURE
2-7 Chest x-ray demonstrating tension pneumothorax; note compressed visceral pleural edge (*arrows*) due to intrapleural air; also note tracheal deviation and mediastinal shift towards the left.

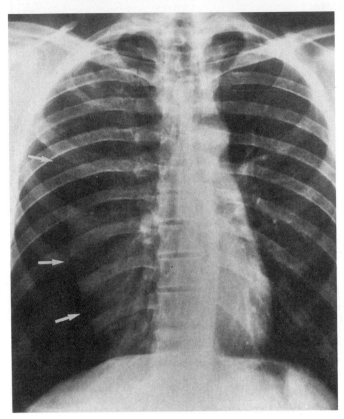

(Taken from Daffner RH. *Clinical Radiology: The Essentials.* 2nd Ed. Philadelphia: Lippincott Williams & Wilkins; 1999.)

3. **H/P** = chest pain, dyspnea
4. **Labs** = pleural biopsy is usually diagnostic
5. **Radiology** = pleural thickening, pleural effusion
6. **Treatment** = radiation and chemotherapy

IX. **Sleep apnea**
   A. Episodic cessation of airflow during sleep
   B. Types
      1. **Obstructive:** obstruction of upper airway during sleep; respiratory effort continues
      2. **Central:** Loss of central respiratory drive leads to cessation of airflow **and** respiratory effort
      3. **Mixed:** Combines both obstructive and central characteristics
   C. **Risk factors** = obesity, sedative use; males >females
   D. Etiology is unknown, but may be linked to abnormal feedback control during sleep or decreased sensitivity of upper airway muscles to stimulation
   E. **H/P** = fatigue, **daytime sleepiness, snoring,** gasping or choking during sleep
   F. **Labs** = sleep studies show episodic decreased Sao_2 and multiple arousals during sleep
   G. **Treatment**
      1. For **obstructive** type, consider weight loss and stop sedative use; continuous positive airway pressure (CPAP) is helpful in chronic cases to maintain airway patency; surgical correction of tonsillar hypertrophy,

polyp removal, correction of congenital upper airway deformities, or tracheostomy may be necessary in severe or refractory cases

2. For **central** type use respiratory stimulants; phrenic nerve pacemaking may be needed in severe cases

X. Pulmonary surgical concerns

A. Atelectasis

1. Localized alveolar collapse; **common after surgery** (especially abdominal) **and anesthesia** (generally **not** clinically serious); may also occur in asthmatics, after foreign body aspiration, or from mass effect of tumors, pulmonary lesions, or lymphadenopathy (more serious atelectasis occurs with **airway obstruction**)
2. **H/P** = asymptomatic if mild or slow development; pleuritic chest pain, dyspnea; fever, decreased breath sounds, dullness to percussion over affected area
3. **Treatment = inspiratory spirometry,** ambulation, and inpatient physical therapy are important for prevention; severe cases require upper airway suctioning or bronchoscopy with deeper suctioning

B. Intubation

1. Placement of tube into trachea to maintain airway patency and control respiration during anesthesia and times of respiratory distress
2. Almost all intubations are performed **orally** (nasal intubation performed for oral surgery, jaw surgery, and in cases when a laryngoscope cannot help to visualize the vocal cords)
3. **Placement**
   a. Appropriate anesthesia and muscle relaxants administered
   b. Patient positioned with moderate cervical flexion
   c. Laryngoscope inserted into mouth and used to lift jaw and visualize lower pharynx (pressure applied to **cricoid** may aid in visualization)
   d. Endotracheal tube inserted past vocal cords (**direct visualization is important**) to depth of 21–23 cm (measured at lips)
   e. Proper placement is checked by measuring **end tidal CO_2** (rise should follow expiration) and confirming bilateral lung expansion with **auscultation**
   f. Endotracheal tube cuff is inflated, and tube is secured
4. **Complications** = dental injury during placement, placement of tube in esophagus, increased risk of infection
5. If intubation is required for longer than three weeks, convert to a **tracheostomy** (surgical insertion of breathing tube through anterior neck into trachea)

C. Ventilation

1. Ventilation is assisted respiration that is required during surgery under anesthesia; may also be required to maintain patent airway or in cases where the patient is not able to breathe without assistance (e.g., neurologic injury, decompensation, oxygenation failure, decreased respiratory drive)
2. Inspiration is ventilator-driven; expiration occurs through natural recoil of lungs
3. Tidal volume (TV), respiratory rate, Fio_2, and inspiratory pressure (pressure forcing each inspiration) may be adjusted
4. Positive end-expiratory pressure (PEEP) helps to prevent alveolar collapse during expiration
5. Patients weaned from ventilator by changing from more patient-independent modes to more patient-dependent modes (e.g., synchronized intermittent mandatory ventilation [SIMV] to CPAP)
6. Extubation (removal of the tube) may be performed when the patient is capable of breathing independently

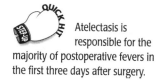
QUICK HIT Atelectasis is responsible for the majority of postoperative fevers in the first three days after surgery.

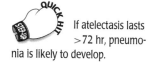
QUICK HIT If atelectasis lasts >72 hr, pneumonia is likely to develop.

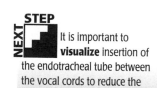
NEXT STEP It is important to **visualize** insertion of the endotracheal tube between the vocal cords to reduce the risk of **esophageal** placement.

TABLE 2-13	Modes of Mechanical Ventilation		
Mode	**Machine Actions**	**Patient Actions**	**Uses**
Controlled mechanical ventilation (CMV)	Determines and automatically delivers tidal volume and rate	No effort	General anesthesia, overdose
Intermittent mandatory ventilation (IMV)	Determines and automatically delivers tidal volume and rate	Can breathe spontaneously between mechanical breaths	Weaning patient from ventilator
Synchronized intermittent mandatory ventilation (SIMV)	Machine tries to synchronize rate with patient-initiated breaths; automatically delivers tidal volume and rate	Can breathe spontaneously between mechanical breaths	More comfortable for patient because of attempted synchronization; frequently used in place of IMV
Assist-control ventilation (AC)	Machine senses patient's attempt to breathe and delivers full preset tidal volume; backup rate if no spontaneous breaths	Patient driven unless no attempts to breathe (backup rate)	Used when patient is more awake and in progressive weaning
Continuous positive airway pressure (CPAP)	Machine maintains airway patency to decrease work of breathing	Patient does all breathing	Used when patient relies less on ventilator; intubation not required

AC, assist-control ventilation; CMV, controlled mechanical ventilation; CPAP, continuous positive airway pressure; IMV, intermittent mandatory ventilation; SIMV, synchronized intermittent mandatory ventilation.

  a. Ventilator is weaned to allow spontaneous breathing by patient
  b. Extubation is appropriate with three out of five of the following: maximum inspiratory pressure <30 cm H_2O, vital capacity >10 mL/kg, arterial pH >7.30, respiratory rate >30/min, tidal volume >5 mL/kg

XI. Pediatric pulmonary concerns
  ### A. Croup
  1. Acute inflammation of larynx
  2. Most commonly between three months to five years of age
  3. Usually due to **parainfluenzae virus type 1;** less commonly due to parainfluenzae virus types 2 and 3, respiratory syncytial virus (RSV) influenza virus, rubeola, adenovirus, or *Mycoplasma pneumoniae*
  4. **H/P** = nasal congestion, **barking cough,** dyspnea, **inspiratory stridor;** fever
  5. **Radiology** = lateral neck radiograph may show subglottic narrowing of airway (**steeple sign**)
  6. **Treatment** = treat symptoms; humidified air, O_2, aerosolized epinephrine, and inhaled corticosteroids may be used in severe cases
  ### B. Epiglottitis
  1. Rapidly progressive infection of epiglottis and surrounding tissues that may cause airway obstruction
  2. Most common in children from 2–7 years of age
  3. Due to *Haemophilus influenzae* **type B** infection; may also be due to streptococcal or other *H. influenzae* bacteria

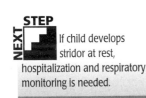

NEXT STEP If child develops stridor at rest, hospitalization and respiratory monitoring is needed.

QUICK HIT In cases of suspected epiglottitis, examine the patient's throat **only** in a setting in which prompt intubation is possible because examination of the patient's throat may lead to additional throat irritation and resulting occlusion.

FIGURE 2-8 Chest x-ray of a child with croup demonstrating subglottic narrowing of the airway, which is reminiscent of the shape of a steeple (steeple sign).

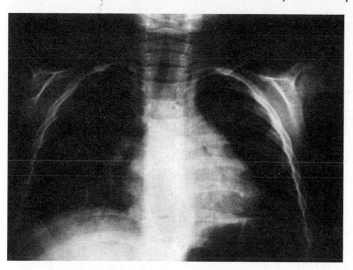

(Taken from Harwood-Nuss A, Wolfson AB, et al. *The Clinical Practice of Emergency Medicine,* 3rd Ed. Philadelphia: Lippincott Williams & Wilkins; 2001.)

4. **H/P = dysphagia,** drooling, soft stridor, **muffled voice;** sudden high fever, inspiratory retractions; children may lean forward with hands on knees to aid breathing
5. **Radiology** = lateral neck radiograph shows swollen opacified epiglottis that partially obstructs the airway (**thumbprint sign**); laryngoscope (only used in controlled situations) can visualize red, swollen epiglottis
6. **Treatment** = keep child calm; promptly intubate and administer IV antibiotics; vaccination is preventative

C. **Bronchiolitis**
   1. Viral infection of bronchioles due to **RSV** (most cases) or parainfluenzae virus type 3 (less common)
   2. Most commonly occurs in winter and spring; usually found in children <2 years of age

FIGURE 2-9 Lateral chest x-ray of a child with epiglottitis demonstrating a swollen epiglottis that resembles a thumbprint (thumbprint sign).

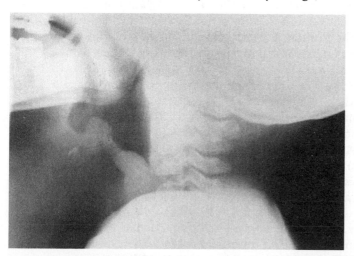

(Taken from Harwood-Nuss A, Wolfson AB, et al. *The Clinical Practice of Emergency Medicine,* 3rd Ed. Philadelphia: Lippincott Williams & Wilkins; 2001.)

PULMONARY DISORDERS

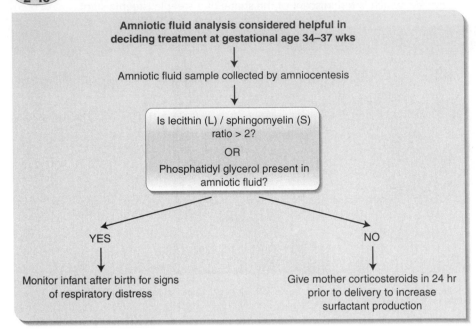

FIGURE 2-10 Amniotic fluid analysis protocol used to determine fetal lung maturity.

3. **H/P** = nasal congestion, cough, **respiratory distress; wheezing,** fever, tachypnea, crackles, prolonged expiration, hyperresonance to percussion
4. **Radiology** = CXR shows hyperinflation of lungs, infiltrates, areas of atelectasis
5. **Treatment** = adequate hydration, humidified air, O_2, nebulizer corticosteroids and β_2-agonists; ribivarin may be used in severe cases; hospitalization may be necessary for infants
6. **Complications** = increased risk of developing asthma

D. **Respiratory distress syndrome of the newborn**
1. Preterm infants (24–37 wks gestation and especially prior to 30 wks gestation) have surfactant deficiency due to lung immaturity that leads to decreased lung compliance, atelectasis, and respiratory failure
2. **H/P** = **presentation within three days of birth;** cyanosis, nasal flaring, expiratory grunting, intercostals retractions; respiratory rate >60/min, hypoxemia, crackles, decreased breath sounds
3. **Labs** = ABG shows increased CO_2, decreased O_2; amniotic fluid analysis may be helpful between 34–37 wks gestation to determine fetal lung maturity with the amniotic lecithin:sphingomyelin ratio (immaturity is rare after 37 wks and results of testing do not change maternal management prior to 34 wks)
4. **Radiology** = CXR shows bilateral atelectasis with **ground glass** appearance and air bronchograms
5. **Treatment** = maternal administration of corticosteroids prior to initiation of labor helps to speed fetal lung maturation; intubation with possible CPAP to aid respiration (keep Pao_2 45–70 mm Hg to prevent retinopathy of prematurity); surfactant replacement therapy

E. **Meconium aspiration syndrome**
1. Aspiration of meconium (fetal stool passed into amniotic sac) pre-delivery causing obstruction of airways and pneumonia
2. **H/P** = cyanosis, intercostals retractions; distended chest, tachypnea, **meconium staining found on umbilical cord**
3. **Radiology** = CXR shows atelectasis, areas of hyperinflation, or pneumothorax

4. **Treatment** = suction nose, mouth, and upper airway at birth; O_2 and ventilation may be required

5. **Complications** = pulmonary hypertension may develop if not promptly treated

F. **Cystic fibrosis (CF)**

1. Autosomal recessive disorder due to defect in chloride-pumping channel in exocrine glands; ducts of exocrine glands (lungs, pancreas, reproductive glands) become clogged with thick secretions

2. Presents in childhood and universally fatal, but proper treatment may allow survival into late 20s or early 30s

3. Affects both pulmonary and gastrointestinal systems (pancreatic enzyme deficiencies and malabsorption)

4. **Risk factors** = Caucasians at higher risk than other races

5. **H/P** = recurrent pulmonary infections (*Pseudomonas, S. aureus*), dyspnea, hemoptysis, chronic sinusitis, cyanosis, cough, meconium ileus at birth, steatorrhea, failure to thrive; digital clubbing, esophageal varices, rectal prolapse, abnormal glucose tolerance

6. **Labs** = decreased serum Na; sweat test shows increased Na and increased Cl (>60 in children, >80 in adults); genetic testing can locate mutation in cystic fibrosis transmembrane conductance regulator (CFTR) gene in suspected patients or in carriers of the gene considering pregnancy

7. **Treatment** = DNase to aid pulmonary disease, bronchodilators, nonsteroidal anti-inflammatory drugs (NSAIDs), antibiotics for any suspected pulmonary infection, and chest physical therapy; supplemental pancreatic enzymes and vitamins A, D, E, and K given for malabsorption

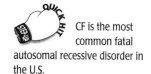

QUICK HIT

CF is the most common fatal autosomal recessive disorder in the U.S.

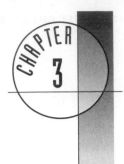

Gastrointestinal Disorders

I. Gastrointestinal (GI) infections

A. **Viral gastroenteritis**

1. Self-limited viral infection of GI tract
2. Common agents include **Norwalk virus,** Coxsackie virus A1, echovirus, and adenovirus; rotavirus is common in children
3. **History and Physical (H/P)** = nausea, vomiting, diarrhea, abdominal pain
4. **Labs** = no fecal white blood cells; viral culture indicates pathogen (usually unnecessary)
5. **Treatment** = self-limited; maintain hydration status

B. **Bacterial gastroenteritis (see Table 3-1)**

C. **Protozoan and parasitic GI infections (see Table 3-2)**

D. **Hepatitis**

1. Inflammatory disease of the liver is most commonly due to viral infection; also may result from alcohol or toxins
2. Acute hepatitis is initial disease; chronic form is disease lasting > 6 months
3. **Risk factors** = intravenous drug abuse (IVDA), alcoholism, travel to developing nations
4. Patterns of transmission vary with virus type
5. **H/P** = malaise, arthralgias, fatigue, nausea, vomiting; jaundice, scleral icterus, tender hepatomegaly, splenomegaly, lymphadenopathy
6. **Labs** = bilirubinuria, **increased AST, increased ALT,** increased bilirubin (total), increased alkaline phosphatase
   a. Hepatitis A virus (HAV)—anti-HAV IgM antibodies present during illness, anti-HAV IgG antibodies present after resolution
   b. Hepatitis B virus (HBV)—antigens and antibodies detected vary with disease state (see Table 3-4)
   c. Hepatitis C virus (HCV)—anti-HCV antibodies and positive HCV polymerase chain reaction indicate infection
7. **Treatment** = rest, frequently self-limited (**except HCV**); α-interferon (α-IFN) or lamivudine for hepatitis B virus (HBV); α-IFN and ribavirin for HCV; hospitalization for hepatic failure; immunoglobulin given to close contacts of patients with HAV; HAV vaccine given to travelers to developing nations; HBV vaccine routinely given to children and healthcare workers

II. Oral and esophageal conditions

A. **Salivary gland disorders**

1. Dysfunction in sublingual, submandibular, or parotid glands resulting from ductal obstruction or inflammation
2. May be due to sialolithiasis (ductal stone) in any salivary gland; parotid disease may also be caused by sarcoidosis, infection, or neoplasm
3. **H/P** = enlarged and painful glands; pain worsens during eating; parotid glands may have painless swelling

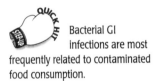
Bacterial GI infections are most frequently related to contaminated food consumption.

Hemolytic uremic syndrome (HUS) is a complication of E. coli 0157 : H7 infection and is characterized by thrombocytopenia, hemolytic anemia, and acute renal failure; it is usually self-limited.

TABLE 3-1 Common Pathogens in Bacterial Gastroenteritis

Pathogen	Source	Signs and Symptoms	Treatment
Bacillus cereus	Fried rice	**Vomiting** within several hours of eating, diarrhea later	Self-limited; hydration
Campylobacter jejuni	Food/water (**most common bacterial GI infection**)	**Bloody** diarrhea, abdominal pain, fever; rare Guillain-Barré syndrome	Hydration, erythromycin; self-limited but may take time to resolve without treatment
Clostridium botulinum	Honey, home-canned foods	Nausea, vomiting, diarrhea, **flaccid paralysis**	Botulism anti-toxin (not given to infants); self-limited
Clostridium difficile	**Antibiotic-induced suppression** of normal colonic flora	**Watery** diarrhea; gray pseudomembranes seen on colonic mucosa	Metronidazole, vancomycin
Escherichia coli	Food/water (**travelers'** diarrhea)	**Watery** diarrhea, vomiting, fever	Hydration; self-limited; TMP-SMX, ciprofloxacin may reduce duration
E. coli type **O157:H7**	Food/water	**Bloody** diarrhea, vomiting, fever, abdominal pain (risk of HUS)	Hydration; self-limited; antibiotics may actually worsen symptoms due to toxin release
Staphylococcus aureus	Room-temperature food	**Vomiting,** within several hours of eating, diarrhea later	Self-limited; hydration
Salmonella species	Eggs, poultry, milk	Nausea, abdominal pain, **bloody** diarrhea, fever, vomiting	Hydration; self-limited
Shigella species	Food/water; associated with overcrowding	Fever, nausea, vomiting, **severe bloody** diarrhea, abdominal pain (risk of HUS)	Hydration; self-limited; ciprofloxacin, TMP-SMX in severe cases
Vibrio cholerae	Water, seafood	**Copious watery** diarrhea, signs of dehydration	**Hydration;** ciprofloxacin, doxycycline
Vibrio parahaemolyticus	Seafood (oysters)	Abdominal pain, **watery** diarrhea within 24 hr of eating	Hydration; self-limited

GI, gastrointestinal; HUS, hemolytic-uremic syndrome; TMP-SMX, trimethoprim-sulfamethoxazole.

4. **Treatment** = warm compresses, massage, or cough drops may help remove ductal stones; antibiotics and hydration for infection; surgery may be required for relief in refractory cases

B. **Dysphagia**
  1. Difficulty swallowing due to oropharyngeal/esophageal transport dysfunction or pain with swallowing (odynophagia)
  2. May be due to neuromuscular disorders (achalasia, motility disorders, scleroderma) or obstruction (peptic strictures, esophageal webs or rings, cancer, radiation fibrosis)
  3. **Obstructive** pathology tends to limit swallowing of **solids; neuromuscular** pathology tends to limit swallowing of **solids and liquids**
  4. **H/P** = feeling of "**food stuck in throat**" when swallowing, cough, solids and/or liquids may be difficult to swallow
  5. **Labs** = manometry measures esophageal pressure; esophageal pH may be abnormal
  6. **Radiology** = barium swallow and esophagogastroduodenoscopy (EGD) may be helpful for diagnosis
  7. **Treatment** = varies with etiology

 NEXT STEP If a patient presents with dysphagia, perform a **barium swallow** before an EGD because of the lower associated risks of the former.

TABLE 3-2 Common Pathogens in Parasitic and Protozoan Gastrointestinal Infections

Pathogen	Source	Signs and Symptoms	Treatment
Giardia lamblia (Color Figure 3-1)	Surface water (usually limited to wilderness or other countries)	**Greasy,** foul-smelling diarrhea; abdominal pain; cysts and trophozoites seen in stool sample	Metronidazole; hydration
Entamoeba histolytica	Water, areas of poor sanitation	Mild to severe **bloody** diarrhea, abdominal pain	Metronidazole, paromomycin
Cryptosporidium parvum	Food/water; immunocompromised patients	**Watery** diarrhea; acid-fast stain of stool shows parasites	Control immune suppression; paromomycin
Trichinella spiralis	Undercooked pork	Fever, **myalgias,** periorbital edema; eosinophilia	Albendazole, mebendazole
Taenia solium	Undercooked pork	Mild diarrhea, **CNS symptoms**	Praziquantel; drainage of cysts

CNS, central nervous system.

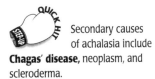

Secondary causes of achalasia include **Chagas' disease,** neoplasm, and scleroderma.

C. **Achalasia**
   1. Neuromuscular disorder of esophagus with **impaired peristalsis and decreased lower esophageal sphincter (LES) relaxation** due to dysfunction of intramural neurons
   2. Idiopathic; most commonly affects 20–40 yr olds
   3. **H/P** = gradually progressive dysphagia of **solids and liquids,** regurgitation, cough, aspiration

TABLE 3-3 Characteristics of Viral Hepatitis

Hepatitis Virus	Virus Type	Spread	Treatment	Prevention	Complications
A (HAV)	Picornavirus (single-stranded RNA)	Food (**shellfish**), fecal-oral	Immune globulin	Vaccine prior to travel	May occur in epidemics
B (HBV)	Hepadnavirus (double-stranded DNA)	**Blood, other body fluids** (including sexual contact)	α-IFN or lamivudine	**Vaccine**	10% adults (80% children) develop chronic hepatitis, cirrhosis, 3–5% develop **hepatocellular carcinoma,** persistent carrier state, 1% develop fulminant hepatic failure
C (HCV)	Flavivirus (single-stranded RNA)	**Blood,** possibly sexual contact	α-IFN and ribavirin	No vaccine	80% patients develop **chronic hepatitis,** 30% develop cirrhosis, slightly increased risk hepatocellular carcinoma, persistent carrier state
D	Delta agent (incomplete single-stranded RNA)	Blood; **requires coexistent Hepatitis B infection**	α-IFN	Hepatitis B vaccine	Severe hepatitis, cirrhosis, persistent carrier state
E	Calicivirus (single-stranded RNA)	Water, fecal-oral	Supportive	No vaccine	High mortality in **pregnant** women

HAV, hepatitis A virus; HBV, hepatitis B virus; HCV, hepatitis C virus; IFN, interferon.

TABLE 3-4 Serologies Seen in Various Disease States of HBV Infection

Course of Disease	HBV Surface Antigen (HBsAg)	HBV e Antigen (HBeAg)	HBV Surface Antibody (anti-HBs)	HBV e Antibody (anti-HBe)	HBV core Antibody (anti-HBc)
Acute infection (4–12 wk postexposure)	Positive	Positive	Negative	Negative	Positive (IgM)
Acute infection window period (12–20 wk postexposure)	Negative	Negative	Negative	Negative	Positive (IgM)
Chronic infection, active viral replication	Positive	Positive	Negative	Negative	Positive (IgG)
Chronic infection, lesser viral replication (good prognosis)	Positive	Negative	Negative	Positive	Positive (IgG)
Past infection (recovered)	Negative	Negative	Positive	Positive	Positive (IgG)
Vaccination	Negative	Negative	Positive	Negative	Negative

HBV, hepatitis B virus.

4. **Labs** = manometry shows increased LES pressure and decreased peristalsis
5. **Radiology** = barium swallow shows "**bird's beak**" sign with tapering at the LES; EGD needed to rule out malignancy
6. **Treatment** = pneumatic dilation, botulinum injections, or myotomy relieve obstruction
7. **Complications** = myotomy may cause gastroesophageal reflux disease (GERD)

D. **Diffuse esophageal spasm**
   1. Neuromuscular disorder in which **nonperistaltic** contractions of esophagus occur
   2. **H/P** = chest pain, dysphagia
   3. **Labs** = manometry shows nonperistaltic, uncoordinated esophageal contractions
   4. **Radiology** = barium swallow shows "**corkscrew**" pattern
   5. **Treatment** = calcium channel blockers, nitrates

E. **Zenker diverticulum**
   1. Outpouching in upper posterior esophagus due to smooth muscle weakness
   2. **H/P** = bad breath, difficulty initiating swallowing, **regurgitation of food several days after eating**
   3. **Radiology** = barium swallow shows outpouching
   4. **Treatment** = cricopharyngeal myotomy or diverticulectomy
   5. **Complications** = EGD can perforate weakness in esophageal wall

F. **Gastroesophageal reflux disease (GERD)**
   1. Low pressure in LES leads to reflux of gastric contents into esophagus
   2. **Risk factors** = obesity, hiatal hernia, pregnancy, scleroderma
   3. Symptoms may worsen with consumption of alcohol and fatty foods or with tobacco use
   4. **H/P** = **burning chest pain** ("heartburn") 30–90 min after eating, sour taste in mouth, regurgitation, dysphagia, cough; pain worsens when lying down and improves with standing
   5. **Radiology** = usually unneeded for diagnosis; EGD, chest radiograph, or barium swallow can help rule out neoplasm, Barrett's esophagus, and hiatal hernia

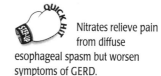
Nitrates relieve pain from diffuse esophageal spasm but worsen symptoms of GERD.

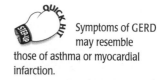
Symptoms of GERD may resemble those of asthma or myocardial infarction.

FIGURE 3-1 Barium swallow in a patient with achalasia; note the distended proximal esophagus with distal tapering and "bird's beak" sign (*white arrow*).

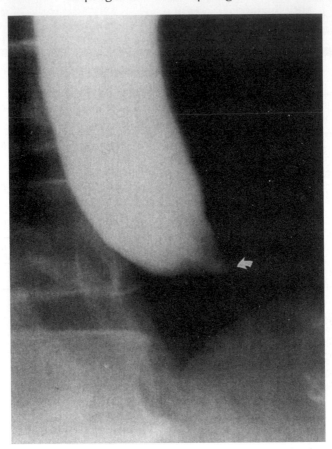

(Taken from Eisenberg RL. *Gastrointestinal Radiology: A Pattern Approach.* 3rd Ed. Philadelphia: Lippincott-Raven Publishers; 1996.)

6. **Treatment** =
  a. Elevation of head of bed, weight loss, dietary modification
  b. Initial medications are antacids followed by H_2 antagonists (10–25% effective), proton pump inhibitors (PPIs) (60–75% effective), and pro-motility agents
  c. Refractory disease may be treated with Nissen fundoplication or hiatal hernia repair
7. **Complications** = esophageal ulceration, esophageal stricture, Barrett's esophagus, adenocarcinoma
G. **Esophageal cancer**
  1. **Squamous cell carcinoma** (more common) or adenocarcinoma (less common) of esophagus
  2. **Barrett's esophagus** (columnar metaplasia of distal esophagus secondary to chronic GERD) commonly precedes adenocarcinoma
  3. **Risk factors** = alcohol, tobacco, chronic GERD
  4. **H/P** = progressive dysphagia (initially solids, later solids and liquids), weight loss, odynophagia, reflux, GI bleeding, vomiting, weakness, cough, hoarseness
  5. **Radiology** = barium swallow shows narrowing of esophagus and abnormal mass; magnetic resonance imaging (MRI) or computed tomography (CT) with contrast can determine extension and metastases; EGD used to identify mass and perform biopsy

FIGURE 3-2 Barium swallow in a patient with diffuse esophageal spasm; notice the "corkscrew" pattern throughout the visible esophagus.

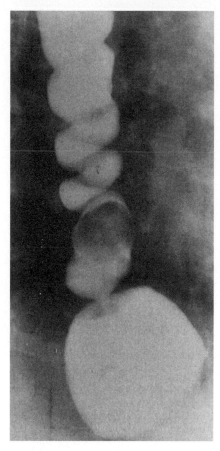

(Taken from Eisenberg RL. *Gastrointestinal Radiology: A Pattern Approach.* 3rd Ed. Philadelphia: Lippincott-Raven Publishers; 1996.)

6. **Labs** = biopsy used to make diagnosis
7. **Treatment** = surgical resection (including total esophagectomy), radiation, chemotherapy
8. **Complications** = poor prognosis; local extension and metastases are frequently present by time of diagnosis

III. Gastric conditions

A. **Hiatal hernia**
  1. Herniation of part of stomach above diaphragm
  2. Types
     a. **Sliding**—gastroesophageal junction and stomach displaced through diaphragm
     b. **Paraesophageal**—stomach protrudes through diaphragm but gastroesophageal junction remains in normal location
  3. **H/P** = possibly asymptomatic; symptoms associated with GERD
  4. **Radiology** = barium swallow shows portion of stomach above diaphragm; chest radiograph may detect hernia without barium swallow if air in stomach is visible above diaphragm
  5. **Treatment** = sliding hernias may be treated with reflux control; paraesophageal hernias may need surgical repair (gastropexy, Nissen fundoplication)
  6. **Complications** = incarceration of stomach in herniation (seen in paraesophageal type)

GASTROINTESTINAL DISORDERS

FIGURE
3-3 Barium swallow in a patient with a small Zenker diverticulum (*white arrow*).

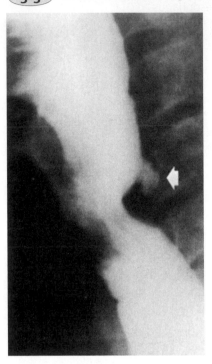

(Taken from Eisenberg RL. *Gastrointestinal Radiology: A Pattern Approach.* 3rd Ed. Philadelphia: Lippincott-Raven Publishers; 1996.)

QUICK HIT

In pernicious anemia, autoantibodies destroy parietal cells leading to low levels of intrinsic factor, vitamin B_{12} malabsorption, and megaloblastic anemia.

B. **Gastritis**
1. Inflammation of gastric mucosa
2. May be **acute (erosive)** or **chronic (nonerosive)**
3. Acute gastritis characterized by rapidly developing, superficial lesions secondary to nonsteroidal anti-inflammatory drug **(NSAID)** use, alcohol, or **stress from severe illness**
4. Chronic gastritis may occur in either antrum or fundus of the stomach
5. **H/P** = possibly asymptomatic; indigestion, nausea, vomiting, hematemesis, melena; symptoms more common for acute form

TABLE 3-5 **Medications Used in Treatment of GERD**

Medication	Mechanism	Adverse Effects	Prescription Strategy
Antacids (calcium carbonate, aluminum hydroxide, etc.)	Neutralize gastric acid	Constipation, nausea, diarrhea	Initial therapy, as needed
H_2 antagonists (cimetidine, ranitidine, etc.)	Reversibly block histamine H_2 receptors to inhibit gastric acid secretion	Headache, diarrhea, rare thrombocytopenia; cimetidine may cause gynecomastia and impotence	Patients not responding to antacids
PPIs (omeprazole, lansoprazole, etc.)	Irreversibly inhibit parietal cell proton pump (H^+/K^+ ATPase) to block gastric acid secretion	Well-tolerated; may increase effects of warfarin, benzodiazepines, phenytoin, digoxin, or carbamazepine in some patients	Patients not responding to antacids
Pro-motility agents (cisapride, etc.)	Promote gastric emptying	Headache, diarrhea, cardiac effects	Patients with poor LES function

GERD, gastroesophageal reflux disease; H^+, hydrogen ion; K^+, potassium ion; LES, lower esophageal sphincter; PPIs, proton pump inhibitors.

FIGURE 3-4 Barium swallow in a patient with squamous cell carcinoma of the esophagus; note the irregularity of the left esophageal wall due to neoplastic mass.

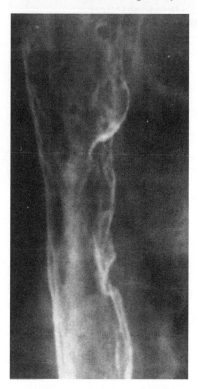

(Taken from Eisenberg RL. *Gastrointestinal Radiology: A Pattern Approach.* 3rd Ed. Philadelphia: Lippincott-Raven Publishers; 1996.)

6. **Labs** – positive urea breath test (detects increase in pH from ammonia-producing bacteria) and positive IgG antibody to *Helicobacter pylori* with existing infection; antral biopsy can detect *H. pylori* infection

7. **Radiology** = EGD allows visualization of gastric mucosa to detect lesions

8. **Treatment** –

    a. Treat acute form like peptic ulcer disease (PUD) and stop alcohol and offending medications; give H_2 antagonists to patients with severe illnesses

    b. Type A chronic gastritis requires vitamin B_{12} replacement

    c. Type B chronic gastritis requires eradication of *H. pylori* through multidrug treatment (e.g., amoxicillin, metronidazole, clarithromycin, PPI)

C. **Peptic ulcer disease (PUD)**

    1. Erosion of gastric and duodenal mucosa secondary to impaired endothelial defenses and increased gastric acidity

TABLE 3-6 Characteristics of Type A and B Chronic Gastritis

Characteristic	Type A	Type B
Frequency	10% of cases	90% of cases
Site	Fundus	Antrum
Pathology	Autoantibodies for parietal cells	Associated with *H. pylori* infection
Labs	Decreased gastric acid level, decreased gastrin	Increased gastric acid level
Associated conditions	Pernicious anemia, achlorhydria, thyroiditis	Peptic ulcer disease, gastric cancer

TABLE 3-7	Distinguishing between Gastric and Duodenal Ulcers	
Characteristic	**Gastric Ulcer**	**Duodenal Ulcer**
Patients	Age >50 yr old, *H. pylori* infection, NSAID users	Younger, *H. pylori* infection
Frequency	25% cases	75% cases
Timing of pain	**Soon after** eating	**2–4 hr after** eating
Gastric acid level	Normal/low	High
Gastrin level	High	Normal
Effect of eating	May **worsen** symptoms and cause nausea and vomiting	**Initial improvement** in symptoms, with **later worsening**

NSAIDs, nonsteroidal anti-inflammatory drug.

Ulcers may also develop secondary to stress from severe burns **(Curling's ulcers)** or intracranial injuries **(Cushing's ulcers).**

In refractory cases of PUD, gastrin level should be determined to detect Zollinger-Ellison syndrome (increased gastrin).

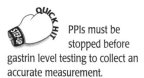
Give COX-2-selective NSAIDs to patients with PUD who require NSAID therapy.

PPIs must be stopped before gastrin level testing to collect an accurate measurement.

2. *H. pylori* is involved in pathology in **most gastric ulcers** and **almost all duodenal ulcers**
3. **Risk factors** = *H. pylori* **infection, NSAIDs,** tobacco, alcohol, corticosteroids; males > females
4. **H/P** = periodic **burning epigastric pain** that may change (better or worse) with eating, nausea, hematemesis, melena, hematochezia; epigastric tenderness; abdominal rigidity, rebound tenderness, and rigidity seen following acute perforation of ulcer
5. **Labs** = positive urea breath test, IgG antibodies, or biopsy detect *H. pylori*; blood count (CBC) can assess degree of GI bleeding
6. **Radiology** = abdominal x-ray (AXR) to detect perforation (free air under diaphragm seen following perforation); EGD used to perform biopsy and detect active bleeding
7. **Treatment** =
   a. **Active bleeding** must be ruled out with CBC and EGD; symptoms lasting >2 months need EGD to rule out gastric adenocarcinoma
   b. Decrease gastric acid levels with **PPI** and **H₂ antagonist;** protect mucosa with sucralfate, bismuth subsalicylate, or misoprostol; **eliminate *H. pylori* infection** with triple antibiotic therapy (metronidazole + clarithromycin + amoxicillin)
   c. Surgery required to repair acute perforations; non-neoplastic refractory cases may require parietal cell vagotomy or antrectomy
8. **Complications** = hemorrhage (posterior ulcers may erode into gastroduodenal artery), perforation (most commonly anterior ulcers), lymphoproliferative disease
D. **Zollinger-Ellison syndrome**
   1. Syndrome secondary to **gastrin-producing tumor** of pancreas (rarely in stomach, duodenum, or spleen)
   2. Associated with malabsorption disorders
   3. **H/P** = **refractory PUD,** diarrhea, steatorrhea, possible other endocrine abnormalities
   4. **Labs** = **increased gastrin;** specific gastrin sampling in several pancreatic or abdominal veins can help localize tumor
   5. **Radiology** = angiography may detect tumor if hypervascular
   6. **Treatment** = few (10%) lesions are resectable; total gastrectomy frequently required to decrease mortality; PPIs and H₂ antagonists may ease symptoms

7. **Complications** = occasionally associated with other endocrine tumors (multiple endocrine neoplasia I [MEN I]) 60% of lesions are malignant

E. **Gastric cancer**

1. **Adenocarcinoma** (common) or squamous cell carcinoma (rare; due to invasion from esophagus) affecting stomach

2. Types
   a. **Ulcerating**—resembles ulcers seen in PUD
   b. **Polypoid**—large intraluminal neoplasms
   c. **Superficial spreading**—mucosal and submucosal involvement only; best prognosis
   d. **Linitis plastica**—all layers of stomach involved; decreased stomach elasticity; poor prognosis

3. **Risk factors** = *H. pylori*, Japanese ancestry, tobacco, vitamin C deficiency, high consumption of preserved foods; males > females

4. **H/P** = weight loss, anorexia, early satiety, vomiting, dysphagia, epigastric pain; enlarged left supraclavicular lymph node (**Virchow's node**)

5. **Labs** = increased carcinoembryonic antigen (CEA), increased 2-glucuronidase in gastric secretions, anemia if active bleeding; biopsy used for diagnosis

6. **Radiology** = barium swallow may show mass or thickened "leather bottle" stomach (linitis plastica); EGD used to perform biopsy and visualize ulcers

7. **Treatment** = surgical resection, chemotherapy; early detection has > 70% survival

8. **Complications** = poor prognosis without early detection (12% 5-year survival)

IV. Intestinal conditions

A. **Malabsorption disorders**

1. **Celiac sprue**
   a. Genetic disorder characterized by gluten intolerance (wheat, barley, rye)
   b. Immune-mediated disorder with antiendomysial and antigliadin antibodies that cause jejunal mucosal damage
   c. **H/P** = failure to thrive, bloating, and abnormal stools in infants; diarrhea, steatorrhea, weight loss, and bloating in adults
   d. **Labs** = positive antiendomysial and antigliadin antibodies in serum; biopsy shows loss of jejunal villi
   e. **Treatment** = removal of gluten from diet (can still eat corn, rice)

The general presentation of malabsorption includes weight loss, **bloating, diarrhea,** possible **steatorrhea,** glossitis, dermatitis, and edema.

2. **Tropical sprue**
   a. Malabsorption syndrome similar to celiac sprue with possible infectious or toxic etiology
   b. Acquired disorder in patients living in **tropical areas**
   c. **H/P** = similar presentation to celiac sprue
   d. **Labs** = no antiendomysial and antigliadin antibodies
   e. **Treatment** = folic acid replacement, tetracycline; removal of gluten from diet has no effect

3. **Lactose intolerance**
   a. Malabsorption syndrome resulting from deficiency of lactase; may also be secondary to Crohn's disease or bacterial overgrowth
   b. Lactose not metabolized in jejunum leading to osmotic diarrhea
   c. **H/P** = diarrhea and bloating after dairy consumption
   d. **Labs** = decreased stool pH
   e. **Treatment** = lactose-restricted or lactose-free diet; adequate dietary protein, fat, calcium, and vitamins; lactase replacement may benefit some patients

Celiac and tropical sprue exhibit the same symptoms, but celiac sprue responds to removal of gluten from diet, and tropical sprue occurs in the tropics.

FIGURE 3-5 Location of absorption of vitamins, minerals, and nutrients throughout the GI tract.

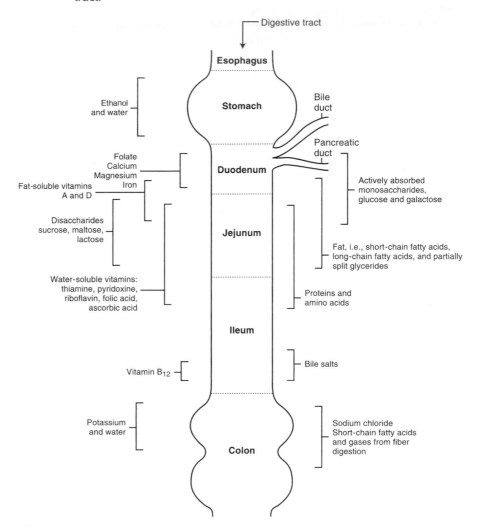

(Modified from Ryan JP. *Physiology*. 1997. Also see Mehta S, Milder EA, Mirachi AJ, Milder E. *Step-Up: A High-Yield, Systems-Based Review for the USMLE Step 1*. 2nd Ed. Philadelphia: Lippincott Williams & Wilkins; 2003.)

4. **Whipple's disease**
   a. Malabsorption disorder secondary to *Tropheryma whippelli* infection (causes intestinal lymphatic obstruction); multiple organs involved
   b. **Risk factors** = Caucasian males with European ancestry
   c. **H/P** = weight loss, joint pain, dementia, cough, bloating, steatorrhea; fever, vision abnormalities, lymphadenopathy, new heart murmur
   d. **Labs** = jejunal biopsy shows foamy macrophages on periodic acid-Schiff (PAS) stain
   e. **Treatment** = trimethoprim-sulfamethoxazole (TMP-SMX) or tetracycline for 6–12 months
   f. **Complications** = high mortality if untreated

B. **Diarrhea**
   1. Increased frequency of bowel movements and increased stool liquidity; **> 200 g/day stool production**

FIGURE
3-6 Diagnostic pathway for suspected malabsorption syndrome.

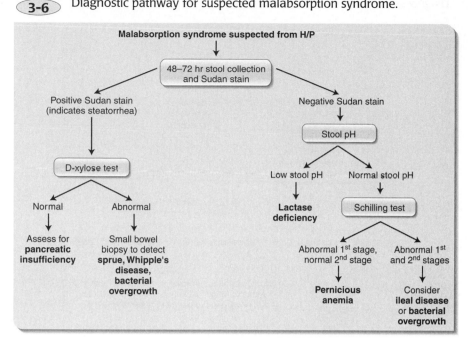

2. **Risk factors** = infection, recent travel
3. Acute diarrhea (< 3 week duration) is usually due to infection
4. Chronic diarrhea has longer duration of symptoms and may be due to malabsorption or motility disorders
   a. **Secretory** diarrheas are usually **hormone-mediated** or due to enterotoxic bacteria

FIGURE
3-7 Diagnostic and treatment pathways for acute diarrhea.

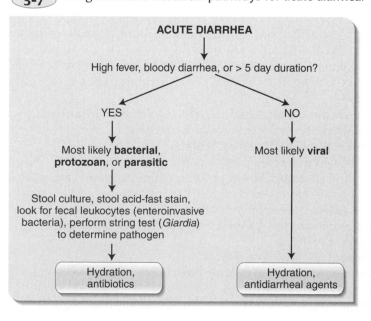

FIGURE
3-8 Diagnostic pathway for chronic diarrhea.

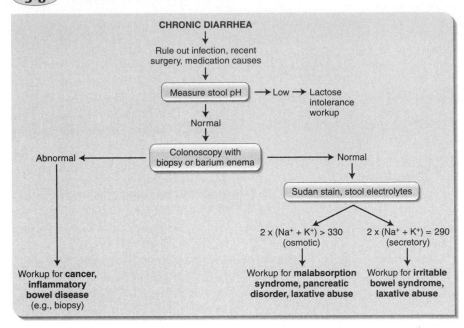

Lactase deficiency is the most common cause of **adult chronic diarrhea.**

Rotavirus is the most common cause of acute diarrhea in **children.**

Half of patients with irritable bowel syndrome have comorbid psychiatric disorders.

Small bowel obstruction is most commonly due to **adhesion** formation, while **large** bowel obstruction is most commonly due to **neoplasm.**

b. **Osmotic** diarrheas are due to **solute collecting in bowel lumen** leading to increased water in bowel; occur after eating, improve with fasting
5. Pediatric diarrhea is most commonly due to infection, antibiotic use, or related to immunosuppression
6. **Treatment** = hydration, **treat underlying cause**

C. **Irritable bowel syndrome**
1. Idiopathic disorder with chronic abdominal pain and **irregular bowel habits**
2. Most commonly begins during **teens** or **young adulthood**
3. **H/P** = abdominal pain, diarrhea, constipation, bloating, possible vomiting or weight loss; mild abdominal tenderness
4. **Labs** = rule out other GI diseases with CBC, electrolytes, stool culture
5. **Radiology** = consider AXR, abdominal CT, or barium studies to rule out other GI causes
6. **Treatment** = assurance from physician, high-fiber diet; antidiarrheal, anticholinergic, or psychiatric medications as needed

D. **Inflammatory bowel disease (IBD) (see Table 3-8)**
1. Disease of small and large bowel with constellation of symptoms associated with inflammatory bowel processes, autoimmune reactions, extraintestinal manifestations, and multiple complications
2. Types = Crohn's disease, ulcerative colitis
3. **Risk factors** = Ashkenazi Jews; Caucasians > African Americans; presents in teens or early 20s

E. **Bowel obstruction**
1. Mechanical obstruction of small or large bowel that can lead to vascular compromise
2. The most common causes of obstruction are **adhesions, hernias,** and **neoplasms**

TABLE 3-8	Comparison of Crohn's Disease and Ulcerative Colitis	
	Crohn's Disease	**Ulcerative Colitis**
Site of involvement	**Entire GI tract may be involved** with multiple **"skipped"** areas; distal ileum most commonly involved; **entire bowel wall affected**	**Continuous disease beginning at rectum** and **extending possibly as far as distal ileum;** only mucosa and submucosa affected
Symptoms	Abdominal pain, weight loss, **watery** diarrhea	Abdominal pain, urgency, **bloody** diarrhea, tenesmus, nausea, vomiting, weight loss
Physical exam	Fever, right lower quadrant **abdominal mass,** abdominal tenderness, **perianal fissures and fistulas,** oral ulcers	Fever, abdominal tenderness, orthostatic hypotension, tachycardia,
Extraintestinal manifestations	Arthritis, ankylosing spondylitis, uveitis, primary sclerosing cholangitis, nephrolithiasis	Arthritis, uveitis, ankylosing spondylitis, primary sclerosing cholangitis, erythema nodosum, pyoderma gangrenosum
Labs	ASCA frequently positive, pANCA rarely positive; biopsy diagnostic	ASCA rarely positive, pANCA frequently positive; biopsy diagnostic
Radiology	Colonoscopy shows colonic ulcers, strictures, **"cobblestoning,"** fissures, and **"skipped"** areas of bowel; barium enema shows fissures, ulcers, and bowel edema	Colonoscopy shows **continuous involvement,** pseudopolyps, friable mucosa; barium enema shows **"lead pipe"** colon without haustra and colon shortening
Treatment	Sulfasalazine, corticosteroids, immunosuppressives; surgical resections of severely affected areas	Sulfasalazine, corticosteroids, immunosuppressives; total **colectomy is curative**
Complications	Abscess formation, fistulas, fissures, malabsorption, toxic megacolon	**Significantly increased risk of colon cancer,** hemorrhage, toxic megacolon

ASCA, anti-yeast *Saccharomyces cerevisiae* antibodies; GI, gastrointestinal; pANCA, perinuclear antineutrophil cytoplasmic antibodies.

F. **Ischemic colitis**
   1. Ischemia and necrosis of bowel secondary to vascular compromise
   2. Due to embolus, bowel obstruction, inadequate systemic perfusion
   3. **Risk factors** = diabetes mellitus (DM), atherosclerosis, congestive heart failure (CHF), peripheral vascular disease, lupus
   4. **H/P** = acute abdominal pain, bloody diarrhea, vomiting; abdominal tenderness (**pain out of proportion to exam**)
   5. **Labs** = increased white cell count (WBC)
   6. **Radiology** = barium enema shows diffuse submucosal changes, "thumb printing"; sigmoidoscopy may show bloody and edematous mucosa; CT may show air within bowel wall
   7. **Treatment** = intravenous (IV) fluids, bowel rest, antibiotics for GI bacteria; surgical resection of necrotic bowel
   8. **Complications** = high mortality in cases of irreversible damage
G. **Appendicitis**
   1. Inflammation of appendix with possible infection or perforation
   2. Due to lymphoid hyperplasia, fibroid bands, or fecaliths

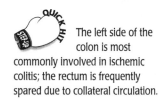 The left side of the colon is most commonly involved in ischemic colitis; the rectum is frequently spared due to collateral circulation.

GASTROINTESTINAL DISORDERS

FIGURE 3-9 Abdominal radiograph in patient with small bowel obstruction; note the multiple loops of dilated bowel with a ladder-like appearance.

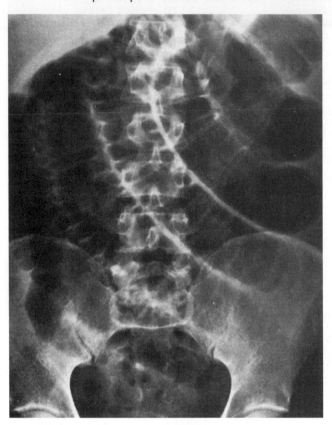

(Taken from Eisenberg RL. *Gastrointestinal Radiology: A Pattern Approach.* 3rd Ed. Philadelphia: Lippincott-Raven Publishers; 1996.)

3. **H/P** = dull periumbilical pain followed by nausea, vomiting, and anorexia; pain gradually moves to right lower quadrant and increases; **tenderness at McBurney's point** (1/3 distance from right anterior superior iliac spine to umbilicus), rebound tenderness, **psoas sign** (psoas pain on hip extension), fever, **Rovsing's sign** (right lower quadrant pain with left lower quadrant palpation); perforation produces severe pain and distention with rebound tenderness, rigidity, and guarding
4. **Labs** = increased WBC with left shift
5. **Radiology** = AXR or chest x-ray may show fecalith or free air under the diaphragm (due to perforation)
6. **Treatment** = **appendectomy** or CT-guided drainage
7. **Complications** = abscess formation, perforation

H. **Ileus**
1. **Paralytic obstruction** of bowel secondary to decreased peristalsis
2. Due to infection, ischemia, **recent surgery,** DM, opioid use
3. **H/P** = vague abdominal pain, nausea, vomiting, bloating, no bowel movements; decreased bowel sounds, no rebound tenderness
4. **Radiology** = AXR shows distention of affected bowel, air-fluid levels; barium enema can help rule out obstruction
5. **Treatment** = stop opioids, make patient NPO (nothing by mouth); colonoscopic decompression if no resolution

I. **Volvulus**
1. **Rotation of bowel** creates obstruction and possible ischemia
2. Tends to occur in **elderly** and **infants**

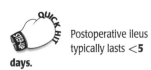 **NEXT STEP** Always get a β-hCG test in a woman of child-bearing age with abdominal pain to **rule out pregnancy.**

NEXT STEP If there is a high clinical suspicion of appendicitis, go right to surgery and do not wait for radiological exams.

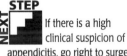 Postoperative ileus typically lasts <**5 days.**

FIGURE 3-10 Abdominal radiograph in patient with large bowel obstruction due to sigmoid volvulus; note the absence of transluminal haustra, which is seen in small bowel obstructions.

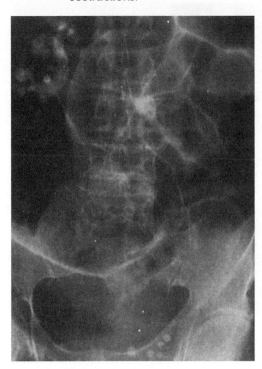

(Taken from Eisenberg RL. *Gastrointestinal Radiology: A Pattern Approach.* 3rd Ed. Philadelphia: Lippincott-Raven Publishers; 1996.)

TABLE 3-9 Comparison of Small and Large Bowel Obstruction

	Small Bowel Obstruction	Large Bowel Obstruction
Causes	**Adhesions, incarcerated hernias,** neoplasm, intussusception, volvulus, Crohn's disease, congenital stricture	**Neoplasm,** diverticulitis, volvulus, congenital stricture
Symptoms	Abdominal pain, **vomiting,** distention, obstipation	Abdominal pain, obstipation, distention, nausea, **late feculent vomiting**
Physical exam	Abdominal tenderness, visible peristaltic waves, high-pitched bowel sounds, absence of bowel sounds, fever	Abdominal tenderness, palpable mass, high-pitched bowel sounds, absence of bowel sounds
Radiology	AXR shows **ladder-like dilated loops of bowel,** air-fluid levels	AXR shows **bowel distention proximal to obstruction;** barium enema may detect obstruction near rectum
Treatment	Make patient NPO, maintain hydration; nasogastric decompression may relieve obstruction but, if unsuccessful, surgery is required	Make patient NPO, maintain hydration; colonoscopy may relieve obstruction but, if unsuccessful, surgery is required

AXR, abdominal x-ray.

FIGURE
(3-11) Barium enema in a patient with diverticular disease; numerous diverticuli can be seen in the left colon.

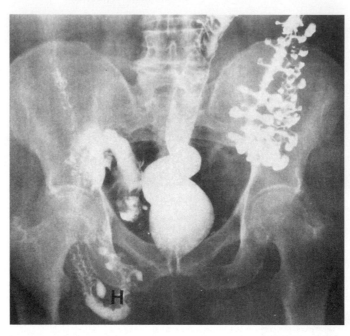

(Modified from Daffner RH. *Clinical Radiology: The Essentials.* 2nd Ed. Philadelphia: Lippincott Williams & Wilkins; 1999.)

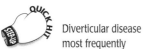
Diverticular disease most frequently occurs in the sigmoid colon and is the most common cause of **acute lower GI bleeding** in patients **over 40 yr old.**

3. **H/P** = distention, abdominal pain, vomiting, obstipation; possible palpable abdominal mass
4. **Radiology** = AXR may show **"double bubble"** proximal and distal to volvulus; barium enema shows **"bird's beak"** for distal volvulus
5. **Treatment** = possibly self-limited; colonoscopic decompression; surgical repair or resection may be required in right-sided pathology

J. **Diverticular disease**
1. Outpouchings of colonic **mucosa** and **submucosa** that herniate through muscular layer **(diverticulosis);** may erode into colonic blood vessel to cause bleeding
2. **Perforation** of diverticuli **results in abscess formation (diverticulitis);** perforation occurs secondary to infection, obstruction, or inflammation
3. **Risk factors** = low fiber diet, high fat diet, >60 yr old
4. **H/P** =
   a. **Generally asymptomatic** during uncomplicated diverticulosis (occasional constipation or mild lower abdominal pain)
   b. In diverticulitis—worse left lower quadrant pain, nausea, vomiting; fever, melena, hematochezia, palpable lower abdominal mass, abdominal tenderness
5. **Labs** = positive stool guaiac test during bleeding; increased WBC for diverticulitis
6. **Radiology** = **diverticuli seen on barium enema** and colonoscopy; free air under the diaphragm indicates perforation
7. **Treatment**
   a. High-fiber diet or fiber supplements for diverticulosis
   b. For diverticulitis—make patient NPO, nasogastric tube, antibiotics (metronidazole, cephalosporins); surgery is required in cases of perforation to resect involved bowel and create a temporary colostomy (bowel repaired at later time)
8. **Complications** = GI bleeding, abscess formation, fistula formation, sepsis

K. **Rectal conditions**
   1. **Hemorrhoids**
      a. Internal and external engorged rectal veins causing mild pain and bleeding (**bright-red blood**)
      b. **Internal** hemorrhoids arise from **superior** rectal veins above the pectinate line (columnar rectal epithelium)
      c. **External** hemorrhoids arise from **inferior** rectal veins below the pectinate line (squamous rectal epithelium)
      d. **Radiology** = sigmoidoscopy used to rule out other causes of bleeding
      e. **Treatment** = increase fiber in diet, avoid prolonged straining; sclerotherapy, ligation, or excision may be performed for worsening symptoms
   2. **Anal fissures**
      a. Painful, bleeding tears in posterior wall of anus secondary to trauma during defecation or anal intercourse
      b. **Treatment** = stool softeners; partial sphincterotomy may be performed for recurrent fissures
   3. **Anorectal abscesses**
      a. Infection of anal crypts, internal hemorrhoids, or hair follicle leading to abscess formation
      b. **H/P** = throbbing rectal pain, tenderness on digital exam
      c. **Treatment** = antibiotics, surgical incision and drainage
   4. **Rectal fistula**
      a. Formation of tract between rectum and adjacent structures secondary to **IBD** or abscess formation
      b. **H/P** = possible visible site draining pus
      c. **Treatment** = fistulotomy
   5. **Pilonidal disease**
      a. Presence of one or more cutaneous sinus tracts in the superior midline gluteal cleft
      b. Obstruction of sinus tract by hair or debris can lead to cyst and abscess formation
      c. **H/P** = usually asymptomatic; obstruction of sinus leads to mildly painful cyst with drainage (possibly purulent), small cysts may progress to larger abscesses
      d. **Treatment** = incision and drainage of abscesses; surgical closure of sinus tracts may prevent recurrence

L. **Carcinoid tumor**
   1. Tumors arising from neuroectodermal cells that function as amine-precursor-uptake and decarboxylation (APUD) cells
   2. Most commonly in **appendix,** ileum, rectum
   3. **H/P** = possibly asymptomatic; possible **carcinoid syndrome** (flushing, diarrhea, bronchoconstriction, tricuspid/pulmonary valvular disease) due to serotonin secretion by tumor (only seen with liver metastases or extragastrointestinal involvement)
   4. **Labs** = increased 5-HIAA in urine
   5. **Radiology** = CT or MRI may detect lesion
   6. **Treatment** = tumors < 2 cm have very low incidence of metastases and should be resected; tumors > 2 cm have high risk of metastases and require extensive resection, chemotherapy, and embolization of separate tumors

M. **Colorectal cancer**
   1. Neoplasm of large bowel or rectum; most commonly adenocarcinoma
   2. **Risk factors** = family history, ulcerative colitis, **colonic polyps,** hereditary polyposis syndromes, low-fiber/high-fat diet, previous colon cancer
   3. Spreads to regional lymph nodes; **metastasizes** most commonly to **lung** and **liver**

TABLE 3-10	Familial Polyposis Syndromes
Hereditary Disease	**Characteristics**
Familial adenomatous polyposis (FAP)	Hundreds of polyps in colon; near-certain development of malignant neoplasm; prophylactic subtotal colectomy recommended
Hereditary nonpolyposis colorectal cancer (HNPCC)	Multiple genetic mutations; cancer arises from normal-appearing mucosa; neoplasms tend to form in proximal colon
Gardner's syndrome	Similar to FAP with addition of common bone and soft tissue tumors
Peutz-Jeghers syndrome	Polyps are hamartomas with low risk of malignancy; mucocutaneous pigmentation of mouth, hands, and genitals
Turcot syndrome	Many colonic adenomas with high malignant potential; comorbid malignant CNS tumors
Juvenile polyposis	Polyps of colon, small bowel, and stomach that frequently are source of GI bleeding; slightly increased risk of malignancy later in life
CNS, central nervous system; GI, gastrointestinal.	

4. **H/P** = change in bowel habits (more common in left-sided disease), weakness, right-sided abdominal pain (in right-sided disease), constipation, hematochezia, malaise, weight loss; abdominal or rectal mass may be palpated

5. **Labs = positive stool guaiac test,** decreased hemoglobin, decreased hematocrit; biopsy is diagnostic; CEA is increased in 70% of patients and is useful for monitoring treatment success and cancer recurrence

6. **Radiology** = barium enema may detect lesion; colonoscopy may detect lesion and obtain biopsy specimens

7. **Treatment** =
   a. **Surgical resection,** regional lymph node dissection; chemotherapy and radiation in cases of positive lymph nodes; palliative resections are helpful in metastatic disease to improve symptoms
   b. Preventative colectomy may be indicated for hereditary syndromes
   c. Duke's classification may be used for prognosis; CEA may be followed after treatment to monitor for recurrence

QUICK HIT

Iron-deficiency anemia in elderly males is considered colon cancer until proven otherwise.

TABLE 3-11	Duke's Classification System for Staging and Corresponding Prognosis of Colorectal Cancer	
Class	**Description**	**Cure Rate**
A	Tumor confined to bowel wall	90%
B	Penetration of tumor into colonic serosa or perirectal fat	80%
C	Lymph node involvement	<60%
D	Distant metastases	<5%

FIGURE 3-12 Diagnostic pathway for GI bleeding. EGD, esophagogastroduodenoscopy; GI, gastrointestinal; IV, intravenous.

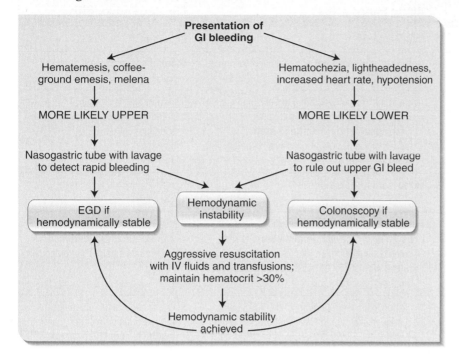

8. **Prevention** =
   a. Annual digital rectal exam starting at 40 yr old
   b. Annual stool guaiac test starting at 50 yr old
   c. Sigmoidoscopy every 5 yr starting at 50 yr old or for new positive stool guaiac test
   d. **Colonoscopy** is more sensitive than sigmoidoscopy but carries a 0.1% risk of perforation; it is now considered preferable over sigmoidoscopy by several expert groups; it should definitely be chosen over sigmoidoscopy for patients with a hereditary high risk of colon cancer

N. **GI bleeding**
   1. May be due to either upper (proximal to ligament of Treitz) or lower (distal to ligament of Treitz) sources
   2. Bright-red blood suggests a rapid or heavy bleed; dark blood (e.g., melena, coffee-grounds emesis) suggests either blood that has passed through much of the GI tract or has been sitting in the stomach for some time
   3. Common causes of upper-GI bleeds are **PUD,** Mallory-Weiss tears (longitudinal esophageal tears secondary to violent retching), **esophageal varices,** gastritis
   4. Common causes of lower-GI bleeds are **diverticulosis, neoplasm,** ulcerative colitis, mesenteric ischemia, arteriovenous malformations (AVMs), hemorrhoids, Meckel's diverticulum
   5. **Radiology** = EGD or colonoscopy shows majority of sources of bleeding; barium studies may detect defects; angiography can help locate AVMs; technetium scan can locate Meckel's diverticulum
   6. **Treatment** = fluid replacement is vital; transfusion for increased blood loss; some small bleeds stop automatically; **treat underlying cause;** sclerotherapy may help stop bleeding from varices; vasopressin may stop bleeding from AVMs and diverticuli; surgical resection of tumors and diverticuli may be needed

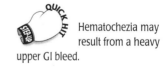
QUICK HIT
Hematochezia may result from a heavy upper GI bleed.

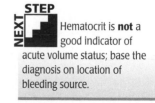
NEXT STEP
Hematocrit is **not** a good indicator of acute volume status; base the diagnosis on location of bleeding source.

TABLE 3-12	Comparison of Acute and Chronic Pancreatitis	
	Acute Pancreatitis	**Chronic Pancreatitis**
Onset	**Sudden,** severe	**Recurrent**
Risk Factors	**Gallstones, alcoholism,** trauma, hypercalcemia, hyperlipidemia, drugs	**Alcoholism,** congenital defect
H/P	Acute epigastric pain radiating to back, nausea, vomiting, **Grey Turner's sign** (bluish discoloration of flank), **Cullen's sign** (periumbilical discoloration), fever; hypotension, shock if severe	Recurrent epigastric pain, steatorrhea, weight loss, nausea, constipation
Labs	Increased amylase and lipase	Increased amylase and lipase, glycosuria
Radiology	Abdominal radiograph may show dilated loop of bowel near pancreas (**sentinel loop**) or right colon distended until near pancreas (**colon cutoff sign**); CT or US may show **pseudocyst** or enlarged pancreas	Abdominal radiograph may show **pancreatic calcifications;** ERCP may be helpful for diagnosis
Treatment	Hydration, pain control with opioids, nasogastric suction, make patient NPO, stop offending agent	Stop alcohol use, opioid analgesia, enzyme supplementation; surgery may be required to repair ductal damage
Complications	Pancreatic abscess, **pseudocyst,** necrosis, fistula formation, renal failure, chronic pancreatitis, hemorrhage, **shock,** DIC, sepsis, respiratory failure	Ductal obstruction, pseudocyst, **malnutrition**

CT, computed tomography; DIC, disseminated intravascular coagulation; ERCP, endoscopic retrograde cholangiopancreatography; US, ultrasound.

V. Pancreatic disorders

A. **Pancreatitis (see Tables 3-12 and 3-13)**
   1. **Acute** or **chronic** inflammation of pancreas associated with anatomical defects, **alcoholism,** acute ductal obstruction, drugs, **gallstones**
   2. Initially results from leak of pancreatic enzymes into pancreatic and surrounding tissues; later due to pancreatic tissue necrosis; prognosis determined by Ranson's criteria

B. **Pancreatic pseudocyst**
   1. Fluid collection arising from pancreas consisting of enzyme-rich fluids contained in sac of inflamed membranous tissue
   2. **H/P = recent acute pancreatitis,** epigastric pain; fever
   3. **Labs** = increased WBC, increased amylase
   4. **Radiology** = pseudocyst visible on ultrasound (US) or CT
   5. **Treatment** = possibly self-resolving; drainage indicated if lasting > 6 weeks, painful, or rapidly growing
   6. **Complications** = rupture, hemorrhage, abscess formation

C. **Exocrine pancreatic cancer**
   1. Adenocarcinoma of pancreas most commonly in head of pancreas
   2. **Risk factors** = tobacco, high-fat diet; male > female
   3. **H/P = abdominal pain radiating to back,** anorexia, nausea, vomiting, weight loss, fatigue; jaundice (if bile duct obstructed), palpable nontender gallbladder (**Courvoisier's sign**), splenomegaly (if in tail)

TABLE 3-13	Ranson's Criteria for Determining Prognosis During Acute Pancreatitis
Increased Mortality Associated with 3 or More of the Following:	
On Admission	**During Initial 48 hr After Admission**
> 55 yr old	Hematocrit decreases > 10%
Serum glucose > 200 mg/dL	BUN increases > 5 mg/dL
Serum LDH > 350 IU/L	Serum calcium < 8 mg/dL
Serum AST > 250 u	Pao$_2$ < 60 mm Hg
WBC > 16000/mL	Base deficit > 4 mEq/L
	Fluid sequestration > 6 L
BUN, blood urea nitrogen; LDH, lactate dehydrogenase; Pao$_2$, partial pressure of arterial oxygen; WBC, white cell count.	

4. **Labs** = possible hyperglycemia; increased CEA; increased bilirubin (total and direct) and increased alkaline phosphatase with bile duct obstruction; biopsy used to make diagnosis

5. **Radiology** = CT or MRI shows mass, dilated pancreas, and dilated bile ducts; endoscopic retrograde cholangiopancreatography (ERCP) locates tumors not seen with CT

6. **Treatment** = nonmetastatic disease may be resected with **Whipple procedure** (removal of pancreatic head, duodenum, proximal jejunum, common bile duct, gallbladder, and distal stomach); enzyme deficiency treated with replacement therapy

7. **Complications** = usually not detected until progressed; **5-year survival < 2%;** migratory thrombophlebitis (**Trousseau's syndrome**)

D. **Endocrine pancreatic cancers**

1. Neoplasms involving glandular pancreatic tissue
2. Frequently difficult to locate; may be seen with CT or MRI
3. **Zollinger-Ellison syndrome**
   a. Gastrin-producing tumors causing increased gastric acid secretion and **refractory PUD**
   b. **Labs = increased gastrin;** secretin administration causes additional increase in gastrin (normally would decrease gastrin)
   c. **Treatment** = surgical resection if able to be isolated; total gastrectomy may be needed for severe PUD
4. **Insulinoma**
   a. Insulin-secreting β-islet cell tumor causing **hypoglycemia**
   b. **H/P** = headache, confusion, weakness, mood instability
   c. **Labs = increased fasting insulin,** hypoglycemia, positive C-peptide
   d. **Treatment** = surgical resection; somatostatin may relieve symptoms in nonresectable disease
5. **Glucagonoma**
   a. Glucagon-secreting α-cell tumor causing hyperglycemia
   b. May present as refractory DM
   c. **H/P** = weight loss; exfoliating rash (**migratory necrolytic erythema**); **symptoms of DM**
   d. **Labs** = hyperglycemia, **increased glucagon**
   e. **Treatment** = surgical resection if localized lesion; somatostatin may improve symptoms
   f. **Complications** = frequently malignant; poor prognosis

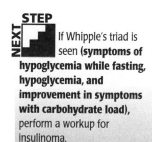

NEXT STEP If Whipple's triad is seen **(symptoms of hypoglycemia while fasting, hypoglycemia, and improvement in symptoms with carbohydrate load),** perform a workup for insulinoma.

FIGURE 3-13 Ultrasound demonstrating multiple gallstones (*white arrows*) in the gallbladder; note the shadow caused by gallstones, which may be more apparent than the gallstones themselves in several cases.

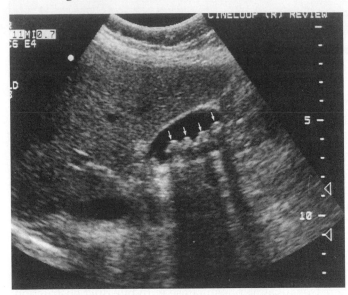

(Taken from Daffner RH. *Clinical Radiology: The Essentials.* 2nd Ed. Philadelphia: Lippincott Williams & Wilkins; 1999.)

6. **VIPoma**
   a. Vasoactive intestinal peptide (VIP)-producing tumor of non-β-islet cells
   b. **H/P = watery diarrhea,** weakness, nausea, vomiting, abdominal pain
   c. **Labs** = decreased K^+, achlorhydria
   d. **Treatment** = surgical resection for localized tumors; corticosteroids, chemotherapy, or somatostatin may improve symptoms

VI. Hepatobiliary disorders
   A. **Cholelithiasis**
      1. Gallstone formation in the gallbladder that may cause cystic duct obstruction
      2. **Risk factors** = older age, obesity, female, multiparity, oral contraceptive use, total parenteral nutrition (TPN), recent rapid weight loss
      3. Majority of stones are composed of **cholesterol;** others are calcium bilirubinate (**pigmented stones**) secondary to chronic hemolysis
      4. **H/P** = possibly asymptomatic; postprandial abdominal pain (**worst in right upper quadrant (RUQ)**), nausea, vomiting, indigestion, flatulence; RUQ tenderness, palpable gallbladder
      5. **Radiology** = US may show gallstones; AXR will only show some pigmented stones (because of high iron content from bilirubin)
      6. **Treatment** = dietary modification (decrease fatty food intake), bile salts (dissolve stones), shock wave lithotripsy (uses sound waves to break up stones); **cholecystectomy** required in many patients
      7. **Complications** = recurrent stones, **acute cholecystitis, pancreatitis**
   B. **Acute cholecystitis**
      1. Inflammation of gallbladder commonly due to **gallstone obstruction of cystic duct;** acalculous cholecystitis may occur in patients on TPN or who are critically ill
      2. **H/P** = RUQ pain radiating to back, nausea, vomiting; fever, palpable gallbladder, RUQ tenderness; symptoms more severe and longer in duration than typical cholelithiasis
      3. **Labs** = increased WBC, increased bilirubin (total and direct), increased alkaline phosphatase

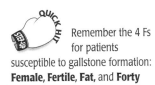

Remember the 4 Fs for patients susceptible to gallstone formation: **Female, Fertile, Fat,** and **Forty** (years old).

STEP
NEXT
If you detect a positive Murphy's sign **(palpation of RUQ during inspiration stops inspiration secondary to pain),** suspect acute cholecystitis and perform an US.

4. **Radiology** = US may show gallstones, sludge, or thickened gallbladder wall; hepatic iminodiacetic acid (**HIDA**) scan will detect cystic duct obstruction (gallbladder fails to fill normally during scan)
5. **Treatment** = hydration, antibiotics, **cholecystectomy;** patients with more mild symptoms may be treated with lithotripsy and bile salts; patients who are not stable for surgery may be treated with ERCP delivery of stone solvents
6. **Complications** = perforation, gallstone ileus, abscess formation

C. **Cholangitis**
1. Infection of bile ducts secondary to ductal obstruction
2. **Risk factors** = cholelithiasis, anatomical duct defect, biliary cancer
3. **H/P** = RUQ pain, chills; **jaundice, fever, RUQ tenderness;** change in mental status or signs of shock seen in severe cases (Color Figure 3-2)
4. **Labs** = increased WBC, increased bilirubin (total and direct), increased alkaline phosphatase, **positive blood cultures**
5. **Radiology** = US or CT may detect obstruction; HIDA scan is more sensitive
6. **Treatment** = hydration, IV antibiotics, cholecystectomy; severe symptoms demand **emergency bile duct decompression** and relief of obstruction

D. **Gallbladder cancer**
1. Adenocarcinoma of gallbladder associated with cholelithiasis and biliary tract disease; generally poor prognosis
2. **H/P** = similar symptoms to acute cholecystitis; anorexia, weight loss, abdominal pain radiating to back; palpable gallbladder, jaundice
3. **Labs** = increased bilirubin (total and direct), increased alkaline phosphatase, increased cholesterol; biopsy provides diagnosis
4. **Radiology** = abdominal radiograph may show **calcified gallbladder;** ERCP can localize lesion and perform biopsy
5. **Treatment** = cholecystectomy, lymph node dissection, partial removal of adjacent hepatic tissue

E. **Alcohol-related liver disease**
1. Progressive liver damage secondary to **alcoholism**
2. Initially characterized by fatty deposits in liver; reversible with alcohol cessation
3. Continued alcoholism causes hepatic inflammation and early necrosis
4. Progressive damage results in cirrhosis
5. **H/P** = asymptomatic for many years of alcoholism; anorexia, nausea, vomiting; abdominal tenderness, ascites, splenomegaly, hepatomegaly, fever, jaundice
6. **Labs** = increased ALT, increased AST, increased GGT, increased alkaline phosphatase, increased bilirubin (total and direct), prolonged PT, increased WBC; biopsy provides diagnosis (**fatty liver,** many PMNs, areas of necrosis)
7. **Treatment** = **cessation of alcohol use,** thiamine, folate, high caloric intake (2500–3000 kcal/day)
8. **Complications** = cirrhosis, hepatic encephalopathy, coagulation disorders

F. **Cirrhosis**
1. **Persistent liver damage** leading to **necrosis** and **fibrosis** of hepatic parenchyma
2. Due to **alcoholism,** chronic **HBV** or **HCV** infection, chronic bile duct obstruction, biliary and hepatic parenchymal diseases, drugs, toxins
3. **H/P** = symptoms follow continuum from early liver diseases; weakness, weight loss, GI bleeding; **hepatomegaly,** splenomegaly, jaundice, **ascites,** abdominal wall varicosities (**caput medusae**), testicular atrophy, gynecomastia, possible mental status changes (due to encephalopathy)
4. **Labs** = decreased albumin, anemia, decreased platelets, prolonged PT; paracentesis of ascites shows fluid with < 2.5 g/dL protein, WBC

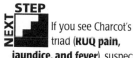
NEXT STEP If you see Charcot's triad (**RUQ pain, jaundice, and fever**), suspect cholangitis and perform an US or HIDA scan.

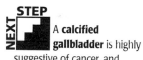
NEXT STEP A **calcified gallbladder** is highly suggestive of cancer, and biopsy should be performed promptly to confirm diagnosis.

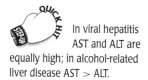
QUICK HIT In viral hepatitis AST and ALT are equally high; in alcohol-related liver disease AST > ALT.

FIGURE
3-14 Portal-systemic anastomoses and common sites of varices in portal hypertension.

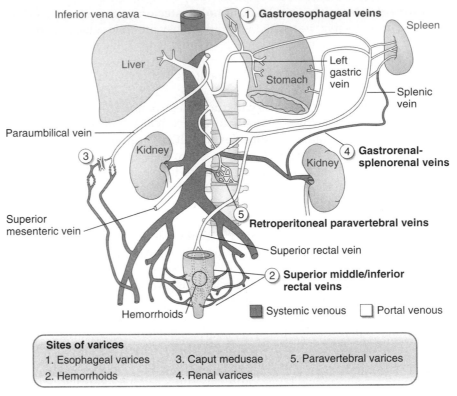

Sites of varices
1. Esophageal varices	3. Caput medusae	5. Paravertebral varices
2. Hemorrhoids	4. Renal varices	

(Modified from Le T, Amin C, Bhushan V, Choo E. *First Aid for the USMLE Step 2.* 4th Ed. New York: McGraw-Hill; 2003.)

$<300/\mu L$, normal glucose level, and decreased amylase; biopsy shows fibrosis and hepatic necrosis

5. **Treatment = nonreversible,** but progression may be halted; stop offending agent; treat varices with vasopressin, somatostatin, or sclerotherapy; lactulose, neomycin, and low-protein diet may improve encephalopathy; **liver transplant** may be needed in progressive cases

6. **Complications = portal hypertension,** varices (due to venous hypertension), ascites, **hepatic encephalopathy** (due to poor filtering of blood), renal failure

G. **Portal hypertension**

1. Increase in portal vein pressure giving it a **higher pressure than the inferior vena cava;** may be due to prehepatic, intrahepatic, or posthepatic causes

2. Prehepatic causes include portal vein thrombosis and schistosomiasis

3. Intrahepatic causes include **cirrhosis** and granulomatous disease

4. Posthepatic causes include **right-sided heart failure,** hepatic vein thrombosis, and Budd-Chiari syndrome (hepatic vein thrombosis secondary to hypercoagulability)

5. Shunting of blood into systemic veins causes **varices** in several locations

6. **H/P = ascites,** abdominal pain, change in mental status (due to hepatic encephalopathy), hematemesis (due to esophageal varices); **hepatomegaly,** splenomegaly, fever, abdominal wall varices, testicular atrophy, gynecomastia

7. **Labs** = increased ammonium (NH_4^+); paracentesis shows ascites with albumin > serum albumin by at least 1.1 g/dL, increased WBC, and normal glucose

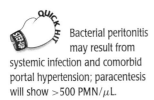

Bacterial peritonitis may result from systemic infection and comorbid portal hypertension; paracentesis will show >500 PMN/μL.

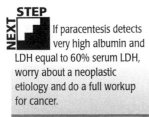

STEP
NEXT If paracentesis detects very high albumin and LDH equal to 60% serum LDH, worry about a neoplastic etiology and do a full workup for cancer.

8. **Radiology** = CT may show ascites and obstructing mass; EGD may show esophageal varices
9. **Treatment** =
   a. Salt restriction and diuretics for ascites
   b. IV antibiotics for bacterial peritonitis
   c. Dialysis for renal failure
   d. Lactulose, neomycin, and low-protein diet for hepatic encephalopathy
   e. Vasopressin or sclerotherapy for bleeding varices
   f. **Hepatic shunting** via laparotomy or transjugular intrahepatic portal-caval shunting (TIPS) is short-term solution for severe disease; **liver transplant** often required as eventual treatment in progressive cases

H. **Hepatic parenchymal and biliary diseases**
1. **Hemochromatosis**
   a. Autosomal-recessive disease of iron absorption
   b. **Excess iron absorption** causes iron deposition in liver, pancreas, heart, and pituitary leading to eventual fibrosis
   c. Rarely is result of chronic blood transfusions or alcoholism
   d. **H/P** = abdominal pain, polydipsia, polyuria, arthralgias; **pigmented rash** (bronze hue), hepatomegaly, testicular atrophy; may see symptoms and signs that resemble DM and CHF
   e. **Labs** = increased iron, increased percentage saturation of iron, increased ferritin, decreased transferrin, slightly increased AST and ALT; biopsy shows increased iron content in liver
   f. **Treatment** = **weekly or biweekly phlebotomy** until normal iron, then monthly phlebotomy; deferoxamine for iron chelation
   g. **Complications** = cirrhosis, hepatoma, CHF, DM, hypopituitarism
2. **Wilson's disease**
   a. Autosomal-recessive disorder of copper secretion, primarily in young adults
   b. **Excess copper deposits** in liver, brain, cornea
   c. **H/P** = psychiatric disturbances (depression, neuroses, **personality changes**), **loss of coordination,** dysphagia; jaundice, tremor, possible green-brown rings in cornea (**Kayser-Fleischer rings**), hepatomegaly; signs may precede symptoms
   d. **Labs** = decreased serum ceruloplasmin, increased urinary copper, slightly increased AST and ALT; biopsy shows increased copper deposits in liver
   e. **Treatment** = **trientine** or penicillamine for copper chelation, life-long zinc for maintenance therapy, dietary copper restriction (no organ meats, shellfish, chocolate, nuts, or mushrooms), supplementary vitamin B_6
3. α_1-**Antitrypsin deficiency**
   a. Autosomal-recessive disorder with decreased α_1-antitrypsin production leading to cirrhosis and panlobular **emphysema**
   b. Most symptoms arise from emphysematic component of disease
   c. **Labs** = increased AST, increased ALT; **pulmonary function tests (PFTs) demonstrate obstructive disease**
   d. **Treatment** = liver transplant or lung transplant may be needed in severe cases; enzyme replacement may be helpful in stopping disease progression
4. **Primary biliary cirrhosis (PBC)**
   a. Autoimmune disease with intrahepatic bile duct destruction leading to accumulation of cholesterol, bile acids, and bilirubin
   b. **Risk factors** = rheumatoid arthritis, Sjögren syndrome, scleroderma; **female > male**
   c. **H/P** = possibly asymptomatic; fatigue, pruritus; jaundice, xanthomas

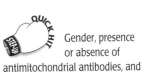

Gender, presence or absence of antimitochondrial antibodies, and ERCP distinguish PBC from PSC.

d. **Labs** = increased alkaline phosphatase, increased GGT, normal AST and ALT, increased cholesterol, increased bilirubin (total and direct); **positive antimitochondrial antibodies;** workup may indicate comorbid autoimmune diseases; biopsy shows inflammation and necrosis in bile ducts

e. **Treatment** = ursodeoxycholic acid improves liver function and symptoms; methotrexate may be added in more severe cases; liver transplant needed in progressive disease

5. **Primary sclerosing cholangitis (PSC)**
   a. Progressive destruction of intrahepatic and extrahepatic bile ducts leading to fibrosis and cirrhosis
   b. **Risk factors** = ulcerative colitis; **male > female**
   c. **H/P** = possibly asymptomatic; fatigue, pruritus; jaundice, xanthomas
   d. **Labs** = increased alkaline phosphatase, increased GGT, normal AST and ALT, increased cholesterol, increased bilirubin (total and direct); biopsy appears similar to that for PBC
   e. **Radiology** = ERCP shows stricturing and irregularity of extrahepatic and intrahepatic bile ducts ("**pearls on string**")
   f. **Treatment** = ursodeoxycholic acid, methotrexate, corticosteroids; surgical resection of affected ducts and liver transplant may be required in progressive cases

6. Hepatic bilirubin transport
   a. Unconjugated bilirubin from red cell (RBC) hemolysis exists in venous circulation
   b. Unconjugated bilirubin enters hepatocytes and is conjugated by **glucuronosyltransferase**
   c. Conjugated bilirubin reenters venous circulation

7. **Gilbert's disease**
   a. Autosomal-recessive or dominant disease with **mild deficiency** of glucuronosyltransferase
   b. **H/P** = mild jaundice following fasting, exercise, or stress
   c. **Labs** = increased indirect bilirubin < 5 mg/dL
   d. **Treatment** = none necessary

Prehepatic conditions cause an increase in **indirect bilirubin; posthepatic** conditions cause an increase in **direct bilirubin; intrahepatic** conditions may cause an increase of **either** or **both** types of bilirubin.

TABLE 3-14	**Causes of Conjugated and Unconjugated Bilirubinemia**		
Increased Total Bilirubin			
Unconjugated (Indirect) Hyperbilirubinemia		**Conjugated (Direct) Hyperbilirubinemia**	
Excess bilirubin production	Hemolytic anemia Disorders of erythropoiesis Internal hemorrhage resorption	Decreased hepatic bilirubin excretion	Impaired bilirubin transport (Dubin-Johnson syndrome, Rotor's syndrome) Hepatocellular disease (cirrhosis, hepatitis) Drug impairment
Impaired conjugation	Physiologic jaundice of newborn Deficiency of glucuronosyltransferase (Gilbert's disease, Crigler-Najjar syndrome) Hepatocellular disease (cirrhosis, hepatitis)	Extrahepatic biliary obstruction	Intrahepatic bile duct disease (PBC, PSC) Gallstone obstruction of bile ducts (choledocholithiasis) Pancreatic or biliary cancer Biliary atresia
PBC, primary biliary cirrhosis; PSC, primary sclerosing cholangitis.			

8. **Crigler-Najjar syndrome**
   a. Autosomal-recessive disease with **severe deficiency** in glucuronosyltransferase
   b. **H/P** = jaundice, CNS symptoms (due to kernicterus)
   c. **Labs** = increased indirect bilirubin > 5 mg/dL
   d. **Treatment** = phenobarbitol may improve symptoms
   e. **Complications** = early kernicterus may cause permanent CNS damage

I. **Hepatic neoplasms**
   1. **Benign tumors** (hepatic adenoma, focal nodular hyperplasia, hemangiomas)
      a. Benign hepatic tumors found more commonly in **women with history of oral contraceptive use**
      b. **H/P** = frequently asymptomatic; possible RUQ fullness
      c. **Radiology** = CT, MRI, or angiography detects hypervascular liver mass
      d. **Treatment** = frequently untreated; larger tumors may be resected or embolized to prevent rupture
   2. **Hepatocellular carcinoma** (hepatoma)
      a. Malignant tumor of liver
      b. **Risk factors** = **HBV or HCV infection,** cirrhosis, hemochromatosis, *Aspergillus* infection, schistosomiasis
      c. **H/P** = RUQ pain, weight loss, malaise, anorexia; jaundice, hepatomegaly, bruit over liver, ascites
      d. **Labs** = slightly increased AST and ALT, increased alkaline phosphatase, increased bilirubin (total and direct), **increased α-fetoprotein;** biopsy provides diagnosis but risks causing substantial hemorrhage
      e. **Radiology** = CT, MRI, or US shows liver mass; angiography may show increased vascularity
      f. **Treatment** = surgical resection of small tumors (lobectomy or partial hepatectomy) and chemotherapy; transplant may be an option for limited disease
      g. **Complications** = poor prognosis; portal vein obstruction, Budd-Chiari syndrome, liver failure

Biopsy of hepatic masses is usually contraindicated because of hypervascularity and risk of hemorrhage.

Liver metastases from breast, lung, or colon cancers are much more common than primary liver cancers.

VII. Pediatric GI disorders

A. **Tracheoesophageal fistula**
   1. Malformation of trachea and esophagus resulting in tract formation between structures
   2. Frequently associated with esophageal atresia
   3. **H/P** = coughing and cyanosis during feeding, food may fill blind pouch, abdominal distention, possible history of aspiration pneumonia
   4. **Radiology** = chest radiograph following nasogastric tube insertion demonstrates malformation (tube in lung or blind pouch)
   5. **Treatment** = surgical repair

B. **Pyloric stenosis**
   1. Hypertrophy of pyloric sphincter causing obstruction of gastric outlet
   2. **H/P** = symptoms begin a few weeks after birth; nonbilious emesis, **projectile emesis; palpable epigastric olive-sized mass**
   3. **Radiology** = barium swallow shows thin pyloric channel (**string sign**); US shows increased pyloric muscle thickness
   4. **Treatment** = pyloromyotomy

C. **Necrotizing enterocolitis**
   1. Idiopathic mucosal necrosis and epithelial cell sloughing
   2. **Risk factors** = preterm birth, low birth weight

FIGURE
3-15 Variations of tracheoesophageal fistulas.

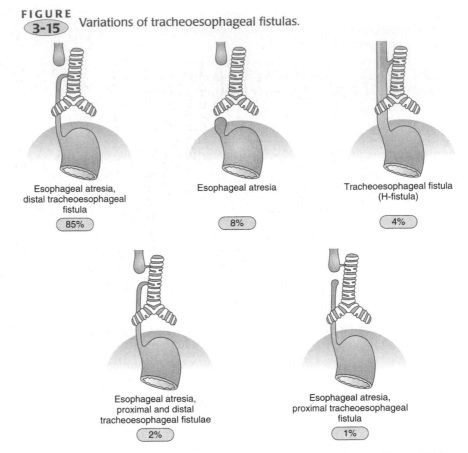

(Modified from Rudolph AM, ed. *Rudolph's Pediatrics.* 19th Ed. Stamford: Appleton and Lange; 1991.)

   3. **H/P** = bilious vomiting; abdominal distention, **bloody stools;** signs of shock in severe cases
   4. **Labs** = metabolic acidosis
   5. **Radiology** = abdominal radiograph shows bowel distention, **air in bowel wall,** or free air under the diaphragm
   6. **Treatment** = TPN, IV antibiotics, surgical resection of affected bowel
D. **Hirschsprung's disease**
   1. Absence of bowel autonomic innervation causing bowel spasm and obstruction
   2. **H/P** = vomiting, **obstipation;** abdominal distention
   3. **Labs** = bowel biopsy shows **absence of ganglia**
   4. **Radiology** = barium enema shows proximal dilation (megacolon) with distal narrowing
   5. **Treatment** = colostomy and resection of affected area
E. **Intussusception**
   1. **Telescoping of bowel into adjacent segment** of bowel leading to obstruction; most frequently proximal to ileocecal valve
   2. **Risk factors** = Meckel's diverticulum, Henoch-Schönlein purpura, adenovirus infection, cystic fibrosis
   3. **H/P** = sudden abdominal pain that lasts < 1 min and is episodic, pallor, sweating, vomiting, bloody mucus in stool (**currant jelly stool**); abdominal tenderness, **palpable sausage-like abdominal mass**
   4. **Labs** = increased WBC
   5. **Radiology** = barium enema will show obstruction

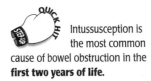

Intussusception is the most common cause of bowel obstruction in the **first two years of life.**

FIGURE
3-16 Abdominal ultrasound demonstrating pyloric stenosis; note the thin pyloric lumen (*L*) and the thicken pyloric musculature (defined by region between *x*'s and +'s).

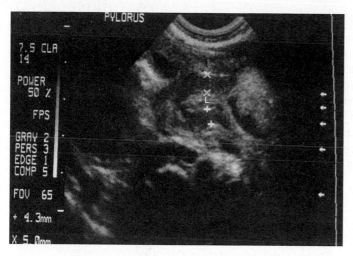

(Taken from Daffner RH. *Clinical Radiology: The Essentials.* 2nd Ed. Philadelphia: Lippincott Williams & Wilkins; 1999.)

6. **Treatment** = barium enema may reduce defect; surgery required for refractory cases
7. **Complications** = bowel ischemia (appendix particularly susceptible)

F. **Meckel's diverticulum**
1. Common **remnant of vitelline duct** that exists as **outpouching of ileum** and may contain **ectopic tissue**
2. **H/P** = asymptomatic; occasionally may present with painless rectal bleeding, **intussusception,** diverticulitis, or abscess formation
3. **Radiology** = gastric mucosa may be detected by technetium radionucleotide scan (**Meckel's scan**)
4. **Treatment** = surgical resection if symptomatic

G. **Neonatal jaundice**
1. Hyperbilirubinemia in the newborn may be due to **physiologic, hepatic,** or **hematologic** causes
   a. Physiologic (**common**)—**physiologic undersecretion,** breast-feeding failure
   b. Increased hemolysis—maternal-fetal ABO incompatibility, hereditary RBC abnormalities, glucose 6-phosphate dehydrogenase (G6PD) deficiency
   c. Bilirubin overproduction without hemolysis—hemorrhage, maternal-fetal transfusion
   d. Hepatic abnormalities—Gilbert's syndrome, Crigler-Najjar syndrome, biliary atresia
2. Physiologic causes frequently resolve within two weeks
3. Kernicterus is deposition of bilirubin in basal ganglia and hippocampus and may cause permanent damage; results from extremely high serum bilirubin and is typically only seen with hepatic abnormalities
4. **H/P** = jaundice, scleral icterus; lethargy, high-pitched cry, seizures, and apnea seen with kernicterus
5. **Labs** = frequently indirect hyperbilirubinemia (due to hemolysis); jaundice developing with initial 24 hours after birth, total bilirubin > 15 mg/dL, or direct bilirubin > 2 mg/dL suggests nonphysiologic cause

Meckel's diverticulum rule of 2's= males **2 times** more common than females, occurs within **2 ft** of ileocecal valve, **2 types** of ectopic tissue (gastric, pancreatic), found in **2%** of the population.

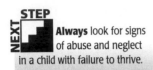

GASTROINTESTINAL DISORDERS

6. **Treatment** = phototherapy used for physiologic jaundice lasting several days; suspected nonphysiologic causes should be worked up and may require exchange transfusion

H. **Failure to thrive**
1. Children below 3rd-percentile weight for age or failure to gain weight appropriate for age
2. May be due to underlying illness or neglect
3. **H/P** = look for leads to organic causes; screen for abuse
4. **Labs** = urinalysis, CBC, blood culture, urine culture, serum electrolytes, cystic fibrosis testing, and caloric intake records may be helpful in making diagnosis
5. **Treatment** = high-calorie diet, treat underlying disorder; educate parents in proper nutrition and feeding; contact social support services in cases of neglect or abuse

CHAPTER 4

Genitourinary Disorders

I. Normal renal function

A. Physiology

1. Kidneys function to filter serum plasma, regulate fluid volume and electrolyte levels, and maintain body fluid homeostasis
2. **Proximal convoluted tubule** (cortex)
   a. Almost all glucose, bicarbonate (HCO_3^-), amino acids, and metabolites are reabsorbed
   b. Two thirds of sodium (Na^+) is reabsorbed; chloride (Cl^-) and water (H_2O) are reabsorbed passively along osmotic gradient
   c. Organic acids (uric acid, etc.) and bases are secreted into tubules
3. **Descending loop of Henle** (medulla)
   a. Increasing interstitial osmotic gradient causes water reabsorption and concentration of tubule fluid
   b. Descending limb is the only segment of the loop that is permeable to H_2O
4. **Ascending loop of Henle** (medulla)
   a. Active reabsorption of Na^+, Cl^-, and potassium (K^+) by $Na^+/K^+/Cl^-$ cotransporter
   b. Reabsorption of magnesium (Mg^{2+}), calcium (Ca^{2+}), and K^+ through paracellular diffusion
5. **Distal convoluted tubule** (cortex)
   a. Cells impermeable to water
   b. Na^+ and Cl^- reabsorbed by Na^+/Cl^- transporter
   c. Ca^{2+} reabsorbed via parathyroid hormone activity
6. **Collecting tubule** (cortex) **and duct** (medulla)
   a. Principal cells drive Na^+ reabsorption and K^+ secretion when stimulated by aldosterone
   b. Intercalated cells secrete H^+ and reabsorb K^+
   c. Antidiuretic hormone (ADH) drives H_2O reabsorption

B. Diuretics (see Table 4-1)

1. Affect electrolyte and fluid resorption at distinct locations along the renal tubular system
2. Renal activity of diuretics affects body fluid composition and volume

II. Disorders of the kidney

A. Pyelonephritis

1. Infection of renal parenchyma most commonly due to *Escherichia coli*; *Staphylococcus saprophyticus*, *Klebsiella*, and *Proteus* are less common pathogens; *Candida* is a potential cause in immunocompromised patients
2. Most commonly occurs as **sequelae of ascending urinary tract infection (UTI)**

 20% of all plasma flow entering the kidney enters Bowman's capsule and is filtered.

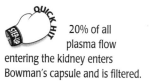 **Carbonic anhydrase** is the catalyst for HCO_3^- resorption in the proximal convoluted tubule.

 Loop diuretics have direct pulmonary vasodilatory activity and are particularly useful in treating **pulmonary edema** due to fluid overload.

FIGURE 4-1 Anatomy of the nephron and major sites of ion, water, and molecule exchange.

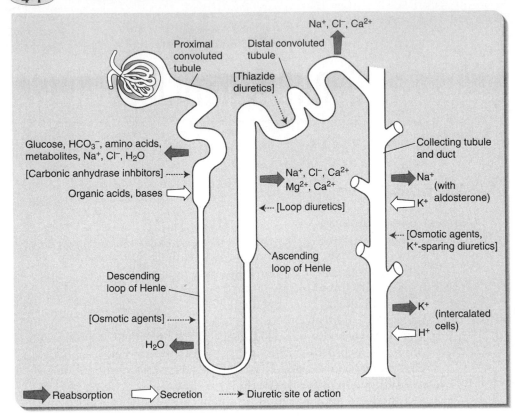

Fluroquinolones have comparable bioavailability for the oral and IV formulations.

The **uretero-vesical junction** is the most common site of renal stone impaction.

Patients with **impacted stones** will be in pain and will **shift position frequently** in unsuccessful attempts to find a comfortable position; patients with **peritonitis** will remain **rigid**.

In an IVP, water-soluble contrast dyes are injected intravenously and excreted by the kidneys; an appropriately timed x-ray will demonstrate excretion of the dye through the urinary tract and may show urinary defects and obstructions.

3. **Risk factors** = urinary obstruction, immunocompromise, history of previous pyelonephritis
4. **H/P** = **flank pain,** chills, nausea, vomiting, urinary frequency, dysuria, urgency; fever, **costovertebral tenderness**
5. **Labs** = **white blood cell casts in urine;** positive urine cultures (possibly negative when due to hematogenous spread)
6. **Treatment** = IV fluroquinolones or cephalosporins (third generation) for 10–14 days; mild cases may be treated with 1–2 days IV antibiotics followed by outpatient oral antibiotics or oral antibiotics alone
7. **Complications** = increased risk of **preterm** labor and acute respiratory distress syndrome (requiring IV antibiotics) in **pregnant** females

B. **Nephrolithiasis (see Table 4-2)**
1. Formation of "kidney" stones; stone formation may also occur elsewhere in urinary tract; symptoms arise when stones become stuck in urinary tract and cause **obstruction**
2. **Risk factors** = family history, low fluid intake, gout, renal tubular acidosis, **hypercalcemia, hyperparathyroidism,** certain drugs (acetazolamide, allopurinol, loop diuretics); males >females
3. **H/P** = **acute severe colicky flank pain** that may extend to inner thigh or genitals, nausea, vomiting, dysuria
4. **Labs** = urinalysis shows hematuria
5. **Radiology** = abdominal x-ray show stones in majority of cases (except uric acid stones); intravenous pyelogram (IVP) shows filling defect; computed tomography (CT) or ultrasound (US) may locate stones
6. **Treatment** = hydration and pain control (possibly narcotics and/or ketorolac); shockwave lithotripsy can break up stones <3 cm diameter so

TABLE 4-1 Common Diuretics and Effects within the Nephron

Diuretic	Site of Action	Mechanism of Action	Indications	Contraindications/ Adverse Effects
Carbonic anhydrase inhibitors (acetazolamide)	Proximal convoluted tubule	Inhibition of carbonic anhydrase causes mild diuresis and prevents HCO_3^- reabsorption	Glaucoma, epilepsy, altitude sickness	Mild metabolic acidosis, hypokalemia, nephrolithiasis
Osmotic agents (mannitol, urea)	Proximal convoluted tubule, loop of Henle, collecting tubule	Increased tubular osmotic gradient increases H_2O excretion	Increased intracranial pressure, acute renal failure (due to shock or drug toxicity)	No effect on Na^+ excretion
Loop diuretics (furosemide, etc.)	Ascending loop of Henle	Inhibit $Na^+/Cl^-/K^+$ cotransporter to decrease reabsorption and indirectly inhibit Ca^{2+} reabsorption	CHF, pulmonary edema, hypercalcemia; rapid onset useful in emergent situations	Ototoxicity, hyperuricemia, hypokalemia, hypocalcemia
Thiazides (hydrochlorothiazide, etc.)	Distal convoluted tubule	Inhibit Na^+/Cl^- transporter to decrease reabsorption and indirectly increase K^+ excretion and increase Ca^{2+} reabsorption	HTN, CHF, hypercalciuria, diabetes insipidus	Hypokalemia, hyperuricemia, hypercalcemia
K^+-sparing (spironolactone)	Collecting tubules	Aldosterone antagonist that inhibits Na^+-K^+ exchange	Secondary hyper-aldosteronism, K^+-preserving diuresis	Gynecomastia, menstrual irregularity, hyperkalemia

CHF, congestive heart failure; HTN, hypertension.

GENITOURINARY DISORDERS

that they pass through the ureters; surgery may be required for larger stones
7. **Complications** = hydronephrosis, recurrent stones
C. **Hydronephrosis**
1. **Dilation of renal calyces** as a result of increased pressure in the distal urinary tract
2. Due to increased intrarenal pressure from urinary tract obstruction (stones, anatomical defects, extra/intra urinary mass)
3. Can lead to permanent damage of renal parenchyma
4. **H/P** = possibly asymptomatic; dull or intermittent flank pain with history of UTI
5. **Radiology** = US or IVP detects dilation
6. **Treatment** = drainage via nephrostomy tube; treat underlying obstruction (balloon dilation of ureter and placement of double-J stent in ureter may allow urine flow)
7. **Complications** = renal failure
D. **Polycystic kidney disease**
1. Hereditary syndrome characterized by the formation of cysts in one or both kidneys leading to eventual kidney functional impairment and failure (Color Figure 4-1)
2. Types
   a. **Autosomal dominant—most common form;** affects **adults;** large multicystic kidneys that function poorly

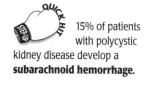

15% of patients with polycystic kidney disease develop a **subarachnoid hemorrhage.**

TABLE 4-2 Types of Nephrolithiasis (Renal Stones)

Type	Frequency	Cause	Radiology	Notes
Calcium phosphate	8%	**Hyperparathyroidism,** renal tubular acidosis	Radiopaque	
Calcium oxalate	72%	**Idiopathic hypercalciuria,** small bowel diseases	Radiopaque	Most patients have no identifiable cause
Uric acid	7%	Chronic acidic/concentrated urine, chemotherapeutic drugs, gout	**Radiolucent**	Treat by alkalinizing urine
Struvite ($Mg\text{-}NH_4\text{-}PO_4$)	12%	**Urinary tract infection**	Radiopaque	More common in **women;** may form staghorn calculi
Cystine	1%	Cystinuria, amino acid transport defects	Radiopaque	May form staghorn calculi

  b. **Autosomal recessive**—rare form; presents in **children;** fatal in initial years of life (without transplant)
3. **H/P** = asymptomatic until adulthood (dominant form); flank pain, chronic UTI, gross hematuria; large palpable kidneys, possible hypertension; symptoms exacerbated by cyst rupture
4. **Labs** = increased blood urea nitrogen (BUN), increased creatinine (Cr), anemia; urinalysis shows hematuria and proteinuria
5. **Radiology** = US or CT will show **large multicystic kidneys;** stones may be a comorbid finding
6. **Treatment** = preserve kidney function by treating UTI and hypertension; dialysis or transplant may be required if function deteriorates into renal failure

TABLE 4-3 Common Causes of Hematuria

Age	Temporary Hematuria	Persistent Hematuria
<20 yr old	Idiopathic UTI Exercise Trauma Endometriosis (women)	Glomerular disease
20–50 yr old	Idiopathic UTI Nephrolithiasis Exercise Trauma Endometriosis (women)	Adult polycystic kidney disease Neoplasm (bladder, kidney, prostate) Glomerular disease
>50 yr old	Idiopathic UTI Nephrolithiasis Trauma	Adult polycystic kidney disease BPH (men) Neoplasm (bladder, kidney, prostate) Glomerular disease

BPH, benign prostatic hyperplasia; UTI, urinary tract infection.

FIGURE 4-2 Intravenous pyelogram demonstrating hydronephrosis in the right kidney (*asterisk*); renal pelvis dilation is evident as is a radiopaque stone in the right ureter (*arrow*); the left kidney appears normal.

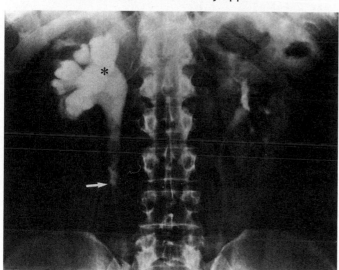

(Taken from Daffner RH. *Clinical Radiology: The Essentials.* 2nd Ed. Philadelphia: Lippincott Williams & Wilkins; 1999.)

7. **Complications** = end-stage renal disease, hepatic cysts, intracranial aneurysms, subarachnoid hemorrhage, mitral valve prolapse; more severe symptoms and quicker deterioration occur in the recessive form

E. **Renal cell carcinoma**
1. Adenocarcinoma of renal parenchyma
2. **Risk factor = tobacco smoking**
3. **H/P** = flank pain, weight loss; abdominal mass, hypertension, fever
4. **Labs** = polycythemia (secondary to increased erythropoietin activity); urinalysis shows hematuria
5. **Radiology** = IVP, US, magnetic resonance imaging (MRI), or CT with contrast may show renal mass
6. **Treatment** = nephrectomy with lymph node dissection; early recognition significantly improves prognosis
7. **Complications** = poor prognosis if not caught in early stages

F. **Interstitial nephropathy**
1. Damage of renal tubules or parenchyma due to **drugs, toxins,** infection, or autoimmune processes
2. Medication causes include β-lactam antibiotics, sulfonamides, **aminoglycosides,** nonsteroidal anti-inflammatory drugs (NSAIDs), and diuretics (in addition to several other drugs)
3. Toxic causes include **cadmium, lead,** copper, mercury, and some poisonous mushrooms
4. Other causes include infection, sarcoidosis, amyloidosis, myohemoglobinuria (due to muscle injury or excessive exercise) and high uric acid levels
5. **H/P** = symptoms of acute renal failure; fever
6. **Labs** = eosinophilia; uranalysis may show granular or epithelia casts; toxin screens may detect offending agents; renal biopsy shows infiltration of inflammatory cells and renal tubular necrosis
7. **Treatment** = stop offending agent; supportive care until renal recovery
8. **Complications** = **acute tubular necrosis (ATN)** (progressive damage of renal tubules), acute or chronic renal failure, renal papillary necrosis (ischemic necrosis of renal parenchyma), end-stage renal disease

Both nephritic and nephrotic syndromes involve diseases of the glomeruli; they are differentiated by the absence (nephritic) or presence (nephrotic) of proteinuria >3 g/day.

Drugs are the most common cause of ARF.

BUN:creatinine ratio is a quick way to help determine the etiology of ARF (**ratio >20 if prerenal cause**).

Fractional excretion of Na^+ may aid in diagnosing a cause of renal failure; **FeNa = (urine Na^+/serum Na^+)/(urine Cr/serum Cr); FeNa <1%** suggests a prerenal cause.

CRF does not occur until >90% renal parenchyma is sclerosed or necrotic.

Kidneys may appear to be normal size in adult polycystic kidney disease, DM, and amyloidosis.

III. Glomerular diseases

A. **Nephritic syndromes** (see Table 4-4)

1. Acute **hematuria** and proteinuria that result secondary to **glomerular inflammation**
2. **H/P** = varies with pathology; oliguria and gross hematuria (evidenced by brown urine) are common
3. **Labs** = vary with pathology; generally increased BUN, increased Cr; hematuria and proteinuria seen on urinalysis; 24-hour urine collection measures protein as <3 g/day
4. **Treatment** = varies with pathology; dialysis or renal transplantation may be required in cases of renal failure

B. **Nephrotic syndromes** (see Table 4-5)

1. Significant proteinuria (**>3 g/day**) associated with hypoalbuminemia and hyperlipidemia
2. Frequently due to glomerulonephritis
3. **H/P** = varies with pathology; generally edema, foamy urine, dyspnea; hypertension, ascites
4. **Labs** = vary with pathology; generally decreased albumin and hyperlipidemia; proteinuria >3 g/day seen on 24-hour urine collection
5. **Treatment** = varies with pathology; frequently includes diuretics and dietary salt and protein restriction

IV. Renal failure

A. **Acute renal failure** (ARF)

1. Sudden decrease in renal function (i.e., glomerular filtering, urine production, or chemical excretion abnormalities with BUN and Cr retention) due to prerenal, intrarenal, or postrenal causes
2. Prerenal causes include **hypovolemia,** sepsis, renal artery stenosis, drug toxicity
3. Intrarenal causes include **ATN** (drugs, toxins), glomerular disease, renal vascular disease
4. Postrenal disease is due to **obstruction** of renal calyces, ureters, or the bladder (stones, tumor, adhesions)
5. **H/P** = fatigue, anorexia, nausea, oliguria; pericardial friction rub, hypertension, fever, possible diffuse rash
6. **Labs** = **increased BUN, increased Cr;** urinalysis and urine or serum electrolyte abnormalities may help diagnosis
7. **Treatment** = prevent fluid overload, stop drugs causing ATN, dietary protein restriction, corticosteroids, dialysis

B. **Chronic renal failure** (CRF)

1. Progressive damage of renal parenchyma that may take several years to develop
2. Hypertension and diabetes mellitus (DM) are most common causes
3. **H/P** = gradual development of uremic syndrome (changes in mental status, decreased consciousness, hypertension, pericarditis, anorexia, nausea, vomiting, gastrointestinal bleeding, peripheral neuropathy, brownish coloration of skin)
4. **Labs** = increased K^+, decreased Na^+, increased phosphate, decreased Ca^{2+}, anemia, metabolic acidosis, increased BUN, increased Cr; urine osmolality is similar to serum osmolality
5. **Radiology** = US may show hydronephrosis or shrunken kidneys
6. **Treatment** = restrict dietary salt and protein, correct electrolyte abnormalities, treat underlying condition; dialysis or renal transplant may be needed in progressive cases
7. **Complications** = end-stage renal disease (CRF with severe symptoms and electrolyte abnormalities requiring dialysis for survival), renal

TABLE 4-4 **Nephritic Syndromes**

Type	Pathology	H/P	Labs	Treatment
Postinfectious glomerulonephritis	Sequelae of systemic infection (most commonly **streptococcus**)	Recent infection, oliguria, edema, brown urine, hypertension; more common in **children**	Hematuria and proteinuria in urinalysis, high antistreptolysin O titer, **bumpy deposits** of IgG and C3 on renal basement membrane on electron microscopy	Self-limited, supportive treatment (decrease edema and hypertension)
IgA nephropathy (Berger's disease)	Uncertain but may be related to infection; deposition of IgA antibodies in mesangial cells	Hematuria	**Increased serum IgA,** mesangial cell proliferation on electron microscopy	Frequently self-limited, severe cases may require corticosteroids; infrequently progresses to renal failure
Goodpasture's syndrome	Deposition of antiglomerular and anti-alveolar basement membrane antibodies	Dyspnea, hemoptysis, myalgias, hematuria	**Serum IgG antiglomerular basement membrane antibodies,** anemia, pulmonary infiltrates on CXR, **linear pattern of IgG antibody deposition** on fluorescence microscopy of glomeruli	Plasmapheresis, corticosteroids, immunosuppressive agents; may progress to renal failure
Alport's syndrome	Hereditary defect in collagen IV in basement membrane	Hematuria, symptoms of renal failure, **high-frequency hearing loss**	Red cell casts, hematuria, proteinuria, and pyuria on urinalysis; **glomerular basement membrane inconsistency** on electron microscopy	Variable prognosis with no therapy identified to halt cases of renal failure; renal transplant may be complicated by Alport-related development of Goodpasture's syndrome
Idiopathic crescentic glomerulonephritis	**Rapidly progressive renal failure** due to idiopathic causes or associated with other glomerular diseases or systemic infection	Sudden renal failure, weakness, nausea, weight loss, myalgias, fever, oliguria	Positive ANCA; inflammatory cell deposition in Bowman's capsule and crescent formation (basement membrane wrinkling) on electron microscopy	Poor prognosis with rapid progression to renal failure; corticosteroids, plasmapheresis, and immunosuppressive agents may be helpful; renal transplant frequently required
Lupus nephritis (mesangial, membranous, focal proliferative, and diffuse proliferative types)	Complication of systemic lupus erythematosus involving proliferation of endothelial and mesangial cells	Possibly asymptomatic, possible hypertension or renal failure; may develop nephrotic syndrome	**ANA, anti-DNA antibodies;** hematuria, and possible proteinuria on urinalysis	Corticosteroids or immunosuppressive agents can delay renal failure
Wegener's granulomatosis (also see Pulmonary chapter)	Similar to crescentic disease with addition of **pulmonary involvement;** granulomatous inflammation of airways and renal vasculature	Weight loss, respiratory symptoms, hematuria, fever	**c-ANCA;** deposition of immune complexes in renal vessels seen on electron microscopy; pulmonary biopsy helpful in diagnosis	Corticosteroids, cytotoxic agents; variable prognosis

ANA, antinuclear antibody; ANCA, antineutrophil cytoplasmic antibody; c-ANCA, cytoplasmic antineutrophil cytoplasmic antibody; CXR, chest x-ray.

TABLE 4-5 Nephrotic Syndromes

Type	Pathology	H/P	Labs	Treatment
Minimal change disease	Idiopathic; may involve fusion of foot processes on basement membrane	Possible hypertension, increased frequency of infections; more common in **young children**	Hyperlipidemia, hypoalbuminemia; proteinuria on urinalysis; fusion of basement membrane foot processes seen on electron microscopy	Corticosteroids, cytotoxic agents
Focal segmental glomerular sclerosis	Frequently idiopathic or associated with drug use or HIV; segmental sclerosis of glomeruli	Possible hypertension; more common in **adults**	Hyperlipidemia, hypoalbuminemia; high proteinuria on urinalysis; sclerotic changes seen in some glomeruli on electron microscopy	Corticosteroids; progressive cases that require renal transplant (uncommon) frequently have recurrence
Membranous glomerulonephritis	Idiopathic or associated with infection, systemic lupus erythematosus, neoplasm, or drugs; thickening of basement membrane	History of infection or medication use may lead to diagnosis	Hyperlipidemia, hypoalbuminemia; proteinuria on urinalysis; **"spike and dome" basement membrane thickening** on electron microscopy	Corticosteroids, cytotoxic agents; variable rates of renal failure and renal vein thrombosis
Membranoproliferative glomerulonephritis	Idiopathic or associated with infection or autoimmune disease; thickening of basement membrane	History of systemic infection or autoimmune condition; gradual progression to renal failure	Hyperlipidemia, hypoalbuminemia, possible hypocomplementemia; proteinuria and possible hematuria on urinalysis; IgG deposits may be seen on basement membrane on fluorescence microscopy; **basement membrane thickening with double-layer "train track" appearance** on electron microscopy	Corticosteroids may delay progression to renal failure
Diabetic nephropathy (diffuse, nodular)	Basement membrane and mesangial thickening related to diabetic vascular changes	History of DM, hypertension, progressive renal failure	Hyperlipidemia, hypoalbuminemia; proteinuria on urinalysis; basement membrane thickening on electron microscopy seen in both types; round nodules **(Kimmelstiel-Wilson nodules)** seen within glomeruli in nodular type	Treat underlying DM, dietary protein restriction, ACE-I therapy

ACE-I, angiotensin converting enzyme inhibitor; DM, diabetes mellitus.

osteodystrophy (bone degeneration secondary to low serum Ca^{2+}), encephalopathy, severe anemia (due to decreased erythropoietin)

  C. **Dialysis**

    1. Induced filtering of blood required when kidney function is inadequate or serum composition increases risk of mortality

    2. Types

      a. **Hemodialysis**—machine filters blood and returns filtered plasma to vasculature; synthetic grafts or surgical arteriovenous fistulas in the forearm are utilized for access

      b. **Peritoneal dialysis**

        (1) Dialysate fluid temporarily pumped into peritoneum via a permanent catheter

TABLE 4-6 Characteristics of Types of Renal Tubular Acidosis			
	Distal (Type 1)	Proximal (Type 2)	Low Renin/Aldosterone (Type 4)
Defect	H^+ secretion leading to secondary hyperaldosteronism	HCO_3^- reabsorption	Primary or secondary aldosterone deficiency
Cause	Idiopathic, autoimmune diseases, drugs, chronic infection, nephrocalcinosis	Fanconi syndrome, Wilson's disease, amyloidosis, hypocalcemia, hepatitis, autoimmune diseases	**DM,** Addison's disease, sickle cell disease, renal failure
Urine pH	>**5.3**	<5.3	<5.3
Serum electrolytes	Low K^+	Low K^+, HCO_3^-	**High K^+, Cl^-**
Radiology	Possible **stones**	**Bone lesions**	
Treatment	Oral HCO_3^-, K^+	Oral HCO_3^-, K^+; thiazide diuretics	Fludrocortisone, K^+ restriction
DM, diabetes mellitus.			

(2) Substances in the blood diffuse across the peritoneum from the surrounding vasculature to the dialysate fluid according to osmotic drive (peritoneum serves as a filter)

(3) Dialysate fluid containing solutes is pumped out of peritoneal cavity

3. **Indications** = severe hyperkalemia, severe metabolic acidosis, fluid overload, uremic syndrome

4. **Complications** = infection at access sites, fluid overload with dyspnea, hypotension (hemodialysis)

5. Frequently precedes renal transplant

V. Acid-base disorders

A. **Renal tubular acidosis (see Table 4-6)**
   1. Abnormalities in renal tubular H^+ secretion or HCO_3^- reabsorption
   2. Leads to non-anion gap metabolic acidosis

B. **Acid-base physiology**
   1. In a healthy person serum pH is regulated by **HCO_3^-** reabsorption (proximal tubule of kidneys) and blood Pco_2 (respiratory activity)
   2. In a healthy person:
      a. pH = 7.40
      b. Pco_2 = 40 mm Hg
      c. Po_2 = 100 mm Hg
      d. HCO_3^- = 24 mEq/L
   3. Pco_2 and pH may be measured with arterial blood gas; HCO_3^- is calculated by Henderson-Hasselbach equation: $pH = pKa + \log\left(\frac{HCO_3}{0.03 Pco_2}\right)$
   4. pH >7.42 = alkalosis; pH <7.3 = acidosis
   5. Disturbances due to **HCO_3^-** abnormalities are **metabolic;** disturbances due to Pco_2 levels are **respiratory**
   6. For any disturbance the body tries to compensate and normalize serum pH

C. **Acid-base disturbances**
   1. **Anion gap**
      a. Difference between serum Na^+ and Cl^- and HCO_3^- ion concentrations

 An easy way to remember the causes of high-anion-gap metabolic acidosis is the mnemonic **MUD PILES: M**ethanol, **U**remia, **D**iabetic ketoacidosis, **P**araldehyde, **I**soniazid (**I**NH), **L**actic acidosis, **E**thanol, **S**alicylates.

TABLE 4-7	Acid-Base Disturbances and Compensatory Mechanisms					
Disorder	**pH**	**[H⁺]**	**[HCO₃⁻]**	**Pco₂**	**Compensation**	**Common Causes**
Metabolic acidosis	↓	↑	↓↓	↓	Hyperventilation	Diarrhea, diabetic ketoacidosis, lactic acidosis, renal tubular acidosis
Metabolic alkalosis	↑	↓	↑↑	↑	Hypoventilation	Vomiting, diuretics, Cushing's syndrome, hyperaldosteronism, adrenal hyperplasia
Respiratory acidosis	↓	↑	↑	↑↑	Increased HCO₃⁻ reabsorption	COPD, respiratory depression, neuromuscular diseases
Respiratory alkalosis	↑	↓	↓	↓↓	Decreased HCO₃⁻ reabsorption	Hyperventilation, high altitude, asthma, aspirin toxicity, pulmonary embolism

COPD, chronic obstructive pulmonary disease; ↑, high; ↓, low; ;↑↑, very high ↓↓, very low.

b. **Anion gap** $= [Na^+] - [Cl^-] - [HCO_3^-]$ (normal $= 8$–12)
c. Normal anion gap acidosis suggests HCO_3^- loss
d. Increased anion gap acidosis suggests H^+ excess
2. **Mixed disorder**
   a. Combination of multiple acid-base disturbances
   b. Detected when corrected HCO_3^- is different from measured value
   c. Corrected HCO_3^- = measured anion gap – normal anion gap + measured HCO_3^- (for which 12 = value of normal anion gap)
   d. If corrected HCO_3^- is:
      (1) Normal, disturbance is solitary high anion gap acidosis
      (2) Increased, disturbance is metabolic alkalosis with high anion gap acidosis
      (3) Decreased, disturbance is non-anion gap acidosis with high anion gap acidosis

TABLE 4-8	Compensation Formulas in Acid-Base Disturbances
Apparent Disturbance	**Compensation**
Metabolic acidosis	Expected Pco_2-1.5 $[HCO_3^-] + (8 \pm 2)$ If $Pco_2 <$expected, then additional respiratory alkalosis If $Pco_2 >$expected, then additional respiratory acidosis
Metabolic alkalosis	If $Pco_2 >50$, then additional respiratory acidosis If $Pco_2 <40$, then additional respiratory alkalosis
Acute respiratory acidosis	Expected pH decrease-(1/10) $\times 0.08 \times (Pco_2 - 40)$
Chronic respiratory acidosis	Expected pH decrease-(1/10) $\times 0.03 \times (Pco_2 - 40)$
Acute respiratory alkalosis	Expected pH increase-(1/10) $\times 0.08 \times (Pco_2 - 40)$
Chronic respiratory alkalosis	Expected pH increase-(1/10) $\times 0.03 \times (Pco_2 - 40)$

FIGURE
4-3 Differentiation of acid-base disturbances and related causes.

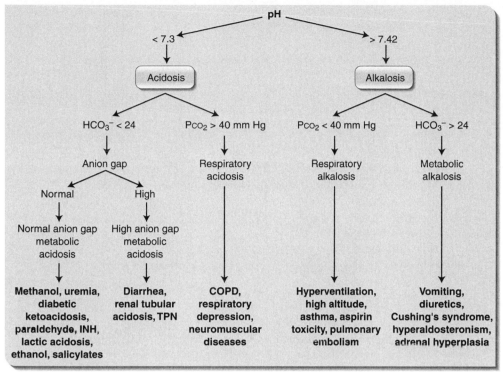

Note: Compensatory mechanisms should be checked to differentiate solitary from mixed disturbances
COPD = Chronic Obstructive Pulmonary Disease   TPN = Total Parenteral Nutrition

VI. Electrolyte disorders

A. **Hypernatremia**
   1. Serum Na^+ >155 mEq/L
   2. Due to **dehydration,** loss of fluid from skin (burns, sweating), loss of fluid from gastrointestinal (GI) tract (vomiting, diarrhea), diabetes insipidus, increased aldosterone
   3. **H/P** = oliguria, thirst, decreased consciousness, mental status changes, seizures
   4. **Treatment** = gradual hydration with hypotonic saline for inadequate fluid intake or excess fluid loss (maximum Na^+ reduction = 12 mEq/day)
   5. **Complications** = seizures, CNS damage; too rapid hydration may cause **cerebral edema**

B. **Diabetes insipidus** (DI)
   1. Disorders of ADH-directed water reabsorption leading to dehydration and hypernatremia
   2. Types
      a. **Central**—failure of posterior pituitary to secrete ADH
      b. **Nephrogenic**—kidneys do not respond to ADH
   3. May be due to drugs, parenchymal renal diseases, or **pituitary tumors**
   4. **H/P** = polydipsia, polyuria, signs of dehydration
   5. **Labs** =
      a. Increased Na^+
      b. Low urine osmolality with large urine volume
      c. Water deprivation test
         (1) Overnight water deprivation followed by ADH administration
         (2) Normal response is no change in urine osmolality

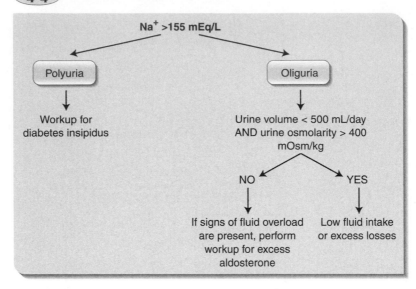

FIGURE 4-4 Evaluation of hypernatremia.

Pseudohypona-tremia is an artifact of hyperlipidemia in which serum Na^+ falsely appears to be low.

STEP NEXT To calculate $[Na^+]$ that will result from correction of hyperglycemia, add 1.6 mEq/L Na^+ for every 100 mg/dL glucose above 100 mg/dL.

STEP NEXT Pseudohyperkalemia occurs from red blood cell hemolysis following blood collection, so K^+ should be measured **immediately** in drawn blood and increased serum K^+ should be confirmed with a **repeat blood sample** using a large gauge needle.

(3) Shows normal result in nephrogenic type

(4) Increased urine osmolality after ADH administration in central type

6. **Radiology** = CT with contrast or MRI may show pituitary tumor

7. **Treatment** =
   a. Treat underlying condition
   b. Central DI—desmopressin (or DDAVP) given as ADH analogues
   c. Nephrogenic DI—salt restriction, increased H_2O intake; treat underlying condition (stop meds, treat tumor or renal disease)

C. **Hyponatremia**
   1. Serum Na^+ <**135** mEq/L
   2. Due to renal **H_2O retention** (congestive heart failure, syndrome of inappropriate ADH secretion [SIADH]), thiazide diuretics (salt wasting), **hyperglycemia** (osmotic hyponatremia), or high fluid intake
   3. **H/P** = confusion, nausea, weakness, decreased consciousness
   4. **Treatment** = treat underlying condition (stop offending agent, correct hyperglycemia or hyperlipidemia, etc.); salt and H_2O restriction unless hypovolemic and serum osmolality <280 mOsm/kg (rehydrate with saline no faster than 12 mEq/day), loop diuretics or hypertonic saline for severe cases (Na^+ <120 mEq/L)
   5. **Complications** = CNS damage; overly rapid correction with hypertonic saline may cause **central pontine myelinolysis**

D. **Syndrome of inappropriate ADH secretion (SIADH)**
   1. **Nonphysiologic release of ADH,** resulting in hyponatremia
   2. Caused by CNS pathology, sarcoidosis, **paraneoplastic syndromes,** psychiatric drugs, major surgery, pneumonia, or HIV
   3. **H/P** = chronic symptoms of hyponatremia
   4. **Labs** = serum hypo-osmolality (<280 mOsm/kg) with urine osmolality >100 mOsm/kg; urine Na^+ >20 mEq/L
   5. **Treatment** = fluid restriction; loop diuretics and hypertonic saline if symptomatic; demeclocycline may help maintain normal Na^+ levels

E. **Hyperkalemia**
   1. Serum K^+ >**5.0** mEq/L
   2. Due to metabolic acidosis, aldosterone deficiency, tissue breakdown, insulin deficiency, adrenal deficiency, K^+-sparing diuretics

FIGURE
4-5 Evaluation of hyponatremia.

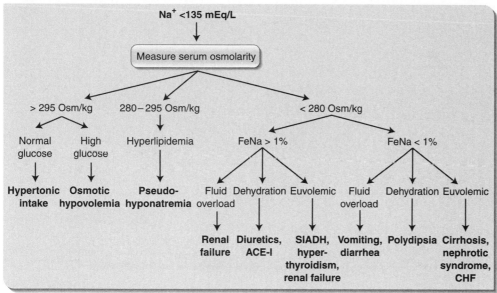

ACE-I = Angiotensin converting enzyme inhibitor   SIADH = Syndrome of inappropriate ADH secretion
CHF = Congestive heart failure   FeNa = Fractional excretion of Na = (Urine [Na$^+$] × serum Cr)/(serum [Na$^+$] × Urine Cr) × 100.

3. **H/P** = weakness, nausea, vomiting; arrhythmias; paralysis or paresthesia in severe cases
4. Electrocardiogram (ECG) = **tall peaked T waves**
5. **Treatment** = calcium gluconate, $NaHCO_3$, or glucose with insulin to encourage K^+ uptake by cells; sodium polystyrene sulfonate binds K^+ and removes it through the GI tract; **dialysis** may be required in severe cases

F. **Hypokalemia**
1. Serum K^+ <**3.5 mEq/L**
2. Due to poor dietary intake, metabolic alkalosis, vomiting, diarrhea, hyperaldosteronism, diabetic ketoacidosis, Cushing's disease, K^+-wasting diuretics, or tubular disease
3. **H/P** = fatigue, weakness, possible paralysis; arrhythmias, hyporeflexia; paralysis, or paresthesia in severe cases
4. ECG = **T wave flattening**, ST depression, **U waves**
5. **Treatment** = treat underlying disorder; give oral or IV KCl (10–20 mEq/hr)
6. **Complications** = overly rapid replacement may lead to **arrhythmias**

G. **Hypercalcemia**
1. Serum Ca^{2+} >**10.5 mg/dL**
2. Due to **hyperparathyroidism, neoplasm,** immobilization, thiazide diuretics, high ingestion of calcium carbonate and milk (milk-alkali syndrome; more often seen in children), sarcoidosis, or hypervitaminosis A or D
3. **H/P** = deep pain, easy fractures, possible nephrolithiasis, nausea, vomiting, constipation, weakness, mental status changes, polyuria
4. **Labs** = increased parathyroid hormone in hyperparathyroidism; very high Ca^{2+} and normal or low parathyroid hormone frequently seen with neoplasm; increased vitamins A or D seen in hypervitaminoses

 Causes of hypercalcemia may be remembered by the mnemonic CHIMPANZEES: **C**alcium supplementation; **H**yperparathyroidism; **I**mmobility; **M**ilk-alkali syndrome; **P**aget's disease; **A**ddison's disease; **N**eoplasms; **Z**ollinger-Ellison syndrome; **E**xcess vitamin A; **E**xcess vitamin D; **S**arcoidosis.

 Hypercalcemia is characterized by **"bones"** (fractures), **"stones"** (nephrolithiasis), **"groans"** (GI symptoms), and **"psychiatric overtones"** (changes in mental status).

 STEP Differentiate between **familial hypocalciuric hypercalcemia** (genetic disorder of Ca^{2+}-sensing receptors) and other causes of hypercalcemia by noting a family history of hypercalcemia, low urine Ca^{2+}, and absence of osteopenia, nephrolithiasis, and mental status changes in the former.

FIGURE
4-6 Evaluation of hypokalemia.

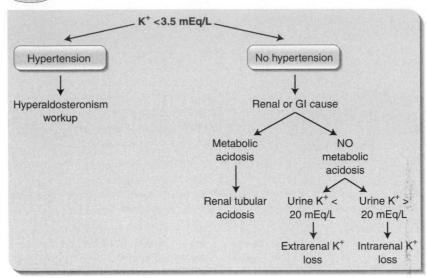

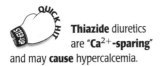

Thiazide diuretics are "Ca^{2+}-**sparing**" and may **cause** hypercalcemia.

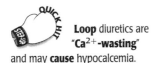

Loop diuretics are "Ca^{2+}-**wasting**" and may **cause** hypocalcemia.

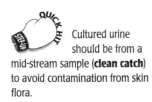

Cultured urine should be from a mid-stream sample (**clean catch**) to avoid contamination from skin flora.

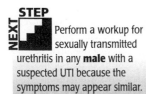

STEP
NEXT
Perform a workup for sexually transmitted urethritis in any **male** with a suspected UTI because the symptoms may appear similar.

5. **Treatment** = hydration, **loop diuretics**; treat underlying disorder; surgery indicated for hyperparathyroidism and resectable neoplasms; glucocorticoids, calcitonin, or bisphosphonates may be required to normalize Ca^{2+} in refractory cases

H. **Hypocalcemia**
   1. Serum Ca^{2+} <**8.5** mg/dL
   2. Caused by hypoparathyroidism, vitamin D deficiency, **loop diuretics,** pancreatitis, or alcoholism
   3. **H/P** = abdominal pain, dyspnea; tetany, **Chvostek's sign** (tapping facial nerve causes spasm), carpal spasm when blood pressure cuff inflated (**Trousseau's sign**)
   4. **Labs** = Ca^{2+} should be adjusted for hypoalbuminemia (lower limit of normal Ca^{2+} decreases 0.8 mg/dL for each 1.0 g/dL albumin below 4.0); decreased corrected Ca^{2+}; increased phosphate seen with hypoparathyroidism and renal failure
   5. **Treatment** = treat underlying disorder; oral Ca^{2+} or IV Ca^{2+} for severe symptoms; vitamin D supplementation if necessary

VII. Bladder and ureteral disorders
   A. **Urinary tract infection** (UTI)
      1. Ascending infection of urethra, bladder, and ureters resulting from inoculation of lower urinary tract (rarely hematogenous spread)
      2. Most commonly due to *E. coli, Proteus, Klebsiella, Enterobacter, Pseudomonas,* and enterococcus
      3. **Risk factors** = **obstruction,** Foley catheter, vesicoureteral reflux, pregnancy, DM, sexual intercourse, immunocompromise; female >male
      4. **H/P** = **urinary frequency, dysuria** (painful urination), suprapubic pain, **urgency**
      5. **Labs** = urinalysis shows increased nitrates, increased leukocyte esterase and white blood cells in urine; urine culture will show >10^5 colonies/mL; blood tests usually not helpful unless due to hematogenous spread
      6. **Treatment** = amoxicillin, trimethoprim-sulfamethoxazole (TMP-SMX), or fluroquinolones for three days; relapsing infection should be treated for 14 days

7. **Complications** = abscess formation, pyelonephritis, renal failure, prostatitis

B. **Bladder cancer**
   1. **Transitional cell carcinoma** (common), squamous cell cancer (uncommon), or adenocarcinoma of the bladder (uncommon)
   2. **Risk factors** = **tobacco,** schistosomiasis, aniline dye, recurrent UTI; male 3 × >female
   3. **H/P** = **painless gross hematuria;** frequency, dysuria, and urgency occur later in disease; palpable suprapubic mass
   4. **Labs** = urinalysis shows hematuria; urine cytology shows malignant cells; biopsy confirms diagnosis
   5. **Radiology** = IVP may show mass; cystoscopy may visualize lesion
   6. **Treatment** = surgical resection, intravesical chemotherapy; radiation used for large tumors
   7. **Complications** = frequent recurrence

VIII. Male reproduction

A. **Urethritis**
   1. Infection of urethra due to sexually transmitted *Neisseria gonorrhoeae* or *Chlamydia trachomatis*
   2. **H/P** = dysuria, frequency, urgency, **burning urination; purulent urethral discharge** seen with *N. gonorrhoeae*
   3. **Labs** = Gram stain shows gram-negative diplococci for *N. gonorrhoeae*; Thayer-Martin culture will detect *N. gonorrhoeae;* negative Gram stain suggests *C. trachomatis*
   4. **Treatment** = single dose ceftriaxone with doxycycline or azithromycin used to treat both possible infections simultaneously; **treat sexual partners**
   5. **Complications** = urethral strictures, frequent reinfection when sexual partners not treated

B. **Prostatitis**
   1. Inflammation of prostate from unknown cause or as complication of UTI
   2. **H/P** = perineal pain, dysuria, frequency, urgency; fever, tender prostate on digital rectal exam
   3. **Labs** = may be suggestive of UTI; possible hematuria; white blood cells seen in prostatic secretions
   4. **Treatment** = TMP-SMX; treat for sexually transmitted diseases (STDs) in sexually active males

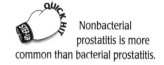

Nonbacterial prostatitis is more common than bacterial prostatitis.

C. **Benign prostatic hyperplasia** (BPH)
   1. **Benign enlargement of prostate** seen with increasing frequency as men age beyond 40 years old
   2. **H/P** = urinary **hesitancy,** straining, **weak or intermittent stream,** dribbling; frequency, urgency, **nocturia,** and urge incontinence develop secondary to incomplete emptying or UTI; digital exam detects uniformly enlarged, rubbery prostate
   3. **Labs** = possible mild increase in prostate-specific antigen (PSA); rule out infection (urinalysis), cancer (biopsy), and renal failure (serum electrolytes, BUN, Cr)
   4. **Radiology** = transrectal US shows enlarged prostate
   5. **Treatment** = α_1-**receptor blockers** improve symptoms; surgery needed for refractory cases (transurethral resection of prostate [TURP])

BPH develops in the **central zone** of the prostate adjacent to the urethra, and does not predispose patients to prostate cancer.

D. **Prostate cancer**
   1. Adenocarcinoma occurring in **peripheral zone** of prostate
   2. **Risk factors** = increased age, family history
   3. **H/P** = frequently asymptomatic; weakened urinary stream, urinary retention, weight loss, back pain in later disease; **nodular or irregular prostate on digital exam,** lymphedema

Prostate cancer is the **most common cancer** in men; however, **lung** cancer is the greatest cause of **cancer-related death** in males, while **prostate** cancer is the **second** highest.

All men >40 years old should receive an annual digital rectal exam to screen for prostate cancer.

4. **Labs** = urinalysis may show hematuria and pyuria; **increased PSA,** increased alkaline phosphatase; biopsy provides diagnosis
5. **Radiology** = transrectal US shows irregular prostate; bone scan, chest x-ray (CXR), and CT may detect metastases
6. **Treatment** =
   a. Good prognosis with early treatment
   b. Radical retropubic prostatectomy and radiation; perineal prostatectomy is a less invasive surgery that may be utilized with low grade tumors
   c. Follow up with PSA post-treatment to monitor for metastases and recurrence
   d. Anti-androgen therapy (hormone therapy or orchiectomy) with chemotherapy may be used to improve symptoms in metastatic disease
   e. Older men may not be treated because tumors are frequently slow-growing
7. **Complications** = **incontinence** and **impotence** are common with radical prostatectomy

E. **Epididymitis**
   1. Inflammation of epididymis associated with testicular inflammation
   2. Due to prostatitis, **STDs,** urinary reflux
   3. **H/P** = epididymal **pain relieved by supporting scrotum;** entire scrotum may be inflamed in severe cases
   4. **Labs** = urinalysis shows white blood cells; urine culture with specialized culture mediums may help diagnose STDs
   5. **Treatment** = treat underlying infection

Supporting the scrotum does **not** relieve pain in testicular torsion but does relieve pain in epididymitis.

F. **Testicular torsion**
   1. **Twisting of spermatic cord** leading to **vascular insufficiency** of testes
   2. **H/P** = very painful and swollen testes, nausea, vomiting; fever, **testes displaced superiorly,** mass in spermatic cord may be felt
   3. **Radiology** = US may show torsion
   4. **Treatment** = **emergent surgical reduction** of torsion within several hours of onset; testes attached to scrotal wall (orchiopexy) to prevent recurrence
   5. **Complications** = testicular ischemia or infarction without prompt treatment

STEP NEXT If testicular torsion is suspected and US is suggestive of the diagnosis, proceed to surgery without waiting for other tests.

G. **Testicular cancer**
   1. Seminomatous (common) or nonseminomatous (uncommon) tumors of testicles
   2. **Risk factors** = prior history of testicular cancer, undescended testes
   3. **H/P** = **painless testicular mass;** GI or pulmonary symptoms may result from metastases
   4. **Radiology** = US may detect dense testicular mass; CXR or CT can detect extent of tumor and metastases
   5. **Labs** = biopsy provides diagnosis; increased β-hCG and increased α-fetoprotein in nonseminomatous tumors
   6. **Treatment** = seminomas treated with radiation and chemotherapy; nonseminomas treated with orchiectomy, lymph node dissection, and chemotherapy; surgical debulking may be used for extensive disease
   7. **Complications** = **prognosis is very good,** but nonseminomas have lower cure rates and increased risk of recurrence

Testicular cancer is the most common cancer in men between 15–35 years old.

H. **Infertility** (male)
   1. Inability of couple to achieve pregnancy following **one year of normal sexual activity without use of contraception**
   2. **H/P** = history of testicular trauma, surgery, chemotherapy, or infection may be contributory; varicocele (collection of veins in scrotum), undescended testes, or penile defects may be seen on exam

Frequent infections in the presence of infertility may necessitate a workup for **cystic fibrosis.**

3. **Labs** = hormone analysis, complete blood count (CBC), and urinalysis may be useful for diagnosis; semen analysis for sperm motility, volume, and concentration may be useful

4. **Treatment** = treat underlying condition; surgical correction of anatomical defects, hormone therapy, education in sexual technique, or *in vitro* fertilization may help in achieving pregnancy

I. **Impotence**

1. Inability to obtain or maintain erection during sexual activity

2. Due to deinnervation, **vascular insufficiency,** endocrine abnormalities, psychological concerns, drugs, or alcoholism

3. **H/P** = history of trauma, surgery, or infection may be contributory; exam should consider vascular (decreased pulses and perfusion), hormonal (testicular atrophy or gynecomastia), and neurologic (decrease anal wink reflex and paresthesias) etiologies

4. **Labs** = possible decreased testosterone, decreased luteinizing hormone (LH), or increased prolactin

5. **Treatment** = treat underlying condition; stop offending agents; psychological counseling and sexual education; papaverine injection or oral phosphodiesterase-5 inhibitors may help maintain penile vascular engorgement

IX. **Pediatric genitourinary concerns**

A. **Wilm's tumor**

1. Malignant tumor of renal origin presenting in **children <4 years old**

2. **Risk factors** = family history, neurofibromatosis, other genitourinary abnormalities

3. **H/P** = weight loss, nausea, vomiting, dysuria, polyuria; palpable abdominal or flank mass, hypertension, fever

4. **Labs** = measure BUN, Cr, and CBC to assess kidney function

5. **Radiology** = CT or US shows renal mass; CXR and CT can show metastases

6. **Treatment** = surgical resection or nephrectomy, chemotherapy, and possible radiation; good prognosis without extensive involvement

B. **Urethral displacement**

1. Urethral opening on top (epispadias) or underside (hypospadias) of penis associated with other penile anatomical abnormalities

2. **H/P** = defect apparent on exam and during urination

3. **Treatment** = surgical correction (ideally during infancy), do not circumcise prior to surgical correction

4. **Complications** = may contribute to infertility

C. **Enuresis**

1. Nocturnal bedwetting seen in young children

2. Seen in all children; **most cases resolve by age four;** rare cases associated with disease

3. **H/P** = **almost always nonpathologic;** unusual findings in history and exam should prompt further workup

4. **Treatment** = education, enuresis alarms, dietary modifications (no fluids near bedtime); desmopressin or imipramine used in refractory cases

D. **Undescended testes (cryptorchidism)**

1. Testes lying in abdominal cavity and not consistently located within scrotum

2. **H/P** = empty scrotal sac, testes inconsistently found in scrotum

3. **Treatment** = if occasionally located in scrotum, may self-resolve; persistent abdominal testes must be corrected surgically before age five to reduce risk of cancer and allow testicular development

4. **Complications** = testicular cancer (risk reduced but not eliminated by surgical correction), infertility

Endocrine Disorders

I. Disorders of glucose metabolism

A. **Normal glucose metabolism**
   1. Regulated by pancreatic enzymes insulin and glucagon
   2. **Insulin**
      a. Secreted by pancreatic β-islet cells in response to glucose intake and feeding (strongest stimuli, but also influenced by other protein and neural input)
      b. Secretion decreases with fasting and exercise (i.e., feedback relationship with nutrient supply)
      c. Induces glucose and amino acid uptake by cells
      d. Drives conversion of glucose to glycogen, fatty acids, and pyruvate
      e. Induces storage of glucose metabolites in tissue (glycogen in liver, fatty acids in adipose cells, protein anabolism)
   3. **Glucagon**
      a. Secreted by α-islet cells primarily in response to decreased glucose and protein intake
      b. Promotes mobilization of glycogen and fatty acids
   4. Insulin:glucagon ratio determines state of glucose metabolism

B. **Diabetes mellitus (DM) type I** (juvenile onset diabetes, insulin-dependent diabetes)
   1. **Loss of ability to produce insulin** most likely due to autoimmune destruction of β-islet cells
   2. Association with human leukocyte antigens HLA-DR3, HLA-DR4, and HLA-DQ genotypes
   3. Usually diagnosed **before 13 years of age**
   4. H/P = polyuria, polydipsia, polyphagia, weight loss; **rapid onset**
   5. **Labs** = hyperglycemia, glycosuria (glucose in urine), serum and urine ketones, increased hemoglobin A_{1c} (indicates hyperglycemia over prior three months)
   6. **Treatment** = scheduled insulin injections, monitoring of serum glucose at home to guide insulin and dietary adjustments, close follow-up to monitor development of complications
   7. **Complications** = **diabetic ketoacidosis (DKA)**, hypoglycemia (secondary to excess insulin administration), retinopathy, neuropathy, nephropathy, atherosclerosis

C. **Diabetes mellitus type II** (adult onset diabetes, non-insulin-dependent diabetes)
   1. Development of **tissue resistance to insulin,** leading to hyperglycemia and gradual decrease in β-islet cells ability to produce insulin
   2. **Risk factors** = family history, obesity

Rubella, Coxsackie virus, and mumps have been associated with onset of β-islet cell destruction leading to DM type I.

Hemoglobin A_{1c} is a good measure for how well therapy is able to control serum glucose over a three-month time period.

ENDOCRINE DISORDERS

TABLE 5-1	Plasma Glucose Diagnostic Criteria for Diabetes Mellitus	
Plasma Glucose Test	**Level (mg/dL)**	**And . . .**
Random plasma glucose	>200	With symptoms of DM
	OR	
Fasting plasma glucose	>126	On 2 separate occasions
	OR	
Plasma glucose	>200	2 hr after 75 g oral glucose load[a]

[a]This is a positive oral glucose tolerance test.
DM, diabetes mellitus.

3. Usually diagnosed **after 40 years old**
4. **H/P** = polyuria, polydipsia, polyphagia; **gradual onset** of symptoms; symptoms related to complications may present prior to actual diagnosis
5. **Labs** = similar to those for DM type I; serum insulin may be increased, normal, or decreased
6. **Treatment** = low-sugar diet, home monitoring of glucose, weight loss, exercise (increases tissue response to insulin), glucose-lowering medications; insulin may be required in cases of insufficient insulin production
7. **Complications** = **hyperosmolar hyperglycemic nonketotic coma** (HHNK), retinopathy, nephropathy, neuropathy, atherosclerosis

D. **Complications of diabetes**
   1. **Diabetic ketoacidosis (DKA)**
      a. Extremely low insulin causes degradation of triglycerides into fatty acids and eventual conversion into **ketoacids**
      b. Occurs in patients with DM type I who do not take prescribed insulin or those who have infections, high stress, myocardial infarction (MI), or high alcohol use
      c. **H/P** = weakness, polyuria, polydipsia, hyperventilation, abdominal pain, vomiting; fruity odor on breath, Kussmaul respirations (slow, deep breathing); mental status changes develop with worsening dehydration
      d. **Labs** = **glucose 300–800 mg/dL**, decreased K+, decreased phosphate, high anion gap metabolic acidosis, **serum and urine ketones**
      e. **Treatment** = IV fluids, insulin, KCl; treat underlying disorder (success of treatment may be confirmed by decreasing ketone levels)

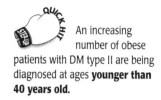 An increasing number of obese patients with DM type II are being diagnosed at ages **younger than 40 years old.**

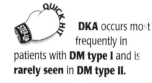 **DKA** occurs most frequently in patients with **DM type I** and is **rarely seen** in **DM type II.**

TABLE 5-2	Formulations of Injected Insulin		
Type of Insulin	**Time of Onset of Action**	**Peak Effect**	**Duration of Action**
Lispro	10 min	1 hr	3–4 hr
Regular	45 min	2–5 hr	8 hr
NPH	2–4 hr	4–10 hr	24 hr
Lente	3–4 hr	6–15 hr	24 hr
Ultralente	6–8 hr	10–30 hr	36 hr

FIGURE 5-1 Examples of insulin regimens in diabetes mellitus: **A.** injection of regular and NPH insulin (in 2:1 ratio) together at breakfast (2/3 total amount) and dinner (1/3 total amount); **B.** adjustment in regimen **A** for patients with nocturnal hypoglycemia (Somogyi effect) and morning hyperglycemia (dawn phenomenon) in which second NPH dose is delayed until bedtime; **C.** tight control regimen used for patients with recurrent hyperglycemia soon after meals.

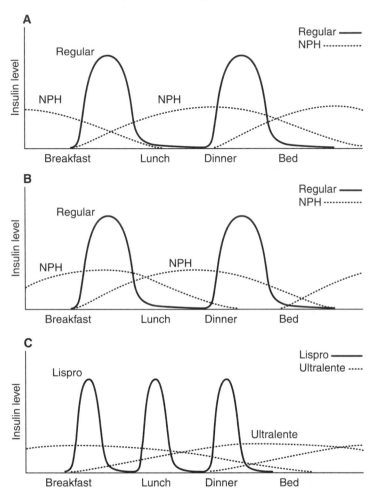

(Modified from Feibusch KC, Breaden RS, Bader CD, Gomperts SN. *Prescription for the Boards: USMLE Step 2.* 3rd Ed. Philadelphia: Lippincott Williams & Wilkins; 2002.)

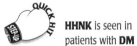

HHNK is seen in patients with **DM type II** and is **not seen** in patients with **DM type I** because sufficient insulin production is required to prevent DKA from occurring first.

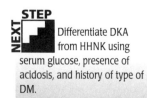

STEP

NEXT Differentiate DKA from HHNK using serum glucose, presence of acidosis, and history of type of DM.

2. **Hyperosmolar hyperglycemic nonketotic coma (HHNK)**
   a. Extremely high glucose with profound dehydration
   b. Occurs in DM type II patients with lengthy infections, stress, or illness; insulin production is sufficient to prevent DKA
   c. **H/P** = polyuria, polydipsia, dehydration, mental status changes; seizures and stroke may occur in severe cases
   d. **Labs** = **glucose** >**600 mg/dL**, **no** acidosis
   e. **Treatment** = IV fluids, insulin, correction of electrolyte abnormalities; treat underlying disorder
3. **Diabetic retinopathy**
   a. Vascular occlusion and ischemia with or without neovascularization in retina leading to visual changes
   b. Associated with microaneurysms, hemorrhages, infarcts, and macular edema
   c. **Background retinopathy** (**no neovascularization**) makes up majority of cases; **proliferative retinopathy** (**with neovascularization**) has increased risk of hemorrhages

TABLE 5-3 Comparisons of Diabetes Mellitus Types I and II

	DM Type I	DM Type II
Cause	Likely autoimmune destruction of β-islet cells	Development of insulin resistance in tissues
Inheritance/genetics	HLA-linked	Strong family history
Age of onset	Usually <13 yr old	Usually >40 yr old
Onset of symptoms	Rapid	Gradual
Pancreatic effects	B-Islet cell depletion	Gradual decrease in β-islet cells
Serum insulin	Low	Increased or normal; low in later disease
Body type	Thin	Obese
Acute complications	DKA	HHNK
Treatment	Insulin	Oral hypoglycemic agents, possibly insulin

DM, diabetes mellitus; HLA, human leukocyte antigen.

> d. **H/P = progressive vision loss**, premature cataracts; retinal changes seen on fundoscopic exam (arteriovenous nicking, hemorrhages, edema, infarcts)
> e. **Treatment = control diabetes**, annual follow-up with ophthalmology, laser photocoagulation for neovascularization
> f. **Complications** = vision loss, early cataracts and glaucoma, retinal detachment

TABLE 5-4 Oral Hypoglycemic Drugs Used in Treatment of Diabetes Mellitus Type II

Drug	Mechanism	Role	Adverse Effects
Sulfonylureas (e.g., tolbutamide, glyburide, glipizide)	**Stimulate insulin release** from β-islet cells, reduce serum glucagon, **increase binding of insulin to tissue receptors**	Frequently first drug used or after metformin	**Hypoglycemia;** contraindicated in patients with hepatic or renal insufficiency (greater risk of hypoglycemia)
Biguanides (metformin)	**Decrease hepatic gluconeogenesis,** reduce hyperlipidemia	Frequently first-line drug	GI disturbance, rare lactic acidosis, possible decreased vitamin B_{12} absorption; contraindicated in patients with hepatic and renal insufficiency
Thiazolidinediones ("glitazones")	Decreases hepatic gluconeogenesis, increases tissue uptake of glucose	Adjunct to other drugs	Weight gain, increase serum LDL, rare liver toxicity in some drugs
α-Glucosidase inhibitors (acarbose)	**Decreases GI absorption** of starch and disaccharides	Monotherapy in patients with good dietary control of DM; adjunct to other drugs; may be used in patients with DM type I	Diarrhea, flatulence, GI disturbance

DM, diabetes mellitus; GI, gastrointestinal; LDL, low-density lipoprotein.

ENDOCRINE DISORDERS

4. **Diabetic nephropathy**
   a. Intercapillary glomerulosclerosis that develops after long-term DM
   b. Slightly greater risk in DM type I than in DM type II
   c. Initially presents with proteinuria; renal insufficiency later develops with nephrotic syndrome
   d. **H/P** = develops after several years with DM (20+); lab abnormalities (proteinuria, increased blood urea nitrogen [BUN] and creatinine [Cr]) may appear well before symptoms; symptoms and signs of renal insufficiency (hypertension [HTN], uremia) develop as renal function deteriorates
   e. **Labs** = microalbuminemia, increased Cr, increased BUN; urinalysis shows proteinuria
   f. **Treatment** = **control diabetes**; angiotensin-converting enzyme **inhibitors (ACE-I)**, low-protein diet, infection prevention; dialysis may eventually be required
   g. **Complications** = end-stage renal disease

5. **Diabetic neuropathy**
   a. Neural damage and conduction defects leading to sensory, motor, and autonomic nerve dysfunction
   b. **Sensory** neuropathy begins in feet and progresses in stocking-glove pattern; symptoms include paresthesias, neural pain, and **decreased vibratory and pain sensation**
   c. **Motor** neuropathy involves infarction of single nerve and most frequently occurs in **cranial nerves**
   d. **Autonomic** neuropathy may cause postural hypotension, impotence, incontinence, and diabetic gastroparesis (delayed gastric emptying)
   e. **Treatment** = **control diabetes**; neural pain may be treated with tri-cyclic antidepressants, phenytoin, carbamazepine, or gabapentin; patients should be taught how to perform regular foot exams
   f. **Complications** = **Charcot joints**, **diabetic foot ulcers**; amputation may be needed to treat progressive infections and deformity

6. **Atherosclerosis**
   a. Incidence greatly increased in diabetic patients secondary to microvascular disease
   b. Increased risk of coronary artery disease and peripheral vascular disease (PVD), leading to increased risk of MI, distal ischemia, and ulcer formation secondary to poor healing and infection
   c. **Treatment** = control HTN and hyperlipidemia
   d. **Complications** = MI (frequently silent), PVD, poor healing of trauma and infections

E. **Hypoglycemia (see Table 5-5)**
   1. Inadequate blood glucose that can result in an inadequate supply of glucose to tissues and brain damage
   2. **H/P** = faintness, weakness, diaphoresis, and palpitations due to responsive excess secretion of epinephrine (attempt to mobilize glycogen); headache, confusion, mental status changes, decreased consciousness due to inadequate supply of glucose to brain

II. **Thyroid disorders**

A. **Thyroid function**
   1. Thyroid hormones induce CNS maturation during growth, increase basal metabolic rate, increase cardiac output, and promote bone growth
   2. Thyrotropin-releasing hormone (TRH) secretion from hypothalamus stimulated by cold and inhibited by stress
   3. TRH induces secretion of thyroid-stimulating hormone (TSH) in anterior pituitary

Patients with sensory neuropathy are at **increased risk** for developing **foot infections** and need to be taught to regularly check their feet to avoid ulcer formation.

Repetitive foot trauma in cases of impaired pain sensation can lead to severe foot deformity and joint destruction (**Charcot joints**).

Diabetic patients are at an increased risk of **silent MI** because of impaired pain sensation.

Cardiac complications are the **greatest cause of death** in diabetic patients.

TABLE 5-5	Causes of Hypoglycemia		
Cause	**Pathology**	**Diagnosis**	**Treatment**
Reactive	Decrease in serum glucose **after eating** (postsurgical or idiopathic)	Hypoglycemia and symptoms improve with carbohydrate meal	**Frequent small meals**
Iatrogenic (excess insulin)	**Excess insulin** administration or adverse effect of **sulfonylurea** use	**Increased insulin in presence of hypoglycemia,** adjustment of drug regimen improves symptoms	Adjust insulin regimen, consider different oral hypoglycemic drug than sulfonylureas
Insulinoma	β-**Islet cell tumor** producing excess insulin	Increased insulin in presence of hypoglycemia, may be detected on CT or MRI	Surgical resection if able to locate
Fasting	**Underproduction of glucose** due to hormone deficiencies, malnutrition, or liver disease	Lab abnormalities and history associated with particular etiology	Proper nutrition, enzyme replacement
Alcohol-induced	Glycogen depletion and **gluconeogenesis inhibition** by high concentrations of alcohol	History of alcohol use, serum ethanol >45 mg/dL	Proper nutrition, stopping alcohol use in high quantities

CT, computed tomography; MRI, magnetic resonance imaging.

4. TSH secretion also controlled by feedback inhibition from thyroxine (T_4) thyroid hormone
5. Metabolic effects are determined by free T_4 and triiodothyronine (T_3); remaining thyroid hormones bound to thyroid-binding globulin (TBG)

B. **Hyperthyroidism**
1. Excess production of thyroid hormones
2. Multiple causes, but **Graves' disease** is most common

 T_4 is converted to T_3 in serum; T_3 is more potent than T_4 but has a shorter half-life.

 If TBG levels increase (e.g., pregnancy, oral contraceptive use), total T_4 increases but free T_4 remains normal.

 Nephrotic syndrome and androgen use decrease TBG levels, leading to decreased total T_4 but normal free T_4.

FIGURE 5-2 Hypothalamopituitary regulation of thyroid hormone production. I⁻, Iodine; T_3, triiodothyronine; T_4, thyroxine; TRH, thyroid-releasing hormone; TSH, thyroid-stimulating hormone.

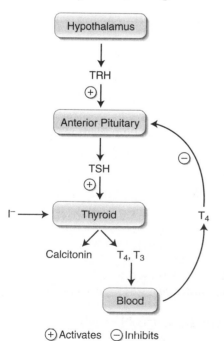

⊕ Activates ⊖ Inhibits

TABLE 5-6   Causes of Hyperthyroidism

Etiology	Pathology	Aids in Diagnosis	Treatment
Graves' disease	Autoimmune **TSI antibodies** bind to TSH receptors in thyroid and stimulate thyroid hormone production	**Exophthalmos, pretibial myxedema,** painless goiter; TSI found in serum; **high uptake on thyroid scan**	Propranolol and PTU for symptomatic relief; **radioablation** with radioactive iodine or **subtotal thyroidectomy** for definitive cure
Nodular toxic goiter (Plummer's disease)	**Multiple hyperactive nodules** produce excess thyroid hormones	Thyroid scan shows **multiple spots of increased uptake**	Radioactive iodine or surgical resection
Subacute thyroiditis (de Quervain's thyroiditis)	Enlarged thyroid due to possible viral stimulus	**Painful goiter,** mild symptoms of hyperthyroidism, neck pain, **fever;** increased ESR; **decreased uptake on thyroid scan**	Self-limited; NSAIDs and β-blockers to treat symptoms; thyroid replacement may be needed if hypothyroidism occurs during gland recovery
Silent lymphocytic thyroiditis	Temporary thyroiditis that **may follow pregnancy**	Painless goiter; **low uptake on thyroid scan; biopsy shows inflammation**	Self-limited; β-blockers to treat symptoms
Factitious hyperthyroidism	Excess thyroid hormone ingestion	**No goiter** in cases of hyperthyroidism; **normal** thyroid scan	Stop excess ingestion

ESR, erythrocyte sedimentation rate; NSAIDs, nonsteroidal anti-inflammatory drugs; PTU, propylthiouracil; TSH, thyroid stimulating hormone; TSI, thyroid-stimulating immunoglobulin.

 NEXT STEP To determine if an enlarged thyroid or thyroid mass is due to excess thyroid activity or a malignant cause, perform a thyroid scan (measures uptake of radioactive iodine to indicate normal, excessive, or absent thyroid function).

 QUICK HIT Hypothyroidism may result from autoimmune processes, **thyroid surgery,** thyroid radioablation, pituitary dysfunction, chronic lithium use, and chronic iodide use.

 QUICK HIT Symptoms of hyperthyroidism may be seen in early Hashimoto's thyroiditis.

 NEXT STEP If decreased TSH and hypothyroidism are seen, suspect a pituitary or hypothalamic etiology.

3. **H/P** = weight loss, increased appetite, **heat intolerance, anxiety,** diaphoresis, palpitations, increased bowel frequency; tachycardia, increased pulse pressure, warm skin, hyperreflexia, possible atrial fibrillation
4. **Labs** = **decreased TSH,** increased total T_4, increased free T_4, increased total T_3, increased T_3 resin uptake
5. **Complications** = thyroid storm

C. **Thyroid storm**
   1. Severe hyperthyroidism induced by infection, surgery, or stress in patients with preexisting hyperthyroidism
   2. **H/P** = existing symptoms of hyperthyroidism, severe diaphoresis, vomiting; tachycardia, fever, **mental status changes**
   3. **Labs** = increased T_4 and T_3, decreased TSH
   4. **Treatment** = β-blockers, propylthiouracil (PTU), methimazole, IV sodium iodine (helps block thyroid hormone release), corticosteroids (inhibit conversion of T_4 to T_3); surgery or radioablation when patient is stable
   5. **Complications** = 25–50% mortality

D. **Hashimoto's thyroiditis**
   1. Most common cause of **hypothyroidism**
   2. Autoimmune condition characterized by chronic thyroiditis; most commonly in middle-aged women
   3. **H/P** = weakness, fatigue, **cold intolerance, weight gain,** constipation, irregular menstruation, **depression,** hoarseness; hyporeflexia, bradycardia, dry skin, edema, **painless goiter**
   4. **Labs** = **increased TSH,** decreased total T_4, decreased free T_4, **antimicrosomal and antithyroglobulin antibodies;** lymphocytic infiltrates and fibrosis seen on biopsy
   5. **Radiology** = **decreased uptake** on thyroid scan ("cold scan")
   6. **Treatment** = life-long levothyroxine

E. **Thyroid carcinoma**
 1. Workup of thyroid nodules
  a. Thyroid nodules are usually benign and increase in frequency with age
  b. Nodules should be evaluated with TSH levels, thyroid function tests, ultrasound (US), and fine needle aspiration (FNA) with biopsy
  c. "Cold" nodules exhibit decreased radioactive iodide (I^-) uptake (from decreased metabolic activity); "hot" nodules exhibit increased iodide uptake (from increased metabolic activity)
  d. Increased risk of malignancy = male, <20 years old, >70 years old, history of neck irradiation, dysphagia, poor iodide uptake on thyroid scan (cold nodule), solid nodule on US
  e. Benign nodules treated with surgery, radioablation, and postoperative levothyroxine to stop thyroid hormone overproduction and decrease risk of malignant conversion
  f. Malignant nodules may arise from a variety of thyroid cell types
 2. **H/P** = nontender solid nodule in anterior neck, dysphagia, hoarseness; cervical lymphadenopathy
 3. **Labs** = biopsy provides diagnosis; thyroid hormones normal or decreased
 4. **Radiology** = US used to determine size and local extension; thyroid scan may show cold nodule
 5. **Treatment** = surgical resection (lobectomy for papillary type, near-total thyroidectomy for other types), radioablation; thyroid replacement (levothyroxine) needed after surgery

III. Parathyroid disorders
 A. **Parathyroid function**
 1. Plasma calcium (Ca^{2+}) regulation
  a. **Parathyroid hormone** (PTH)—secreted in response to low serum Ca^{2+}; induces osteoclasts to reabsorb bone and increase plasma Ca^{2+}; induces kidneys to increase 1,25-$(OH)_2$ vitamin D production, decreases phosphate reabsorption, and increases distal tubule Ca^{2+} reabsorption
  b. **1,25-$(OH)_2$ vitamin D**—metabolite of dietary vitamin D; production in kidneys increases with PTH secretion, increases intestinal Ca^{2+} absorption; increases renal proximal tubule phosphate reabsorption
  c. **Calcitonin**—secreted by thyroid parafollicular cells; inhibits bone reabsorption

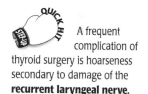

A frequent complication of thyroid surgery is hoarseness secondary to damage of the **recurrent laryngeal nerve.**

TABLE 5-7	Types of Thyroid Carcinoma			
Type	**Cells Affected**	**Frequency**	**Characteristics**	**Prognosis**
Papillary	Columnar cells of gland	**Most common form;** most common in younger patients	Begins as slow-growing nodule; eventually metastasizes to local cervical lymph nodes	**Good;** few recurrences
Follicular	Cuboidal cells in follicles	25% of thyroid cancers; more common in **older patients**	May function like normal thyroid tissue; metastasizes to liver, bone, brain, and lung	Not as good as papillary type; 50% 10-yr survival
Medullary	Parafollicular C cells	5% of thyroid cancers	**Produces calcitonin;** may present with other endocrine tumors (MEN 2a)	Poor; metastases common at diagnosis
Anaplastic	Poorly differentiated neoplasm	10% or less of thyroid cancers	**Very aggressive;** local extension causes hoarseness, dysphagia	Poor
MEN 2a, multiple endocrine neoplasia type 2a				

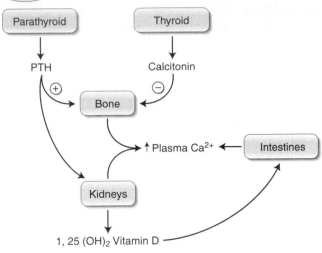

FIGURE 5-3 Plasma Ca²⁺ regulation. PTH, parathyroid hormone.

$\oplus$ Induces resorption of bone
$\ominus$ Inhibits resorption of bone

QUICK HIT

Remember the "**bones**," "**stones**," "**groans**," and "**psychiatric overtones**" of hypercalcemia in cases of hyperparathyroidism.

QUICK HIT

Decreased Ca²⁺ with increased PTH suggests a hyperparathyroidism secondary to **malnutrition**, malabsorption, **renal disease**, or calcium-wasting drugs.

B. **Primary hyperparathyroidism**
   1. **Excess PTH secretion,** leading to **hypercalcemia**
   2. Majority of cases result from **single adenoma;** most remaining cases occur with hyperplasia of all four glands; parathyroid cancer is rare
   3. **H/P** = usually asymptomatic; symptoms of hypercalcemia may be present (bone pain, nausea and vomiting, mental status changes, renal stones, constipation, weakness, increased risk of fracture) (see Chapter 4, Genitourinary disorders for further discussion of hypercalcemia)
   4. **Labs** = increased Ca²⁺, decreased phosphate, increased urine Ca²⁺, increased PTH
   5. **Treatment** = surgical resection (parathyroidectomy) of single adenoma; for four-gland hyperplasia, all glands are removed, and portion of one gland is implanted in muscle of forearm to maintain some PTH production; treat hypercalcemia with IV fluids and loop diuretics

C. **Hypoparathyroidism**
   1. PTH deficiency due to **surgical removal** of parathyroids or abnormal development of glands, leading to hypocalcemia
   2. **H/P** = tingling in lips and fingers, dry skin, weakness, symptoms of hypocalcemia (abdominal pain, tetany, dyspnea); possible tachycardia and positive Trousseau's (carpal spasm when blood pressure cuff inflated) and Chvostek's signs (tapping of facial nerve causes spasm) (see Chapter 4, Genitourinary disorders)
   3. **Labs** = decreased Ca²⁺, increased phosphate, decreased PTH
   4. **Treatment** = Ca²⁺ and vitamin D supplementation

D. **Pseudohypoparathyroidism**
   1. Hypocalcemia resulting from tissue **nonresponsiveness to PTH**
   2. Associated with developmental and skeletal abnormalities (**Albright's hereditary osteodystrophy**)
   3. **H/P** = symptoms of hypocalcemia, short stature, poor mental development in children
   4. **Labs** = decreased Ca²⁺, increased phosphate, **increased PTH;** administration of PTH causes no change in serum or urine Ca²⁺
   5. **Treatment** = Ca²⁺ and vitamin D supplementation

IV. Pituitary and hypothalamic disorders

A. **Hypothalamic-pituitary function**

1. Hypothalamus responds to stimuli by modulating pituitary activity; hormones are released into the hypophyseal portal system to regulate subsequent hormone release from the anterior pituitary; impulses sent through the hypothalamo-hypophyseal tract regulate hormone release from the posterior pituitary; anterior pituitary hormone secretion is regulated by feedback mechanisms in addition to hypothalamus

2. Posterior pituitary is a neural extension of the hypothalamus and is responsible for antidiuretic hormone (ADH) and oxytocin secretion

B. **Hyperprolactinemia**

1. Excess **prolactin** secretion by anterior pituitary

FIGURE 5-4

Hypothalamopituitary axis. ACTH, adrenocorticotropic hormone; ADH, antidiuretic hormone; CRH, corticotrophin-releasing hormone; GH, growth hormone; GHRH, growth hormone-releasing hormone; GnRH, gonadotropin-releasing hormone; FSH follicle-stimulating hormone; LH, luteinizing hormone; PRH, prolactin-releasing hormone; T_3, triiodothyronine; T_4, thyroxine; TRH, thyrotropin-releasing hormone; TSH, thyroid-stimulating hormone.

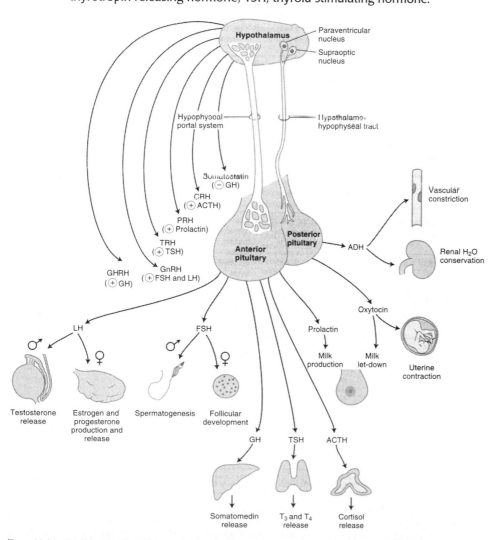

(From Mehta S, Milder EA, Mirachi AJ, Milder E. *Step-Up: A High-Yield, Systems-Based Review for the USMLE Step 1.* 2nd Ed. Philadelphia: Lippincott Williams & Wilkins; 2003.)

ENDOCRINE DISORDERS

Prolactinoma is the most common pituitary tumor.

STEP Compare current appearance of adult patients to multiple pictures at younger ages to aid in the detection of a gradual enlargement in features seen in acromegaly.

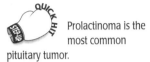

STEP If you see a child with extremely **advanced growth for the given age** (gigantism), perform a workup for increased GH.

Patients with acromegaly have **insulin resistance** (similar to DM type II) but rarely develop diabetes.

ACTH and MSH arise from the same precursors and follow the same trend in their serum concentrations.

a. Causes decreased luteinizing hormone (LH) and follicle-stimulating hormone (FSH) secretion, galactorrhea (milk secretion) and amenorrhea in women
b. Causes gynecomastia in men
2. May result from **prolactinoma,** drugs that block dopamine synthesis (e.g., phenothiazines, risperidone, haloperidol, methyldopa, verapamil), dopamine-depleting drugs, or hypothalamic damage
3. **H/P = amenorrhea** and **galactorrhea (women);** decreased libido, decreased potency, and **gynecomastia (men);** bilateral hemianopsia may result from mass effect of tumor in sella turcica
4. **Labs** = increased prolactin; if adenoma, prolactin > 300 ng/mL and TRH administration causes no additional prolactin secretion
5. **Radiology** = CT or MRI may detect pituitary tumor
6. **Treatment** = bromocriptine, surgical resection of tumor, stopping offending agents, or radiation

C. **Acromegaly**
1. Excess secretion of **growth hormone** (GH) by anterior pituitary due to adenoma
2. **H/P = enlargement** of hands and feet, coarsening of facial features (enlargement of nose, jaw, and skin folds), joint pain (due to osteoarthritis), neural pain (due to nerve entrapment); changes may be gradual
3. Heart, lungs, spleen, liver, and kidneys become enlarged and may cause symptoms secondary to dysfunction
4. **Labs** = increased GH, increased GH 1–2 hr following 100 g glucose load (GH decreases in normal cases)
5. **Radiology** = CT or MRI may detect tumor
6. **Treatment** = surgical resection of adenoma; bromocriptine or octreotide to lessen effects of GH
7. **Complications = cardiac failure,** DM (rare), spinal cord compression, vision loss secondary to pressure of tumor on optic nerve

D. **Hypopituitarism**
1. **Deficiency of all anterior pituitary hormones** due to tumor, hemorrhagic infarction (pituitary apoplexy), surgical resection, trauma, sarcoidosis, tuberculosis, postpartum necrosis (Sheehan syndrome)
2. Some pituitary hormones are kept in storage, and target organs may maintain some autonomous function, so symptoms specific to deficiency of each type of hormone appear at various times

TABLE 5-8 Progression of Hormone Deficiency in Hypopituitarism

Order of Loss	Hormone(s)	Symptoms
1	LH, FSH	Infertility, decreased libido, and decreased pubic hair; amenorrhea and genital atrophy in women; impotence and testicular atrophy in men
2	GH	Growth failure and short stature in children
3	TSH	Hypothyroidism leading to fatigue and cold intolerance; no goiter
4	Prolactin	No postpartum lactation
5	ACTH, MSH	Adrenal insufficiency leading to fatigue, weight loss, decreased appetite, and poor response to stress; decreased skin pigment due to low MSH

ACTH, adrenocorticotropic hormone; FSH, follicle-stimulating hormone; GH, growth hormone; LH, luteinizing hormone; MSH, melanocyte-stimulating hormone; TSH, thyroid stimulating hormone.

ENDOCRINE DISORDERS

3. **Labs =**
   a. Decreased LH, FSH, estrogen (women), and testosterone (men); hypoglycemia
   b. Decreased GH, no increase in GH after administration of insulin
   c. Decreased TSH, T_4, and T_3 uptake
   d. Decreased prolactin (most noticeable postpartum)
   e. Decreased adrenocorticotropic hormone (ACTH) and cortisol does not increase following administration of insulin (normally should increase at least 10 μg/dL)
4. **Treatment** = treat underlying cause if possible; **recombinant hormone replacement therapy** consisting of GH replacement for children (used occasionally in adults), levothyroxine, cortisol, estrogen-progesterone for women (combination pill), testosterone for men; gonadotropin-releasing hormone (GnRH) may be useful for restoring fertility in women

E. **Disorders of posterior pituitary**
   1. Syndrome of inappropriate ADH secretion (SAIDH) (see Chapter 4, Genitourinary disorders)
   2. Diabetes insipidus (see Chapter 4, Genitourinary disorders)

V. Adrenal disorders
A. **Adrenal function (see Table 5-9)**
B. **Cushing's syndrome**
   1. Syndrome of **excess cortisol** due to **excess corticosteroid administration, pituitary adenoma** (Cushing's disease), paraneoplastic ACTH production, or adrenal tumor

> **QUICK HIT**
> **Excess corticosteroid administration** is the **most common** cause of Cushing's syndrome; excess ACTH production by a **pituitary adenoma** is the **second most common** cause.

TABLE 5-9 Function of Zones In Adrenal Cortex and Medulla

Region	Stimulation	Secretory Products	Action of Secretory Products
Zona glomerulosa (cortex)	Renin-angiotensin system	Epinephrine, norepinephrine	Conserve body sodium, maintain body fluid volume
Zona fasciculata (cortex)	ACTH	Cortisol	Maintain glucose production from proteins, aids in fat metabolism, aids in vascular regulation, influences immune response, aids in nervous regulation
Zona reticularis (cortex)	ACTH	Androgens	Development of secondary sexual characteristics, increase bone and muscle mass, promote male sexual differentiation and sperm production
Medulla	Preganglionic sympathetic neurons	Epinephrine, norepinephrine	Postsynaptic neurotransmitter in sympathetic autonomic system, induce sympathetic effects (glucose mobilization, increase heart contractility and rate, etc.)

ACTH, adrenocorticotropic hormone.

FIGURE 5-5 Evaluation of a patient with suspected Cushing's syndrome due to cortisol excess. ACTH, adrenocorticotropic hormone.

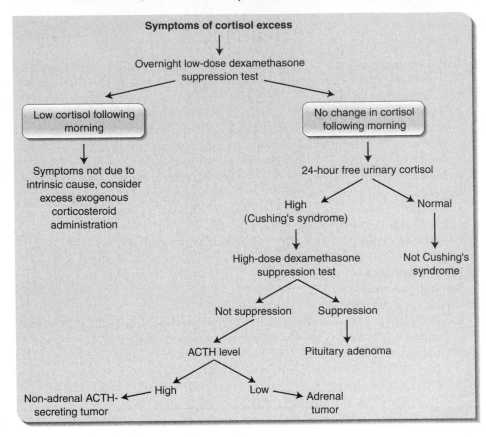

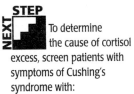

STEP NEXT To determine the cause of cortisol excess, screen patients with symptoms of Cushing's syndrome with:
- **low dexamethasone suppression test**—1–2 mg dexamethasone given at night; low cortisol normally found next morning; no decrease in cortisol seen in Cushing's syndrome;
- **high dose dexamethasone suppression test**–8 mg/day for 2 days; used to **determine cause** of cortisol excess.

2. **H/P** = weakness, depression, menstrual irregularities, polydipsia, polyuria, decreased libido, impotence; HTN, **acne, increased hair growth,** central obesity, **"buffalo hump"** (hunchback-like hump on back), **"moon facies"** (rounded face due to increased fat deposition), **purple striae** on abdomen
3. **Labs** = (in addition to those depicted in Figure 5-5) hyperglycemia, glycosuria, decreased K^+
4. **Treatment** = in cases of excess administration adjust corticosteroid dosing; for pituitary or adrenal tumor perform surgical resection; for paraneoplastic syndromes octreotide may improve symptoms; cortisol replacement may be needed after surgery
5. **Complications** = increased infection risk, **avascular necrosis of hip,** hypopituitarism or adrenal insufficiency after surgery
C. **Hyperaldosteronism**
  1. **Excess aldosterone secretion** due to unilateral **adrenal adenoma** (Conn's syndrome) or **increased renin-angiontensin system activity** secondary to low blood pressure in kidney
  2. **H/P** = polyuria, headache, weakness, paresthesias; HTN, tetany, possible edema
  3. **Labs** = **decreased K^+, increased Na^+,** metabolic alkalosis, decreased renin (Conn's syndrome only), **increased 24-hr urine aldosterone**
  4. **Radiology** = CT or MRI may detect adrenal mass
  5. **Treatment** = **spironolactone;** surgical resection of tumor; treat underlying disorder causing renin-angiotensin system hyperactivity

D. **Adrenal insufficiency**
   1. **Mineralocorticoid** (i.e., aldosterone) or **glucocorticoid** (i.e., cortisol) **deficiency** due to adrenal disease or ACTH insufficiency
   2. Type
      a. **Addison's disease** (primary insufficiency)—autoimmune destruction of adrenal cortices; may occur with other endocrine autoimmune processes
      b. **Secondary corticoadrenal insufficiency**—due to decreased ACTH secondary to chronic corticosteroid use (adrenal atrophy) or insufficient ACTH production by pituitary
      c. May also be due to infection or adrenal hemorrhage
   3. **H/P** = weakness, **fatigue,** anorexia, nausea, vomiting; hypotension, possible **increased skin pigmentation** (due to feedback influence of melanocyte-stimulating hormone [MSH])
   4. **Labs** =
      a. Decreased Na^+ and increased K^+ secondary to low aldosterone, eosinophilia, decreased cortisol
      b. Increased ACTH with Addison's disease, decreased ACTH with secondary insufficiency
      c. Decreased cortisol that increases following ACTH analogue administration in secondary insufficiency, but not in Addison's disease
   5. **Treatment** = **cortisol, mineralocorticoid replacement,** and hydration to achieve adequate volume status; titrate cortisol levels for periods of stress (increased need) and to avoid exacerbating secondary adrenal insufficiency
   6. **Complications** = **Addisonian crisis** (severe weakness, fever, mental status changes, and vascular collapse due to stress and increased cortisol need; treat with IV glucose and hydrocortisone or pressors), secondary insufficiency due to excess cortisol replacement

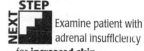

NEXT STEP Examine patient with adrenal insufficiency for **increased skin pigmentation;** this finding is **seen in Addison's disease** (secondary to increased MSH production accompanying increased ACTH production) but **not in secondary insufficiency.**

FIGURE 5-6 Steroid hormone synthesis and causes of congenital adrenal hyperplasia. NADPH, nicotinamide adenine dinucleotide phosphate (reduced form).

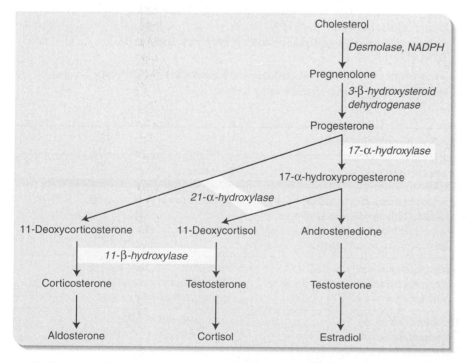

(Modified from Champe PC, Harvey RA. *Lippincott's Illustrated Reviews: Biochemistry.* 2nd Ed. Philadelphia: Lippincott-Raven; 1994.)

E. **Congenital adrenal hyperplasia (CAH)**
1. Enzymatic defect in synthesis of cortisol, resulting in decreased cortisol, reactive increase in ACTH production, adrenal hyperplasia, and androgen excess
2. **17-α-hydroxylase deficiency**
   a. Deoxycorticosterone overproduction; cortisol, androgen, and estrogen deficiencies
   b. **H/P = amenorrhea (women), ambiguous genitalia (men)**; HTN
   c. **Labs = decreased K$^+$, increased Na$^+$,** decreased testosterone, **decreased androstendione,** decreased 17-α-hydroxyprogesterone
3. **21-α-hydroxylase deficiency**
   a. (Usually) partial deficiency of enzyme resulting in excess androstenedione, insufficient cortisol and aldosterone
   b. **H/P =** ambiguous genitalia (female infants), virilization (women), macrogenitosomia and precocious puberty (men); dehydration and **hypotension** in more severe cases
   c. **Labs = decreased Na$^+$, increased K$^+$,** decreased testosterone, increased androstenedione
4. **11-β-hydroxylase deficiency**
   a. Enzyme deficiency resulting in **excess deoxycorticosterone,** deoxycortisol, and androgen and insufficient cortisol and aldosterone
   b. **H/P =** ambiguous genitalia (female infants), virilization (women), macrogenitosoma and precocious puberty (men); **HTN** (secondary to deoxycorticosterone)
   c. **Labs =** increased deoxycorticosterone, increased deoxycortisol, increased androstenedione, decreased testosterone
5. **Treatment =** cortisol administration decreases ACTH production and secondary androgen excess; fludrocortisone used in severe 21-α-hydroxylase deficiency to inhibit salt-wasting; surgical repair of genitalia in infants
F. **Pheochromocytoma**
1. Adrenal gland tumor that secretes epinephrine and norepinephrine, leading to stimulation of sympathetic nervous system
2. **H/P =** sudden palpitations, chest pain, diaphoresis, headache, anxiety; intermittent tachycardia, HTN
3. **Labs =** increase 24-hr urinary catecholamines and vanillylmandelic acid (VMA)
4. **Treatment =** surgical resection; α- and β-blockers used prior to and during surgery to control blood pressure

TABLE 5-10 **Types of Multiple Endocrine Neoplasia (MEN)**

Type	Endocrine Involvement	Characteristics	Treatment
1	Parathyroid Pancreas Pituitary	Hyperparathyroidism, hypercalcemia, **possible Zollinger-Ellison syndrome,** various **pituitary disorders** (e.g., acromegaly, Cushing's syndrome, galactorrhea)	Subtotal parathyroidectomy, surgical resection of pancreatic tumor or octreotide, surgical resection of pituitary tumor
2a	Medullary thyroid Pheochromocytoma Parathyroid	**Medullary carcinoma,** increased calcitonin, **hyperparathyroidism,** hypercalcemia, increased serum and urine catecholamines	Total thyroidectomy, surgical resection of pheochromocytoma, subtotal parathyroidectomy
2b	Medullary thyroid Pheochromocytoma Neuroma	**Medullary carcinoma,** increased calcitonin, **hyperparathyroidism,** hypercalcemia, **Marfanoid body habitus,** mucosal nodules	Total thyroidectomy, surgical resection of pheochromocytoma

VI. Multiple endocrine neoplasia (MEN)

    A. Autosomal dominant syndromes involving dysfunction of multiple endocrine glands

    B. Gland dysfunction may be secondary to hyperplasia or neoplasm

VII. Pediatric endocrine concerns

    A. Cretinism

       1. Congenital hypothyroidism due to severe iodide deficiency or hereditary disorder of thyroid hormone synthesis that leads to abnormal mental development and growth retardation

       2. **H/P** = poor feeding, large fontanelles that remain open, thick tongue, constipation; umbilical hernia, poor growth and mental development

       3. **Labs** = decreased T_4, increased TSH

       4. **Radiology** = x-ray shows poor bone development; thyroid scan shows decreased uptake and decreased thyroid tissue

       5. **Treatment** = levothyroxine started soon after birth to avoid permanent developmental delays

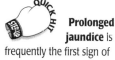

Prolonged jaundice is frequently the first sign of cretinism.

ENDOCRINE DISORDERS

Hematology and Oncology

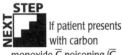

NEXT STEP If patient presents with carbon monoxide $\overline{C}$ poisoning ($\overline{C}$ displaces O_2 on Hgb, leading to insufficient delivery of O_2 to tissues), administer **100% O_2** via face mask to increase alveolar concentration of O_2 and decrease the opportunities for $\overline{C}$ to bind to Hgb.

Mean RC lifespan is 120 days.

I. Anemias

A. **Red blood cell (RBC) physiology**
1. RBCs serve to transport O_2 from alveoli to tissues via the blood stream and transport CO_2 from tissue to lungs
2. Normal hemoglobin (Hgb) A serves as a binding protein for O_2 and CO_2, and its affinity for O_2 follows the Hgb-O_2 dissociation curve
    a. **Metabolic alkalosis,** decreased body temperature, and increased Hgb F (fetal) shift curve to left
    b. **Metabolic acidosis,** increased body temperature, **high altitude,** and exercise shift curve to **right**
3. Circulating RBCs, myeloid cells, and lymphoid cells all originate from the same stem cells in bone marrow
4. RBCs become enucleated during maturation in bone marrow and depend upon glycolysis for survival
5. Normal Hgb concentration and hematocrit (Hct):
    a. 4–18 g/dL and 40–54% in men
    b. 12–16 g/dL and 37–48% in women
    c. Low Hgb and Hct (i.e., anemia) result in insufficient supply of O_2 to tissues and cause ischemia
6. Types of anemia are characterized by mechanism of pathology and mean corpuscular volume (MCV)

B. **Hemolytic anemia**
1. Anemia that results when RBC lifespan is shortened and marrow production of RBCs is not capable of meeting demand for new cells
2. May be due to defects in RBC membrane, RBC interior, or extracellular effects
3. **H/P** = possibly asymptomatic; weakness, fatigue, dyspnea on exertion; **pallor,** tachycardia, tachypnea, increased pulse pressure, possible systolic murmur, **jaundice;** severe cases may have palpitations, syncope, angina, chills, abdominal pain, **hepatosplenomegaly,** and **brownish discoloration of urine**
4. **Labs** = decreased Hgb, decreased Hct, **increased reticulocyte count, increased bilirubin (indirect),** increased lactate dehydrogenase (LDH), **normal MCV,** decreased serum haptoglobin; Coombs' test is helpful for making diagnosis
5. **Coombs' test**
    a. Coombs' reagent (rabbit IgM directed against human IgG and complement) is mixed with RBCs to aid in diagnosis of hemolytic anemia
    b. Direct test—Coombs' reagent mixed with RBCs; agglutination indicates presence of IgG and complement on RBC membranes (e.g., warm and cold agglutinin disease)

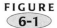

FIGURE 6-1 Hemoglobin-oxygen dissociation curve.

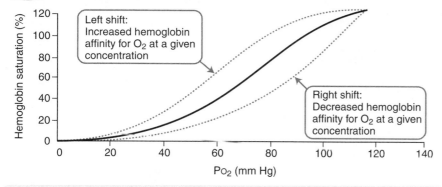

Left shift: metabolic alkalosis, decreased body temperature, increased Hgb F concentration
Right shift: metabolic acidosis, increased body temperature, high altitude, exercise

(Modified from Mehta S, Milder EA, Mirachi AJ, Milder E. *Step-Up: A High-Yield, Systems-Based Review for the USMLE Step 1*. 2nd Ed. Philadelphia: Lippincott Williams & Wilkins; 2003.)

    c. Indirect test—patient serum mixed with type O RBCs which, in turn, are mixed with Coombs' reagent; agglutination indicates presence of anti-RBC antibodies in serum (e.g., Rh alloimmunization)
  6. **Blood smear = schistocytes** (RBC fragments), spherocytes, and/or burr cells (Color Figure 6-1)

C. **Iron-deficiency anemia**
  1. Anemia resulting from insufficient heme production secondary to **iron deficiency**
  2. Iron deficiency results from **blood loss,** poor dietary intake or absorption from the gastrointestinal (GI) tract, pregnancy, or menstruation
  3. **H/P** = fatigue, weakness, dyspnea on exertion, **pica** (craving to eat ice, dirt, etc.); pallor, tachycardia, tachypnea, increased pulse pressure, possible systolic murmur; **angular chelitis** (irritation of lips and corners of mouth), **spooning of nails** in severe cases
  4. **Labs** = decreased Hgb, decreased Hct, decreased MCV, decreased or normal reticulocyte count, **decreased ferritin,** decreased iron, decreased transferrin (i.e., total iron-binding capacity), positive stool guaiac possible if secondary to GI losses
  5. **Blood smear = hypochromic microcytic RBCs** (Color Figure 6-3)
  6. **Treatment** = iron supplementation (several months of treatment required to replete stores), determine cause of iron loss
  7. **Complications** = constipation and nausea common with iron supplementation (e.g., transfusion)

D. **Lead-poisoning anemia** (acquired sideroblastic anemia)
  1. Anemia resulting from heme synthesis inhibition by lead ingestion (more common in **children,** especially those in urban environments)
  2. Similar presentation may be seen in anemia caused by alcoholism or isoniazid use
  3. **H/P** = fatigue, weakness; pallor, mental developmental delays, **gingival lead lines, peripheral neuropathy** (decreased motor control of extremities)
  4. **Labs** = decreased Hgb, decreased Hct, decreased MCV, increased serum lead
  5. **Blood smear** = microcytic RBCs, **basophilic stippling of RBCs,** ringed sideroblasts (Color Figure 6-4)
  6. **Treatment** = remove source of lead; EDTA for lead chelation

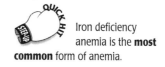
Iron deficiency anemia is the **most common** form of anemia.

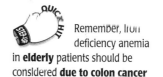
Remember, iron deficiency anemia in **elderly** patients should be considered **due to colon cancer** until ruled out.

HEMATOLOGY AND ONCOLOGY

FIGURE
6-2 Development of myeloid and lymphoid cell lines from pluripotent stem cells in bone marrow.

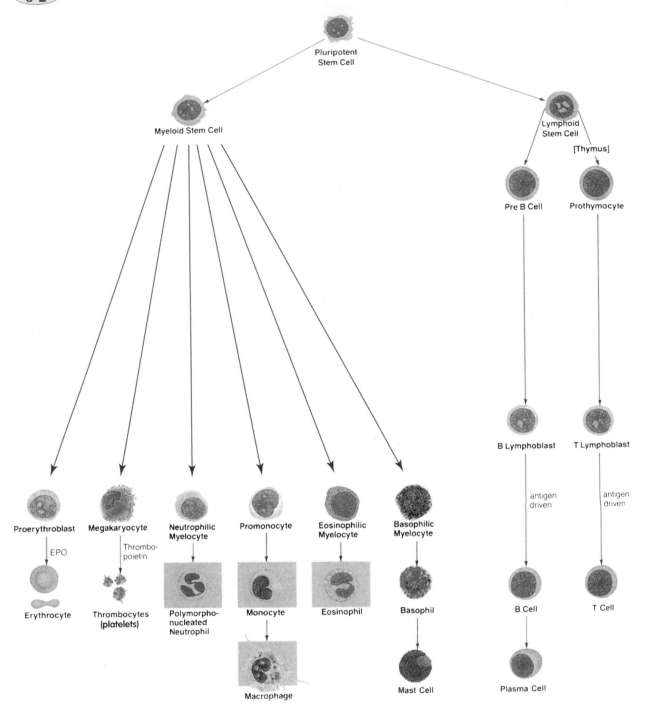

(Modified from Turgeon M. *Clinical Hematology: Theory and Procedures.* 2nd Ed. Boston: Little, Brown; 1993.)

Folate deficiency is the most common cause of **megaloblastic** anemia.

Inadequate folate intake is seen with **alcoholism** and in the elderly because of poor nutrition.

E. **Folate-deficiency anemia**
1. Anemia resulting from inadequate folate intake or increased folate need (e.g., poor nutrition, chemotherapy)
2. **H/P** = fatigue, weakness, dyspnea on exertion, diarrhea, **sore tongue;** pallor, tachycardia, tachypnea, increased pulse pressure, possible systolic murmur; **no neurologic symptoms**
3. **Labs** = decreased Hgb, decreased Hct, **increased MCV,** decreased serum folate; bone marrow biopsy shows increased erythroblasts

TABLE 6-1 Classification of Anemias by Mean Corpuscular Volume (MCV) and Common Etiologies

Microcytic (MCV <80 μL)	Normocytic (MCV 80–100 μL)	Macrocytic (MCV >100 μL)
Iron deficiency	Hemolytic	Folate deficiency
Lead poisoning	Chronic disease	Vitamin B_{12} deficiency
Chronic disease	Hypovolemia	Liver disease
Sideroblastic		
Thalassemias		

TABLE 6-2 Types of Hemolytic Anemias

Type	Pathology	Blood Smear	Coombs' Test	Other Diagnostic Aids	Treatment
Drug-induced	Bind to RBC membrane and induce production of **anti-drug antibodies,** form **immune complexes** that fix complement, or induce **anti-Rh antibodies**	Burr cells, schistocytes	**Direct +**	Recent penicillin, L-dopa, quinidine, other drug use	Stop offending agent
Immune	**Anti-RBC antibodies,** autoimmune disease, possibly drug induced	Spherocytes	**Direct +**	**Warm-reacting antibodies** (IgG) or **cold-reacting antibodies** (IgM)	Corticosteroids, **avoid cold exposure** (with cold-reacting antibodies), stop offending agent; splenectomy may be needed in persistent cases
Mechanical	RBCs broken by force or **turbulent flow**	**Schistocytes**	Negative	**Prosthetic heart valve,** HTN, coagulation disorder	Treat underlying cause
Hereditary spherocytosis (Color Figure 6-2)	Genetic **defect of RBC membranes** resulting in spherical RBCs	**Spherocytes**	Negative	**Hepatosplenomegaly**	Splenectomy
G6PD deficiency	Deficiency of G6PD (enzyme required to repair oxidative damage to RBCs); ingestion of oxidant (fava beans, ASA, sulfa drugs)	RBCs with **"bites"** taken out of them, **Heinz bodies** (small densities of Hgb in RBC)	Negative	**Low G6PD;** dizziness, fatigue begins within days of ingesting oxidant; mild form in African Americans, more severe form in people of Mediterranean decent	Avoid oxidants; transfusion may be needed in severe cases

ASA, aspirin; G6PD, glucose 6-phosphate dehydrogenase; HTN, hypertension; RBC, red blood cell.

HEMATOLOGY AND ONCOLOGY

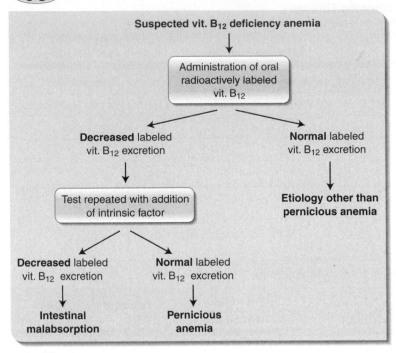

FIGURE 6-3 Schilling test protocol. vit., vitamin.

vit. = Vitamin

4. **Blood smear = macrocytic RBCs, hypersegmented neutrophils**
5. **Treatment** = oral folate supplementation

F. **Vitamin B_{12} deficiency anemia**
1. **Pernicious anemia** (autoimmune anemia due to lack of intrinsic factor) or anemia resulting from inadequate vitamin B_{12} intake, ileal resection, bacterial overgrowth in gastrointestinal (GI) tract, or *Diphyllobothrium latum* infection (a worm)
2. **H/P** = fatigue, weakness, dyspnea on exertion; pallor, tachycardia, tachypnea, increased pulse pressure, possible systolic murmur, **symmetric paresthesias, ataxia,** possible psychosis
3. **Labs** = decreased Hgb, decreased Hct, **increased MCV,** decreased vitamin B_{12}; **Schilling test** useful to diagnose pernicious anemia
4. **Blood smear = macrocytic RBCs, hypersegmented neutrophils** (Color Figure 6-6)
5. **Treatment** = monthly intramuscular vitamin B_{12} injections, dietary supplementation of vitamin B_{12}

G. **Anemia of chronic disease**
1. Anemia occurring in patients with neoplasia, diabetes mellitus, autoimmune disorders, or long-standing infections
2. Frequently associated with production of lactoferrin (iron storage protein with greater iron affinity than transferrin)
3. **H/P** = history of appropriate disease state, fatigue, weakness, dyspnea on exertion; tachycardia, pallor
4. **Labs = mildly decreased Hgb and Hct,** normal or decreased MCV, decreased iron, decreased transferrin, increased ferritin
5. **Blood smear** = normocytic RBCs
6. **Treatment = treat underlying disorder**

H. **Aplastic anemia**
1. **Pancytopenia** resulting from bone marrow failure
2. Due to drugs (including chloramphenicol, sulfonamides, phenytoin, chemotherapeutics) or toxins

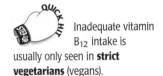

Inadequate vitamin B_{12} intake is usually only seen in **strict vegetarians** (vegans).

3. **H/P** = fatigue, weakness, **persistent infections, poor clotting** with possible uncontrolled bleeding, easy bruising; pallor, tachycardia, tachypnea, systolic murmur, increased pulse pressure
4. **Labs** = decreased Hgb, decreased Hct, decreased white blood cells (WBCs), decreased platelets; bone marrow biopsy shows **hypocellularity**
5. **Treatment** = stop offending agent; transfusions, immunosuppressive agents, or bone marrow transplant may be required

II. Genetic disorders of hemoglobin
A. **Sideroblastic anemia**
1. Anemia due to **defective heme synthesis** resulting in decreased Hgb levels in cells
2. May be genetic disorder or due to alcohol, isoniazid, or lead poisoning (patient history is useful for differentiating cause)
3. **H/P** = fatigue, weakness, dyspnea on exertion; pallor, tachycardia, tachypnea, increased pulse pressure, possible systolic murmur
4. **Labs** = decreased Hgb, decreased Hct, increased ferritin, increased iron, possible decreased MCV
5. **Blood smear** = **multiple sizes of RBCs** with normocytic, **microcytic,** and macrocytic cells possible; **ringed sideroblasts** (RBC precursors) (Color Figure 6-5)
6. **Treatment** = pyridoxine helpful for hereditary cases; erythropoietin helpful in minority of patients; transfusion may be required in severe cases
7. **Complications** = 10% patients progress to **acute leukemia**
B. **Thalassemia**
1. Hgb defects resulting from abnormal production of heme α-globin or β-globin subunits
2. Disease state arises from **unbalanced production** ratio of α and β chains
3. **Normal Hgb**
   a. Composed of two α chains and two β chains
   b. Four genes determine α chain synthesis; two genes determine β chain synthesis
4. **α-thalassemia**
   a. More prevalent in Asians
   b. Variants have between 1–4 defective genes
5. **β-thalassemia**
   a. More prevalent in patients of Mediterranean descent
   b. Variants have either one or two defective genes
6. **Labs** = **decreased MCV,** increased reticulocyte count, increased hemoglobin Bart's (Hgb that binds O_2 but is unable to release it to tissues in α-thalassemia), increased hemoglobin A_2 or F in β-thalassemia; Hgb electrophoresis can detect genetic abnormalities and severity of defects
7. **Blood smear** =
   a. α-thalassemia—abnormally shaped microcytic RBCs, target cells (Color Figure 6-7)
   b. β-thalassemia—RBCs in variable size and shape (including microcytic cells) with basophilic stippling
8. **Treatment** = transfusions for more severe variants, folate supplementation may be helpful in all symptomatic forms and in mild forms during stress; iron chelation may be required in patients receiving chronic transfusions; bone marrow transplant may be helpful in children with minimal hepatomegaly, no portal fibrosis, and adequate iron chelation therapy
9. **Complications** = **chronic iron overload** from repeat transfusions causes damage to heart and liver; patients with hemoglobin H disease and β-thalassemia major frequently die in childhood and require frequent transfusions for survival; children of parents with carrier state are at increased risk for developing disease

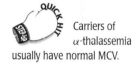

Carriers of α-thalassemia usually have normal MCV.

STEP Differentiate between causes of microcytic anemia using the ratio of MCV:RBC count (Mentzer index):
• MCV:RBC count >13 suggests iron deficiency
• MCV:RBC count <13 suggests thalassemia

STEP If microcytic anemia is found on blood smear, rule out thalassemia before administering supplemental iron to prevent iron overload.

TABLE 6-3	Variants of α- and β-Thalassemias		
Thalassemia Type	Variant	Number of Abnormal Genes	Characteristics
α	Hydrops fetalis	4	No α-globin production; **fetal death** occurs
	Hemoglobin H disease	3	Minimal α-globin production; **chronic hemolytic anemia,** pallor, splenomegaly; **hemoglobin Barts** in serum; microcytic RBCs on blood smear; decreased lifespan
	α-thalassemia minor	2	Reduced α-globin production; **mild anemia;** microcytic RBCs and target cells on blood smear
	α-thalassemia carrier	1	Generally **asymptomatic;** children of carriers at increased risk for thalassemia pending genotype of other parent
β	β-thalassemia major	2	No β-globin production; asymptomatic until decline of fetal hemoglobin; growth retardation, developmental delays, bony abnormalities, hepatosplenomegaly, anemia; increase in hemoglobin A2 and F; microcytic RBCs on blood smear; patients die in childhood without transfusions
	β-thalassemia minor	1	Reduced β-globin production; mild anemia; patients can lead normal lives; transfusions may be needed during periods of stress

RBC, red blood cell.

The β-globin defect in sickle cell disease causes production of **defective β chains;** the β-globin defect in β-thalassemia causes **decreased production** of normal β chains. β-globin defect:
- In sickle cell disease causes production of **defective β chains**
- In β-thalassemia causes **decreased production** of normal β chains

Heterozygous **carriers** of sickle cell defect (sickle cell trait) are **asymptomatic** and carry **improved resistance to malaria.**

Presence of fetal hemoglobin in newborns delays presentation of sickle cell symptoms until after six months of age when fetal hemoglobin levels have decreased.

C. **Sickle cell disease**
1. Autosomal recessive defect in β-globin chain of Hgb, leading to production of **abnormal Hgb S**
2. Acidosis, hypoxia, and dehydration cause Hgb S molecules to polymerize and distort RBCs into a **sickle shape** that is **more susceptible to hemolysis** and **vascular clumping** than normal cells
3. More common in people of African heritage
4. **H/P** = stressful events (infection, illness, trauma, hypoxia) induce **sickle cell crisis** characterized by **deep bone pain,** chest pain, new stroke onset, painful swelling of hands and feet, dyspnea, priapism (painful, prolonged erection); splenomegaly, jaundice, fever, tachypnea seen on exam
5. **Labs =**
   a. Decreased Hct, increased reticulocyte count, increased polymorphonuclear cells (PMNs)
   b. Hemoglobin electrophoresis detects Hgb S without normal Hgb A
   c. Sickledex® solubility test can detect Hgb abnormalities but cannot differentiate between carrier trait and homozygous disease state
6. **Radiology** = "fish-mouth" vertebrae; lung infiltrates in acute chest syndrome (radiological findings in setting of chest pain and dyspnea)
7. **Blood smear** = target cells, nucleated RBCs; **deoxygenation of blood produces sickle cells** (Color Figure 6-8)
8. **Treatment =**
   a. **Hydration, supplemental O$_2$,** and **analgesics** (frequently narcotics required) **during sickle cell crises**

b. Hydroxyurea (increases Hgb F production) and avoidance of crisis stimuli decrease frequency of crises

c. Pneumococcal vaccine reduces risk of infection in asplenic patients; prophylactic penicillin should be given until five years of age to help prevent pneumococcal infection in asplenic children

d. Transfusions may be required in severe cases

9. **Complications** =

a. Chronic anemia, pulmonary hypertension (HTN), heart failure, **aplastic crisis** (usually secondary to parvovirus B19 infection), **acute chest syndrome**

b. Autosplenectomy, stroke, osteonecrosis, and multiple organ ischemia may result secondary to **vascular occlusion**

c. Increased risk of infection by **encapsulated organisms**

III. Leukocyte disorders and hypersensitivity

A. **Lymphopenia without immune deficiency**

1. Decreased lymphocyte count seen in diseases with **increased cortisol** levels or after **chemotherapy,** radiation, or lymphoma; antibody production not affected

2. **H/P** = repeated infections with possible recent history of chemotherapy or radiation

3. **Labs** = decreased WBCs especially B and T lymphocytes

4. **Treatment** = if possible, stop offending agents; bone marrow transplant may be needed

B. **Eosinophilia**

1. Abnormally high levels of eosinophils seen in Addison's disease, neoplasm, asthma, allergic drug reactions, collagen vascular diseases, and parasitic infections

2. **H/P** = asymptomatic; history of predisposing condition

3. **Labs** = increased eosinophil count

4. **Treatment** = treat underlying disorder, stop offending agent

C. **Neutropenia without immune deficiency** (agranulocytosis)

1. Decreased neutrophil count seen with some viral infections (hepatitis, influenza), drugs (fluoxetine, antithyroid medications, chloramphenicol, sulfonamides), collagen vascular diseases, chemotherapy, and aplastic anemia

2. **H/P** = weakness, chills, fatigue, recurrent infections; fever

3. **Labs** = decreased neutrophil count

4. **Treatment** = treat underlying disorder, stop offending agents, granulocyte colony-stimulating factor, corticosteroids

D. **Hypersensitivity reactions**

1. Allergen-induced immunologic response by body involving cellular or humoral mechanisms

2. **Labs** = skin allergen testing or radioallergosorbent test (RAST) may be useful in determining specific allergies

3. **Treatment** = **contact prevention** and **avoidance** of offending agents is important; antihistamines and corticosteroids may improve symptoms after reaction; if anaphylaxis is a concern, epinephrine injections should be kept readily available

E. **Anaphylaxis**

1. Severe type I hypersensitivity reaction after re-exposure to allergen (penicillins, insect stings, latex, eggs, nuts, and seafood are common causes)

2. **H/P** = tingling in skin, itching, cough, chest tightness, **difficult swallowing and breathing** (secondary to angioedema), syncope; tachycardia, wheezing, urticaria, **hypotension,** arrhythmias

3. **Labs** = skin testing or RAST can confirm allergic response

Patients with sickle cell disease are particularly susceptible to **_Salmonella_ osteomyelitis** (although _Staphylococcus aureus_ is still the most common etiology) and **sepsis** by **encapsulated organisms** (_Streptococcus pneumoniae, Haemophilus influenzae, Neisseria meningitides, Klebsiella_).

The types of hypersensitivity reactions may be remembered by the mnemonic **ACID: A**naphylactic, **C**omplement-mediated, **I**mmune complex-mediated, **D**elayed.

TABLE 6-4	Types of Hypersensitivity Reactions		
Type	**Mediated By**	**Mechanism**	**Examples**
I	IgE antibodies attached to mast cells	Allergens react with antibody to cause **mast cell degranulation** and histamine release	Allergic rhinitis, asthma, **anaphylaxis**
II	IgM and IgG antibodies	Allergens react with antibodies to initiate **complement cascade** and cell death	**Immune hemolytic anemia,** hemolytic disease of the newborn, Goodpasture's syndrome
III	IgM and IgG immune complexes	Antibodies form **immune complexes** with allergens which are then deposited in tissue and initiate complement cascade	Arthus reaction, serum sickness, glomerulonephritis
IV	T cells and macrophages	**T cells** present allergens to macrophages and secrete lymphokines that induce macrophages to destroy surrounding tissue	Transplant rejection, **allergic contact dermatitis**

STEP NEXT Epinephrine should be given **immediately** to a person undergoing an anaphylactic reaction, without waiting for additional tests.

STEP NEXT Monitor **heparin** anticoagulation with **PTT.**

QUICK HIT Low molecular weight heparins do **not** require monitoring by PTT.

STEP NEXT Monitor **warfarin** anticoagulation with a normalized PT (i.e., **international normalized ratio [INR])** to track relative effect on the extrinsic pathway.

STEP NEXT Treat warfarin overdose with **vitamin K.**

4. **Treatment = subcutaneous epinephrine, intubation** (if closed airway), antihistamines, recumbent positioning, IV hydration; vasopressors may be needed for severe hypotension; avoidance of stimuli is key to prevention; desensitization therapy may be successful depending on allergen

IV. **Clotting disorders**
   A. **Normal clotting function**
      1. **Platelets**
         a. Circulate in plasma
         b. Important in **primary control** of bleeding
         c. Cause local vasoconstriction and form platelet plug at site of vascular injury in response to adenosine diphosphate (ADP) secreted by injured cells
         d. Bleeding time may be used to assess platelet function but is poorly reproducible and time consuming
      2. **Coagulation cascade**
         a. Responsible for formation of **fibrin clot** at site of injury
         b. **Intrinsic pathway** induced by exposure to negatively charged foreign substances; measured by partial thromboplastin time (**PTT**)
         c. **Extrinsic pathway** induced by exposure to tissue factor; measured by prothrombin time (**PT**)
      3. **Antithrombotic drugs**
         a. Used to prevent or treat pathologic clot (thrombus) formation (deep vein thrombosis [DVT], thromboembolic stroke, mural thrombus, pulmonary embolism [PE], postsurgical or traumatic thrombus, etc.)
         b. May affect platelet function, intrinsic pathway, or extrinsic pathway
   B. **Thrombocytopenia**
      1. Decreased number of platelets (<100,000) leading to abnormal bleeding
      2. May be idiopathic, autoimmune, or due to external causes (e.g., drugs, infection, nutrition)

FIGURE 6-4 Coagulation cascade. Neg., negatively. INR, international normalized ratio; PT, prothrombin time; PTT, partial thromboplastin time.

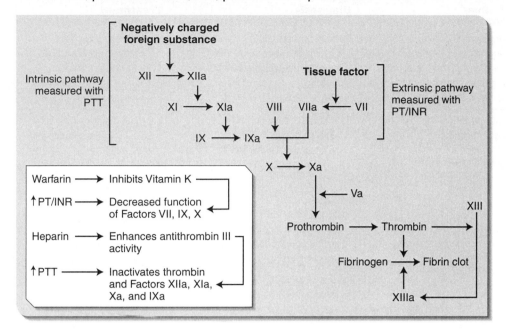

C. **von Willebrand's disease**
1. Autosomal dominant disease with deficiencies of **factor VIII** and **von Willebrand's factor** (vWF), leading to abnormal clotting and platelet function
2. **H/P** = easy bruising, mucosal bleeding (nose, gums), menorrhagia; multiple sites of bruising and mucosal bleeding on exam
3. **Labs** = **increased PTT, increased bleeding time,** decreased factor VIII antigen, decreased vWF

 vWF and Factor VIII are the only clotting factors not synthesized by the liver and remain at normal levels while other factor levels decrease in liver failure.

TABLE 6-5 Common Anticoagulant Drugs

Drug	Mechanism	Role	Adverse Effects
ASA	Inhibits platelet aggregation through suppression of thromboxane A_2 synthesis	Decreases thrombus risk in CAD and post-MI, decreases postoperative thrombus risk	Increased risk of hemorrhagic stroke, **GI bleeding**
Heparin	Binds to **antithrombin III** to increase activity and prevent clot formation	Postoperative prophylaxis for DVT and PE, dialysis, decreases post-MI thrombus risk, safer than warfarin during pregnancy	Hemorrhage, hypersensitivity, **thrombocytopenia**
Low molecular weight heparin	Binds to **factor Xa** to prevent clot formation	Postoperative prophylaxis for DVT and PE, safest option during pregnancy	Hemorrhage
Warfarin	Antagonizes vitamin K action	**Long-term** anticoagulation (CAD, stroke, post-surgery)	Hemorrhage, **drug interactions, teratogenicity**
Other antiplatelet drugs (clopidogrel, ticlopidine)	Inhibits platelet aggregation by mechanism different from ASA	Anticoagulation in patients that cannot tolerate ASA	**Prolonged bleeding,** neutropenia

ASA, aspirin; CAD, coronary artery disease; DVT, deep vein thrombosis; GI, gastrointestinal; MI, myocardial infarction; PE, pulmonary embolism.

TABLE 6-6	Causes of Thrombocytopenia		
Cause	**Pathology**	**Diagnosis**	**Treatment**
Impaired production (drugs, infection, aplastic anemia, folate/Vitamin B₁₂ deficiency)	**Absent or reduced megakaryocytes** due to offending agent or **abnormal megakaryocytes** due to metabolic deficiency	Findings consistent with precipitating condition; **bone marrow biopsy** helpful for diagnosis	Stop offending agent, treat underlying disorder, bone marrow transplantation
Abnormal pooling	**Splenic platelet sequestration**	Splenomegaly, normal bone marrow biopsy, platelets <40,000	May not be required; splenectomy if symptomatic
Idiopathic thrombocytopenia purpura (ITP)	**Autoimmune** disease with anti-platelet antibodies	**Platelets <10,000**	Self-limited in children; adults require corticosteroids, splenectomy, IV immunoglobulin, or plasmapheresis
Thrombotic thrombocytopenic purpura (TTP)	Unknown mechanism; platelets react with endothelial cells to cause **arterial occlusion**	**Neurologic deficits,** low Hct, increased reticulocyte count	Corticosteroids, ASA, plasmapheresis, splenectomy
Hemolytic-uremic syndrome	Massive RBC hemolysis (frequently due to **E. coli O157:H7** infection) causes renal failure, end-arteriole occlusion	**Schistocytes** on blood smear, flu-like symptoms, diarrhea, HTN, high LDH	FFP, plasmapheresis, treat infection

ASA, acetylsalicylic acid; FFP, fresh frozen plasma; Hct, hematocrit; HTN, hypertension; IV, intravenous; LDH, lactate dehydrogenase; RBC, red blood cell.

Green vegetables are a good supply of vitamin K.

Patients using **warfarin** may present with a clinical picture similar to that of vitamin K deficiency.

4. **Treatment** = desmopressin, fresh frozen plasma (FFP) or cryoprecipitate, factor VIII concentrate prior to surgery, avoidance of aspirin (ASA)

D. **Vitamin K deficiency**
   1. Inadequate vitamin K supply due to poor intake, malabsorption, or eradication of vitamin K-producing GI flora (secondary to prolonged antibiotic use)
   2. Vitamin K required in synthesis of factors II, VII, IX, and X
   3. **H/P** = easy bruising, delayed clot formation
   4. **Labs** = increased PT, increased PTT
   5. **Treatment** = vitamin K injections, FFP

E. **Hemophilia**
   1. X-linked recessive disease with deficiency of either factor VIII (hemophilia A) or factor IX (hemophilia B)
   2. **H/P** = **uncontrolled bleeding** occurring spontaneously or after minimal trauma, excessive bleeding following surgical or dental procedures; **hemarthroses** (bleeding in joints), intramuscular bleeding, and GI or genitourinary bleeding may be evident on exam
   3. **Labs** = **increased PTT, normal PT, normal bleeding time,** decreased factor VIII or IX antigen
   4. **Treatment** = factor VIII or IX concentrate or FFP, desmopressin (may increase factor VIII production in hemophilia A), transfusions frequently needed in cases of large blood loss
   5. **Complications** = death due to severe uncontrolled bleeding, **HIV infection** common in patients receiving frequent transfusions prior to mid 1980s

HEMATOLOGY AND ONCOLOGY

F. **Disseminated intravascular coagulation** (DIC)
  1. Widespread abnormal coagulation due to sepsis, severe trauma, neoplasm, or obstetric complications
     a. Initial coagulopathy with widespread clot formation occurs because of extensive activation of the clotting cascade by endothelial tissue factor released during bacteremia
     b. Deficiency in clotting factors results from extensive clotting
     c. Abnormal bleeding results from clotting factor deficiencies
  2. **H/P** = appropriate history of precipitating condition; uncontrolled bleeding from wounds and surgical sites, hematemesis, dyspnea; digital cyanosis, hypotension, tachycardia, possible neurologic or renal insufficiency signs, possible shock
  3. **Labs** = decreased platelets, increased PT, increased PTT, decreased fibrinogen, **increased fibrin split products, increased D-dimer,** decreased Hct
  4. **Blood smear** = schistocytes, few platelets
  5. **Treatment** = **treat underlying disorder,** platelets, FFP, cryoprecipitate; heparin may be needed for thrombi
  6. **Complications** = poor prognosis without early treatment; thrombi cause numerous infarcts

V. Hematological infections
  A. **Sepsis**
    1. Bacteremia with an associated systemic response
    2. Common agents include *Escherichia coli, Klebsiella, Pseudomonas, Streptococcus,* and *Staphylococcus*
    3. **H/P** = malaise, chills, nausea, vomiting; fever, mental status changes, tachycardia, tachypnea; may progress to **septic shock** with hypotension, cool extremities (initially warm), and petechiae
    4. **Labs** = increased WBCs; positive urine, blood, or sputum cultures needed to diagnose infection; labs may detect signs of DIC
    5. **Radiology** = chest x-ray may show infiltrates and pneumonia
    6. **Treatment** = hydration, broad-spectrum antibiotics **initially** then pathogen-specific antibiotics when agent identified by culture; remove (or change) possible routes of infection (Foley catheter, IV, etc.); progression to septic shock may require intubation and vasopressors
    7. **Complications** = septic shock, DIC
  B. **Malaria**
    1. Parasitic infection by ***Plasmodium*** spp. (*P. vivax, P. falciparum, P. ovale, P. malariae*) transmitted by *Anopheles* mosquito
    2. **H/P** = **periodic fever and chills** at approximately two-day intervals, splenomegaly; *P. falciparum* infection may include decreased consciousness, pulmonary edema, and renal insufficiency
    3. **Blood smear** = Giemsa stain shows *Plasmodium* spp. (Color Figure 6-9)
    4. **Treatment** = **antimalarials** (chloroquine, etc.); mefloquine used in chloroquine-resistant *P. falciparum*
  C. **Mononucleosis**
    1. Infection by **Epstein-Barr virus** (EBV) affecting B cells and oropharyngeal epithelium
    2. Transmitted by **intimate contact** (e.g., kissing, intercourse)
    3. **H/P** = **fatigue,** sore throat, malaise; **lymphadenopathy,** splenomegaly, fever
    4. **Labs** = positive heterophile antibodies, positive EBV serology (i.e., MonoSpot test), increased WBCs
    5. **Treatment** = self-limited

Bleeding in **DIC** occurs because **pathologic clotting uses up supplies** of platelets and coagulation factors; bleeding in other clotting disorders occurs because of insufficient production, abnormal production, or early destruction of platelets or coagulation factors.

Encapsulated organisms are a more common cause of sepsis in **asplenic** patients (e.g., sickle cell disease) than in other patients.

S. aureus is a common cause of sepsis in **intravenous drug abusers.**

STEP Do not start antibiotics until **after** first blood culture has been collected to avoid false-negative cultures.

While rare in the United States, malaria is extremely common in other countries, especially in **sub-Saharan Africa.**

Travelers to sub-Saharan Africa, tropical South America, or southwest Asia should take **prophylactic** chloroquine or mefloquine during their stay.

Symptoms of mononucleosis do not appear until 2–5 weeks after infection with EBV.

HEMATOLOGY AND ONCOLOGY

HIV infection has greatest prevalence in Africa, where transmission is typically through heterosexual contact.

While the rate of HIV transmission through needle sticks (i.e., health care workers) is very low (0.3%), prophylactic zidovudine and lamivudine should be started immediately if there is an appreciable risk of transmission; HIV antibody tests should be performed immediately, six weeks, three months, and six months after exposure to determine if transmission occurred and treatment should be continued until transmission is determined to not have occurred.

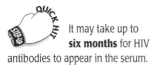

It may take up to **six months** for HIV antibodies to appear in the serum.

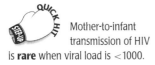

Mother-to-infant transmission of HIV is **rare** when viral load is <1000.

HIV-positive mothers should **not** breast feed to reduce risk of transmission.

D. **Human immunodeficiency virus (HIV)**
  1. RNA retrovirus that infects CD4 lymphocytes (**helper T cells**) and destroys them, eventually leading to **acquired immune deficiency syndrome (AIDS)**
  2. Virus uses reverse transcriptase to incorporate genetic material into host cell genome and produce copies of DNA
  3. Transmitted via **bodily fluids** (blood, semen, vaginal secretions, breast milk)
  4. **Risk factors** (United States) = homosexual or bisexual males, intravenous drug abuse (IVDA), blood transfusions prior to mid 1980s (e.g., hemophiliacs), heterosexual partners of other high-risk individuals, infants born to infected mothers, accidental exposure to bodily fluids (e.g., needle sticks, fluid splashes) among health care workers (low probability but possible); higher rate among African American and Latino populations
  5. **Acute H/P = flu-like symptoms,** sore throat, myalgias, fatigue; fever, lymphadenopathy, viral rash; symptoms typically last <2 months
  6. Following acute infection, patient enters **latent phase** with few or no symptoms and low viral load that lasts months to years (time increases with treatment)
  7. **Late H/P** (i.e., AIDS) = **opportunistic infections** and **AIDS-defining illnesses** begin to present, weight loss, night sweats, dementia
  8. **Labs =**
     a. Enzyme-linked immunosorbent assay (**ELISA**) detects HIV antibodies and is 99% sensitive
     b. Positive ELISA is confirmed with repeat test and/or **Western Blot** (lower sensitivity but high specificity) to rule out false positives; **CD4 count** is used to track extent of disease progression (AIDS is defined by CD4 count <200);
     c. **Viral load** indicates the rate of disease progression (low during latent phase and high once AIDS diagnosed)
  9. **Treatment =**
     a. **Antiretroviral therapy** should be initiated for **CD4 count <350** or **viral load >20,000**
     b. Common initial regimens
        (1) 1–2 protease inhibitors with two nucleoside analogs
        (2) One non-nucleoside reverse transcriptase inhibitor with two nucleosides
        (3) Combination therapy (multiple drugs combined in one pill)
     c. Compliance with therapy is vital to delaying disease progression
     d. Antibiotic prophylaxis for opportunistic infections is started when CD4 count <200; opportunistic infections treated as they occur
        (1) Trimethoprim-sulfamethoxazole (TMP-SMX) for *Pneumocystis carinii* pneumonia (PCP) and toxoplasmosis
        (2) Clarithromycin or azithromycin for *Mycobacterium avis* complex (MAC)
        (3) Isoniazid when close contacts have tuberculosis
     e. Close following of serology is important for dictating the direction of care
     f. Pregnant mothers with HIV should be treated to keep viral load low and should be given zidovudine during labor; newborns to HIV-positive mothers should be given zidovudine for six weeks after birth and should be tested for presence of virus (anti-HIV antibodies will always be present in these children) in initial six months of life

TABLE 6-7 Common Opportunistic Infections, Neoplasms, and Complications Seen in AIDS

Condition/Infection	When Seen	H/P	Diagnosis	Treatment
Candida esophagitis	CD4 <100	Dysphagia, **odynophagia**	Endoscopy with biopsy	Fluconazole, ketoconazole
Infectious diarrhea (bacterial, parasitic, viral)	Up to **60%** of patients	Prolonged diarrhea (presentation varies with etiology)	Stool culture, parasite evaluation, *Clostridium difficile* toxin test	Depends on etiology (see Chapter 3, GI Disorders)
Bacterial pneumonia (*S. pneumoniae, H. influenzae*)	CD4 <500	**Rapid onset,** productive cough, high fevers	Gram stain, lobar consolidation on CXR	Cephalosporins
Pneumocystis carinii pneumonia (PCP)	CD4 <200	**Gradual onset, nonproductive cough,** dyspnea on exertion, fever	Bilateral infiltrates on CXR, increased LDH, sputum Gram stain	TMP-SMX, corticosteroids
Tuberculosis	CD4 <500, high risk populations (e.g., crowded living, prisons)	Cough, night sweats, weight loss, fever	**Acid-fast bacilli,** cavitary defects and hilar adenopathy on CXR, positive PPD (must be checked with anergy test)	Isoniazid, rifampim, pyrazinamide, ethambutol
Cryptococcal meningitis	CD4 <100	Headache, neck stiffness, fever, mental status changes	Elevated pressure on lumbar puncture, **yeast seen with India ink** stain of CSF, **positive cryptococcal antigen** in CSF or serum	Amphotericin B, fluconazole
Cerebral toxoplasmosis	CD4 <100	Headache, confusion, possible **focal neurologic symptoms**	**Positive *toxoplasma* IgG antibody,** ring-enhancing lesions on CT or MRI	Pyrimethamine, sulfadiazine, clindamycin **(chronic treatment may be needed)**
Lymphoma (frequently in CNS)	**CD4 <50**	Headache, confusion, possible **focal neurologic symptoms**	CT or MRI shows lesion	Chemotherapy, radiation
AIDS dementia	CD4 <200	Confusion, mental status changes, **generalized neurologic symptoms** including tremor	History of declining mental function, generalized neurological symptoms, elevated β-2 microglobulin in CSF, cerebral atrophy on CT or MRI	May improve with antiretroviral therapy
Cytomegalovirus (CMV)	**CD4 <50**	**Vision loss,** esophagitis, diarrhea	Viral titer, yellow infiltrates with hemorrhage on fundoscopic exam	Ganciclovir, foscarnet
Mycobacterium avium complex (MAC)	**CD4 <50**	Fatigue, weight loss, fever, diarrhea, abdominal pain, lymphadenopathy, hepatosplenomegaly	Blood cultures	Clarithromycin, azithromycin, ethambutol, rifabutin, rifampin
Kaposi's sarcoma	CD4 <500	**Purple subcutaneous nodules** on face, chest, or extremities	Biopsy of lesions	Chemotherapy, radiation, α-interferon
Herpes zoster/simplex	CD4 <500	Shingles, oral or genital lesions	Tzanck smear, viral culture	Acyclovir, foscarnet

CNS, central nervous system; CSF, cerebral spinal fluid; CT, computed tomography; CXR, chest x-ray; GI, gastrointestinal; H/P, history and physical; LDH, lactate dehydrogenase; MRI, magnetic resonance imaging; PPD, purified protein derivative of tuberculin; TMP-SMX, trimethoprim-sulfamethoxazole.

FIGURE 6-5 Serologic profile of HIV infection.

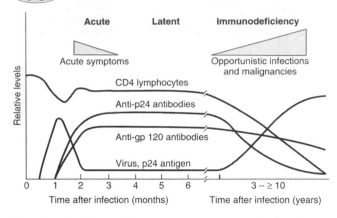

Note: p24 and gp 120 are viral proteins that serve as markers for HIV infection.

(Taken from Mehta S, Milder EA, Mirachi AJ, Milder E. *Step-Up: A High-Yield, Systems-Based Review for the USMLE Step 1.* 2nd Ed. Philadelphia: Lippincott Williams & Wilkins; 2003.)

10. **Complications** = opportunistic infections, neoplasms, cardiomyopathy, neuropathy, arthritis, polymyositis, anemia; while several advancements in treatment have been made, no cure or effective vaccine has been developed

VI. Hematological neoplastic conditions
A. Polycythemia vera
1. Myeloproliferative disorder of bone marrow stem cells leading to **increased production** of RBCs, WBCs, and platelets
2. Tends to occur after age 60; many progress to leukemia
3. **H/P** = fatigue, headache, **pruritus** (especially after contact with warm water), tinnitus, blurred vision, epistaxis; **splenomegaly,** hepatomegaly, large retinal veins on fundoscopic exam

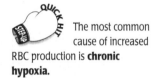

The most common cause of increased RBC production is **chronic hypoxia.**

TABLE 6-8 **Antiviral Medications Used in Treatment of HIV**

Drug Class	Examples of Drug	Mechanism	Adverse Effects
Nucleoside reverse transcriptase inhibitors	Abacavir (ABC) didanosine (ddI) lamivudine (3TC) zidovudine (AZT)	Inhibit production of viral genome, prevent incorporation of viral DNA into host genome through reverse transcriptase inhibition	Some have risk of bone marrow toxicity, neuropathy, pancreatitis, or hypersensitivity
Non-nucleoside reverse transcriptase inhibitors	delavirdine (DLV) efavirenz (EFV) nevirapine (NVP)	Inhibit reverse transcriptase activity to prevent viral replication	Possible hepatic toxicity, neurologic effects, rash
Protease inhibitors	indinavir (IDV) nelfinavir (NFV) ritonavir (RTV)	Interferes with viral replication to cause production of nonfunctional viruses	Hyperglycemia, hypertriglyceridemia, drug interactions, lipodystrophy
Combination agents	Combivir Trizivir	Combines multiple medications into same pill; ideal to reduce confusion of dosing schedules or to improve compliance	Consistent with component drugs

4. **Labs = increased Hgb, increased Hct,** increased RBC mass, increased or normal WBCs and platelets, decreased erythropoietin; biopsy shows hypercellular marrow

5. **Treatment** = serial phlebotomy, antihistamines (for pruritus), ASA (thrombus prophylaxis), hydroxyurea (bone marrow suppression)

6. **Complications** = thrombus formation, **leukemia** (acute and chronic myelogenous), stroke

B. **Multiple myeloma**

1. Malignant proliferation of **plasma cells;** increased incidence with prior monoclonal gammopathy of undetermined significance (MGUS)

2. Abnormal monoclonal protein (**M protein**) produced from IgG and IgA heavy chains, and κ and λ light chains (these light chains are known as **Bence Jones proteins**)

3. **H/P = bone pain,** weakness, weight loss, constipation, **pathologic fractures,** frequent infections; pallor, bone tenderness

4. **Labs** = decreased Hgb, decreased Hct, decreased WBCs, increased BUN and creatinine (secondary to renal insufficiency); serum protein electrophoresis (SPEP) and urine protein electrophoresis (UPEP) detect high M protein and Bence Jones proteins; bone marrow biopsy shows increased plasma cells

5. **Radiology = "punched-out"** lesions in long bones and skull

6. **Treatment** = radiation, chemotherapy, bone marrow transplant, repair of fractures, treat infections

7. **Complications** = renal failure, recurrent infections, hypercalcemia; poor prognosis with survival for 2–3 years after diagnosis

C. **Lymphoma (see Table 6-9)**

1. Malignant transformation of lymphocytes primarily in **lymph nodes** that may also involve bloodstream or nonlymphatic organs

2. Categorized as Hodgkin's and non-Hodgkin's variants

D. **Leukemia**

1. Malignant transformation of myeloid or lymphoid cells involving bloodstream and bone marrow

2. **Acute** leukemia tends to involve immature cells while **chronic** leukemia involves more mature cells

3. Bone marrow involvement may cause pancytopenia

4. **Acute lymphocytic leukemia** (ALL)

   a. **Most common in children** (3–7 years old); whites >African Americans

   b. Proliferation of cells of **lymphoid** origin (lymphocytes)

   c. **H/P = bone pain,** frequent infections, fatigue, dyspnea on exertion, easy bruising; fever, pallor, purpura, hepatosplenomegaly, lymphadenopathy

   d. **Labs** = decreased Hgb, decreased Hct, decreased platelets, decreased WBCs, increased uric acid, increased LDH; bone marrow biopsy shows **abundant blasts;** Philadelphia chromosome (translocation of chromosomes 9 and 22) found in 15% **adult** cases

   e. **Blood smear** = numerous blasts (Color Figure 6-11)

   f. **Treatment** = chemotherapy, bone marrow transplant

   g. **Complications** = while cure rates are good (60–85%) in children, adults have worse prognosis; presence of Philadelphia chromosome carries poor prognosis

5. **Acute myelogenous leukemia** (AML)

   a. Proliferation of **myeloid** cells; both children and adults affected

   b. **H/P** = fatigue, easy bruising, dyspnea on exertion, frequent infections; fever, pallor, hepatosplenomegaly

ALL is the **most common cancer** in **children.**

Most ALL originates in **B cells.**

TABLE 6-9	Characteristics of Hodgkin's and Non-Hodgkin's Lymphomas	
Characteristic	**Hodgkin's Lymphoma**	**Non-Hodgkin's Lymphoma**
Cells of origin	Macrophages	Lymphocytes (**most commonly B cells**)
Classification (low to higher grade)	Lymphocytic (rare, best prognosis), mixed cellularity (**most common**), nodular sclerosis (**women,** fibrosis of lymph nodes), lymphocytic depletion (rare, worst prognosis)	Small lymphocytic (B cells, indolent), follicular small cell (B cells, most common, chromosomes 14 and 18 translocation), large cell (B cells), lymphoblastic (**T cells,** children), Burkitt's (**EBV-related,** chromosomes 8 and 14 translocation), cutaneous T cell (skin lesions)
Risk factors, patient population	20–40 yr old or >60 yr old	EBV, HIV, <65 yr old
H/P	Painless lymphadenopathy (**neck**), weight loss, pruritus, night sweats, fever, hepatosplenomegaly	Painless lymphadenopathy (**generalized**), weight loss, fever, night sweats
Labs	Lymph node biopsy shows **Reed-Sternberg cells** (Color Figure 6-10)	Lymph node or bone marrow biopsy shows lymphocyte proliferation (**cleaved cells in follicular small cell variant**)
Treatment	Radiation, chemotherapy	Palliative radiation, chemotherapy
Prognosis	**Good,** 80% cure rate unless far-progressed	**Poor** (months for aggressive types, years for less aggressive variants)

EBV, Epstein-Barr virus; H/P, history and physical.

    c. **Labs** = decreased Hgb, decreased Hct, decreased platelets, decreased WBCs; bone marrow biopsy shows **blasts** and staining with **myeloperoxidase** and **para-aminosalicylic acid**

    d. **Blood smear** = large myeloblasts with **notched nuclei** and **Auer rods** (Color Figure 6-12)

    e. **Treatment** = chemotherapy, retinoic acid, bone marrow transplant

    f. **Complications** = relapse common, DIC; long-term survival is poor despite frequently successful remissions

6. **Chronic lymphocytic leukemia** (CLL)

    a. Proliferation of **mature B cells** in patients >65 years old

    b. **H/P** = fatigue, frequent infection (secondary to no plasma cells); lymphadenopathy, hepatosplenomegaly

    c. **Labs** = increased WBCs; bone marrow shows lymphocyte infiltration

    d. **Blood smear** = numerous small lymphocytes, **smudge cells** (Color Figure 6-13)

    e. **Treatment** = supportive therapy, chemotherapy, radiation, splenectomy, leukophoresis

    f. **Complications** = malignant B cells may form autoantibodies, leading to severe hemolytic anemia; poor prognosis with mean six-year survival

Patients with CLL are frequently asymptomatic and are commonly diagnosed following a workup for an abnormal CBC performed for an unrelated reason.

HEMATOLOGY AND ONCOLOGY

7. **Chronic myelogenous leukemia** (CML)
   a. Proliferation of **mature myeloid** cells seen in middle-aged adults; may be associated with radiation exposure
   b. Follows stable course for several years before progressing into **blast crisis** (rapid worsening of neoplasm) that is usually fatal
   c. **H/P** = possibly asymptomatic prior to progression; fatigue, weight loss, night sweats; fever, splenomegaly; blast crisis presents with worsening symptoms and bone pain
   d. **Labs** = increased WBCs, increased uric acid, increased vitamin B_{12}, positive **Philadelphia chromosome,** decreased leukocyte alkaline phosphatase
   e. **Treatment** = chemotherapy, bone marrow transplant, palliative therapy with α-interferon or hydroxyurea
   f. **Complications** = blast crisis signals rapid progression and is usually fatal
8. **Hairy cell leukemia**
   a. Proliferation of B cells most frequently in middle-aged men
   b. May appear similar to CLL; carries better prognosis than CLL
   c. **H/P** = fatigue, frequent infections; splenomegaly, **no lymphadenopathy**
   d. **Labs** = decreased Hgb, Hct, platelets, and WBCs (rarely WBCs increased); bone marrow biopsy shows lymphocyte infiltration
   e. **Blood smear** = numerous lymphocytes with **"hairy"** projections
   f. **Treatment** = chemotherapy

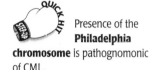

Presence of the **Philadelphia chromosome** is pathognomonic of CML.

VII. Oncologic therapy

A. **Treatment strategy**
   1. **Eradication** of neoplastic cells is ultimate goal
   2. When eradication is not possible, therapy seeks to **delay disease progression** or serve **palliative** role
   3. Mass effect of tumors and paraneoplastic syndromes may cause effects that are treated with surgery, radiation, or chemotherapy to relieve symptoms even when overall prognosis is bleak

B. **Cancer surgery**
   1. Performed to **reduce mass** of solid tumors or **remove** well-contained tumors
   2. Removal of substantial surrounding tissue frequently performed to increase chances of removing microscopic extensions of tumor
   3. Many procedures carry significant morbidities and prolonged recoveries due to size of surgery or organ removal (e.g., Whipple procedure for pancreatic cancer, gastrectomy for gastric cancer)

C. **Radiation therapy**
   1. Performed to **necrose** tumor cells and **decrease tumor size**
   2. May be curative in some cancers (some head and neck tumors); serves palliative role in several cases (e.g., Pancoast tumor)
   3. Adverse effects include impaired surgical wound healing, fibrosis of tissue, skin irritation, esophagitis, gastritis, pneumonitis, neurologic deficits, and bone marrow suppression
   4. May be related to later development of certain cancers (e.g., thyroid, CML)

D. **Chemotherapy**
   1. Aims to eradicate smaller populations of neoplastic cells and destroy cells not removed through surgery or radiation
   2. May sensitize neoplastic cells to radiation therapy (i.e., radiosensitizers)
   3. May be primary treatment modality in certain cancers particularly receptive to pharmacological therapy

TABLE 6-10 **Common Chemotherapeutic Drugs**

Drug Class	Mechanism	Applications	Adverse Effects
Nitrogen mustard alkylating agents (cyclophosphamide, chlorambucil, ifosfamide, mechlorethamine)	React with nucleophiles to form free radicals and alkylate DNA, RNA, and proteins; activity interferes with replication and transcription and results in cytotoxic effects; activity not cell cycle specific	HL, NHL, CLL, multiple myeloma, small cell lung cancer, breast cancer, ovarian cancer, cervical cancer, testicular cancer, sarcomas	Bone marrow suppression, alopecia, nausea, vomiting, infertility, rash, hemorrhagic cystitis, CNS toxicity
Nitrosourea alkylating agents (carmustine, streptozocin)	Similar to nitrogen mustards	Brain cancer, HL, multiple myeloma, renal cell cancer, pancreatic endocrine cancers, carcinoid tumors	Bone marrow suppression, nausea, vomiting, GI ulcers, hepatotoxicity, glucose intolerance
Alkyl sulfonate alkylating agents (busulfan)	Similar to nitrogen mustards	CML	Bone marrow suppression, infertility, skin pigmentation, pulmonary fibrosis
Ethyleneimine/ methylmelamine alkylating agents (thiotepa, hexamethylmelamine)	Similar to nitrogen mustards	Bladder cancer, breast cancer, ovarian cancer, endometrial cancer, cervical cancer, small cell lung cancer	Bone marrow suppression, infertility, nausea, vomiting, neurotoxicity
Triazene alkylating agents (dacarbazine)	Similar to nitrogen mustards	Melanoma, sarcomas, HL	Bone marrow suppression, fatigue, nausea, vomiting
Vinca alkaloids (etoposide, vinblastine, vincristine)	Interact with spindle proteins to stop cellular mitosis	Testicular cancer, small cell and non-small cell lung cancers, HL, NHL, testicular cancer, renal cell cancer, ALL	Leukopenia, anorexia, nausea, vomiting, diarrhea, bone marrow suppression, neurotoxicity, alopecia
Antibiotics (bleomycin, dactinomycin, daunorubicin, doxorubicin, mitomycin)	Inhibit DNA and RNA synthesis; affect multiple cell stages	NHL, HL, AML, ALL, testicular cancer, cervical cancer, breast cancer, choriocarcinoma, sarcomas, Wilm's tumor, gastric cancer, thyroid cancer, pancreatic cancer, colon cancer, lung cancer	Hypersensitivity, pulmonary fibrosis, alopecia, bone marrow suppression, nausea, vomiting, cardiomyopathy, infertility, renal toxicity, hepatotoxicity
Antimetabolites (cytarabine, 5-flurouracil, methotrexate, mercaptopurine)	Interfere with enzyme regulation or DNA and RNA activity; function during S phase of cell cycle	NHL, AML, ALL, CML (blast crisis), breast cancer, gastric cancer, colon cancer, pancreatic cancer, head/neck cancers, esophageal cancer, basal cell carcinoma, choriocarcinoma, bladder cancer, osteosarcoma	Bone marrow suppression, anorexia, hepatotoxicity, cerebellar dysfunction, cardiac ischemia, GI ulceration, nausea, diarrhea, desquamation of hands and feet, alopecia, neurotoxicity
Platinum analogues (carboplatin, cisplatin)	Cross-link DNA and cytoplasmic proteins to decrease activity	Testicular cancer, ovarian cancer, head/neck cancers, lung cancer, bladder cancer, cervical cancer, esophageal cancer	Vomiting, myelosuppression, renal toxicity, ototoxicity, neurotoxicity, alopecia
Steroid hormones and antagonists (prednisone, tamoxifen, estrogens, leuprolide)	Hormones or their removal may induce tumor remission	ALL, HL, NHL, estrogen-sensitive breast cancer, prostate cancer	Cushing's syndrome, cataracts, adrenal insufficiency upon discontinuation, nausea, vomiting, rash, vaginal bleeding, hot flashes, thrombus formation, hypercalcemia, stroke, MI, gynecomastia, impotence
Procarbazine	Inhibits DNA and RNA synthesis	Hodgkin's and non-Hodgkin's lymphomas	Bone marrow suppression, nausea, vomiting, diarrhea, neurotoxicity
Paclitaxel	Binds to spindle proteins to induce polymerization and cause cell death	Ovarian cancer, breast cancer, small cell lung cancer, head/neck cancers	Hypersensitivity, neutropenia, neurotoxicity

ALL, acute lymphocytic leukemia; AML, acute myelogenous leukemia; CLL, chronic lymphocytic leukemia; CML, chronic myelogenous leukemia; CNS, central nervous system; GI, gastrointestinal; HL, Hodgkin's lymphoma; MI, myocardial infarction; NHL, non-Hodgkin's lymphoma.
Do not memorize the table of chemotherapeutic drugs because this is not a high-yield study plan. Focus on the common mechanisms, uses, and adverse effects of the various drug classes and remember that multiple drugs are frequently used simultaneously to treat a given condition.

4. **Multiple drugs** with different cell cycle-specific targets are frequently combined to increase neoplastic cell death while minimizing toxicity to normal tissues, to have an effect against a broader range of cells, and to slow development of resistance
5. Adverse effects include cancer resistance and toxic effects against healthy cells

VIII. Other pediatric hematological and oncologic concerns (not addressed in other sections)

A. **Hemolytic disease of the newborn**
1. If Rh^+ fetal cells enter circulation of Rh^- mother, **anti-Rh antibodies** may develop
2. Antibodies do not affect pregnancy with initial Rh interaction but cause severe fetal RBC hemolysis in subsequent pregnancies with Rh^+ fetuses (fetal hydrops)
3. **Risk factors** = Rh^- mother with abortion, amniocentesis, or third-trimester bleeding
4. Hemolysis will likely cause death of fetus
5. **Treatment** = administration of Rho(D) immune globulin (**RhoGAM**) with 72 hours of delivery of initial Rh^+ fetus or at any time maternal and fetal blood may have mixed will prevent development of anti-Rh antibodies and protect future pregnancies by suppressing maternal formation of anti-Rh antibodies; transfusion may be required if condition develops in newborn

B. **Fanconi anemia**
1. Autosomal recessive disorder with **bone marrow failure** and pancytopenia
2. **H/P** = fatigue, dyspnea on exertion, frequent infections; frequently associated with **short stature, abnormal skin pigmentation,** horseshoe kidney, and bone abnormalities
3. **Labs** = decreased Hgb, Hct, platelets, and WBCs; bone marrow biopsy shows hypocellularity; chromosome analysis detects multiple strand breakages
4. **Treatment** = antibiotics, transfusions, bone marrow transplant; androgens and corticosteroids may increase bone marrow activity
5. **Complications** = death in childhood is common

C. **Diamond-Blackfan anemia**
1. Congenital **pure RBC anemia**
2. **H/P** = fatigue, dyspnea, cyanosis, and pallor detected early in life; occasionally associated with renal and bone abnormalities
3. **Labs** = decreased Hgb, decreased Hct, decreased reticulocyte count, increased MCV; bone marrow biopsy shows decreased activity but increased presence of erythropoietin
4. **Treatment** = transfusions, corticosteroids, bone marrow transplant

D. **Neuroblastoma**
1. Tumors of neural crest cell origin that may arise in adrenal glands or sympathetic ganglia
2. **Risk factors** = neurofibromatosis, tuberous sclerosis, pheochromocytoma, Beckwith-Wiedemann syndrome
3. **H/P** = abdominal distention, weight loss, malaise, bone pain, diarrhea; abdominal mass, HTN, possible Horner's syndrome, movement disorders, hepatomegaly, fever, periorbital bruising
4. **Labs** = possible increased vanillylmandelic and homovanillic acids in 24-hour urine collection
5. **Radiology** = CT may locate adrenal or ganglion tumor

Prognosis for neuroblastoma is good if diagnosed before one year old.

Rhabdomyosarcoma is the **most common soft tissue sarcoma** in children.

6. **Treatment** = surgical resection, chemotherapy, radiation
7. **Complications** = poor prognosis if presenting after two years old; metastasizes to bone and brain

E. **Rhabdomyosarcoma**
   1. Tumor of striated muscle in children
   2. **H/P** = painful soft tissue mass with swelling; large tumors frequently cause mass effect on nearby structures
   3. **Labs** = biopsy is diagnostic
   4. **Radiology** = CT or MRI, shows extent of tumor
   5. **Treatment** = surgical debulking, radiation, chemotherapy

Selected Topics in Emergency Medicine, Critical Care, and Surgery

● EMERGENCY MEDICINE

I. Accidents and injury

A Burns

1. Injury to epithelial surface and deeper tissues due to exposure to significant heat or radiation, caustic chemicals, or electrical shock

2. Classified by depth of involvement
   a. **1st degree**—epidermis only involved
   b. **2nd degree**—partial-thickness dermal involvement
   c. **3rd degree**—full-thickness dermal involvement

3. Extent of burns are estimated by "rule of 9s"

4. H/P = dependent upon degree:
   a. 1st- and 2nd-degree burns have erythema and are painful; blisters are also seen in 2nd-degree burns
   b. 3rd-degree burns are painless and skin appears charred, leathery, or gray
   c. Electrical burns may appear like 3rd-degree burns, may show severe damage at entrance and exit sites of electrical current, and may have cardiac and neurologic symptoms (ventricular fibrillation, seizures, loss of vision)

5. Treatment =
   a. **Outpatient** treatment is sufficient for **1st degree** and minor 2nd-degree burns
   b. **Inpatient** treatment required for **2nd-degree** burns >10% body surface area, **3rd-degree** burns >2% body surface area; or 2nd- and 3rd-degree burns affecting face, hands, genitalia, or major skin flexion creases
   c. 2nd- and 3rd-degree burns >25% body surface area or involving the face require **airway management** (frequently intubation), IV fluids, and careful control of body temperature (increased risk of hypothermia)

Burns secondary to **electrical shock** are sometimes called 4th-degree burns because they may involve muscles, bones, and other internal structures.

STEP Determine IV fluid resuscitation need with **Parkland's formula:** lactated Ringer's solution given in total volume of [**(2–4 mL)** × **(kg body weight)** × **(% body surface area burned)**]. Half of volume is given during the initial 8 hours, and the remaining half is given over the following 16 hours.

FIGURE 7-1 "Rule of 9s" for calculating extent of burns. The surface anatomy of body is divided into sections of 9% body surface area (genitals are considered 1% surface area).

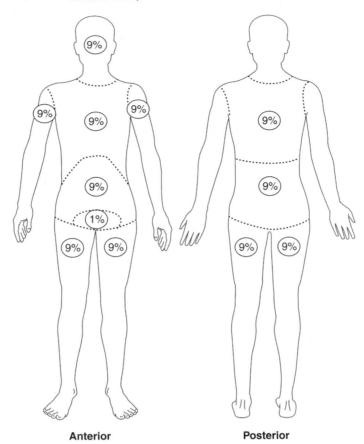

Anterior   Posterior

   d. Patients with significant **smoke inhalation** (diagnosed by increased carboxyhemoglobin levels) should receive high-flow O_2 and close monitoring for respiratory compromise requiring intubation
   e. Cardiac and neurologic issues in **electrical** burns should be managed to decrease mortality
   f. Nasogastric tube should be placed when there is gastrointestinal (GI) involvement
   g. Chemicals should be diluted or neutralized, and garments with any chemicals on them should be removed to prevent additional injury
   h. Generous use of analgesics and/or regional anesthesia for **pain control**
   i. **Antimicrobial agents** (topical silver sulfadiazine or bacitracin) should be used in dressings to decrease risk of infection, and tetanus toxin should be administered if immunization status unknown or not up to date
   j. Non-adherent bandaging or biologic dressings should be applied directly to severe burns; dressings should not be wrapped around affected areas because of potential swelling and constriction
   k. Surgical debridement and exploration should be performed to remove necrotic tissue and to determine extent of deeper tissue involvement; plastic reconstruction surgery may be needed
6. **Complications** =
   a. **Infection** (especially *Pseudomonas*, sepsis), stress ulcers (Curling's), aspiration, dehydration, ileus, renal insufficiency (due to

rhabdomyolysis), compartment syndrome, epithelial contractions (may limit range of motion)

   b. Electrical burns are associated with myocardial infarction (MI), cataracts, and seizures

   c. Risk factors for **mortality** may be defined as age >60 years, >40% body surface area involvement, and inhalation injury; patients carry a 0.3%, 3%, 33%, or 90% chance of death if they have 0, 1, 2, or 3 of these risk factors, respectively

B. Drowning

1. Hypoxemia resulting from **submersion** in some type of fluid, usually water
2. Fluid types
   a. **Fresh water**—hypotonic fluid is absorbed from alveoli into vasculature resulting in decreased electrolyte concentrations and red blood cell (RBC) lysis
   b. **Salt water**—hypertonic fluid creates an osmotic gradient that draws fluid from pulmonary capillaries into alveoli and causes **pulmonary edema** and increased serum electrolyte concentrations
   c. **Both** types of fluid cause **pulmonary damage** and **cerebral hypoxia**
3. H/P = prolonged submersion in liquid (pools, bathtubs, and buckets are frequent sites); cyanosis, decreased consciousness, patient may not be breathing or may have cardiac arrest
4. **Treatment** = secure airway and perform resuscitation; **supplemental O$_2$**, nasogastric tube placement, maintenance of adequate body temperature
5. **Complications** = correlate with degree and length of hypoxemia, and include brain damage and hypothermia

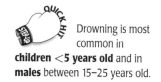

QUICK HIT

Drowning is most common in **children <5 years old** and in **males** between 15–25 years old.

C. Choking

1. **Aspiration of foreign body** into trachea or bronchi preventing normal gas exchange
2. Food is common cause in all ages; toys, coins, and other small objects are common in children
3. H/P = patient eating or child playing with small objects, gagging, coughing, or wheezing that progresses to stridor with increased severity of obstruction
4. **Radiology** = Chest x-ray (CXR) may be useful in identifying item and determining location; bronchoscopy may visualize item
5. **Treatment** =
   a. Actively coughing patients should be encouraged to remain calm and to keep coughing to dislodge object
   b. Patients unable to breathe should be given the **Heimlich maneuver**
   c. Emergent tracheotomy may be required in a patient with continued obstruction
   d. Bronchoscopy may be required to remove objects
7. **Complications** = atelectasis, pneumonia, lung abscess; hypoxemia may cause complications similar to those seen with drowning

QUICK HIT

The right middle bronchus is most common location of aspirated items that pass beyond the trachea because of its greater vertical orientation compared to the left main bronchus.

D. Heat emergencies (see Table 7-1)

1. **Exertional** disorders (due to **physical exertion**, not pathology innate to body) that result from elevated body temperature
2. Categorized as heat stroke or heat exhaustion

E. Hypothermia

1. Body temperature <**95° F** (35° C) due to cold exposure
2. **Risk factors** = alcohol intoxication, elderly
3. H/P = lethargy, weakness, severe shivering; decreased body temperature, possible arrhythmias
4. **Electrocardiogram (ECG)** = **J waves**, possible Vtach or Vfib

TABLE 7-1 Heat Emergencies due to Exertional Causes

Disorder	Heat Exhaustion	Heat Stroke
Symptoms	Weakness, headache, substantial sweating	Confusion, blurred vision, nausea, no sweating
Body temperature	Slightly increased	Substantially elevated
Labs	Usually normal	Increased WBC, increased BUN, increased creatinine
Treatment	Hydration (oral unless progressive symptoms), electrolyte replacement	Cool environment, spray patient with water and then fan
Complications	Progression to heat stroke	Rhabdomyolysis, seizures, brain damage, death

BUN, blood urea nitrogen; WBC, white blood cell count.

5. **Treatment** = warm patient externally (warm bed, bath, blankets) or internally (warm IV fluids or ingested fluids); treat arrhythmias as appropriate (see Chapter 1, Cardiovascular Disorders)

F. **Venomous bites and stings (see Table 7-2)**
   1. Injection of venom from bite or sting of snakes (in U.S.: rattlesnake, copperhead, water moccasin, coral snake), spiders (black widow, brown recluse), or other animal (e.g., scorpion)
   2. Venom contains neurotoxins, cardiotoxins, or proteolytic enzymes that can potentially be fatal

II. Toxicology

A. **General principles**
   1. Initial evaluation must focus on **determining type of poison ingested;** patient history, witness input, and clues found near patient (empty bottles of medications, other medications, etc.) help in making diagnosis
   2. The sooner treatment is begun after toxic exposure, the better the outcome
   3. Types of poisoning therapy
      a. Induced vomiting—only useful in initial 1–2 hours after ingestion and only for noncaustic agents; **rarely** used
      b. **Charcoal**—blocks absorption of poisons; repeat doses every few hours; not useful for alcohols or metals
      c. Gastric lavage—usually reserved for intubated patients within initial hour after ingestion

FIGURE 7-2 Diagram of electrocardiogram demonstrating a J wave (*arrow*), a characteristic finding in hypothermia.

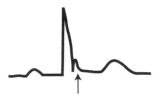

TABLE 7-2 Common Types of Venomous Bites and Stings

Type of Bite	Symptoms	Treatment	Complications
Snake (rattlesnake, copperhead, water moccasin, coral snake)	Pain and swelling at bite, progressive dyspnea, toxin-induced DIC	Antivenin	Effects more severe in children. Death in 6–8 hrs
Scorpion	Severe pain and swelling at bite, increased sweating, vomiting, diarrhea	Antivenin, atropine, phenobarbitol	Acute pancreatitis, myocardial toxicity, respiratory paralysis
Spider (black widow, brown recluse)	Abdominal pain, vomiting, jaundice, DIC	Black widow: calcium gluconate, methocarbamol; Brown recluse: dexamethasone, colchicines, dapsone	Brown recluse bites more severe DIC
Mammals	Pain and swelling at bite, penetrating trauma depending on size of bite	Saline irrigation, debridement, tetanus and rabies prophylaxis, antibiotics for infection	Infection (staphylococci, *Pasteurella multocida*, rabies virus)
Human	Pain and swelling at bite, tender local lymphadenopathy	Saline irrigation, broad coverage antibiotics, thorough documentation	High incidence of infection with primary closure or delayed presentation

DIC, disseminated intravascular coagulation.

d. **Antidotes**—reverse or inhibit poison activity; use is dependent upon identification of agent
e. Diuretics—may help in cases where increased urination helps remove toxin (salicylates, phenobarbitol)
f. Dialysis—used in cases of severe symptoms or when other treatments are unsuccessful

B. **Ingested poisons**
1. Poisoning through oral ingestion of a particular toxin
2. May occur in children from accidental ingestion of cleaning products, medications, or personal care products
3. May occur in elderly patients from accidental repeat dosing of usual medications
4. May be intentional (i.e., suicide attempt)

C. **Carbon monoxide poisoning**
1. Hypoxemia that results from inhalation of carbon monoxide from car fumes, smoke, or paint thinner
2. Carbon monoxide displaces O_2 on hemoglobin (Hgb) and prevents O_2 delivery to tissues
3. **H/P** = sufficient exposure, headache, dizziness, nausea, myalgias; generalized erythema, mental status changes, possible hypotension
4. **Labs** = increased carboxyhemoglobin
   Treatment = 100% O_2 (displaces carbon monoxide from Hgb); patients with smoke inhalation may require intubation secondary to upper airway edema

III. Cardiovascular emergencies

This section only discusses emergent cardiovascular conditions that require resuscitation and immediate treatment—refer to Chapters 1 and 8 on Cardiovascular and Neurologic Disorders for additional information regarding MI, arrhythmias, and stroke.

A. **Cardiac arrest**
1. Abnormal cardiac function resulting in acutely insufficient cardiac output

NEXT STEP Beware the alcohol abuser that comes into the emergency department **fictitiously** saying that he has ingested ethylene glycol and needs ethanol for treatment; check for sweet breath and a toxin screen before giving ethanol.

NEXT STEP Organophosphates may also be absorbed through the **skin,** so all contaminated clothing must be removed from patients with this type of poisoning.

NEXT STEP Any patient with significant **thermal burns,** burns of the **face,** exposure to large quantities of **smoke** (e.g., house fires) should be worked up for **carbon monoxide poisoning** and **thermal airway injury.**

QUICK HIT Pulse oximetry may appear **normal** in carbon monoxide poisoning.

TABLE 7-3 Common Poisons and Antidotes

Substance	Symptoms	Treatment
Drugs		
Acetaminophen	Nausea, hepatic insufficiency	N-acetylcysteine
Anticholinergics	Dry mouth, urinary retention, QRS widening on ECG	Physostigmine
Benzodiazepines	Sedation, respiratory depression	Flumazenil
β-Blockers	Bradycardia, hypotension, hypoglycemia, pulmonary edema	Glucagon, atropine
Cocaine	Tachycardia, agitation	Supportive care
Cyanide	Headache, nausea, vomiting, altered mental status	Nitrates, hydroxycobalamin
Digoxin	Nausea, vomiting, visual changes, arrhythmias	Digoxin antibodies
Heparin	Excessive bleeding, easy bruising	Protamine sulfate
Isopropyl alcohol	Decreased consciousness	Maintain respiratory function (intubation), supportive care
Methanol	Headache, visual changes, dizziness	Ethanol, dialysis
Opioids	Pinpoint pupils, respiratory depression	Naloxone
Salicylates	Nausea, vomiting, tinnitus, hyperventilation, anion gap metabolic acidosis	Charcoal, dialysis
Strychnine	Convulsions	Supportive care
Tricyclic antidepressants	Tachycardia, dry mouth, urinary retention, QRS widening on ECG	Sodium bicarbonate, diazepam
Warfarin	Excessive bleeding, easy bruising	Vitamin K, FFP
Industrial Chemicals		
Caustics (acids, alkali)	Severe oropharyngeal and gastric irritation or burns, drooling, odynophagia, abdominal pain, gastric perforation symptoms	Copious irrigation (do not induce emesis or attempt neutralization), activated charcoal
Ethylene glycol	Ataxia, hallucinations, seizures, sweet breath	Ethanol, dialysis
Organophosphates (insecticides, fertilizers)	Salivation, lacrimation, vomiting, diarrhea, increased urination, paralysis, decreased consciousness	Atropine, pralidoxime, supportive care
Metals		
Lead	Peripheral neuropathy, anemia	EDTA, dimercaprol
Mercury	Renal insufficiency, tremor, mental status changes	Dimercaprol

ECG, electrocardiogram; FFP, Fresh frozen plasma.

FIGURE
7-3

Initial treatment protocol for the unresponsive patient. CPR, cardiopulmonary resuscitation; EMS, emergency medical services; Vfib, ventricular fibrillation; Vtach, ventricular tachycardia.

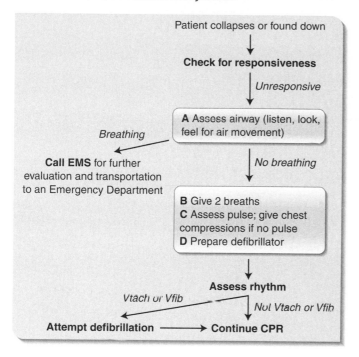

2. Requires immediate treatment to prevent ischemic morbidity and death
3. Strict application of the **ABCs** is needed to appropriately assess the unresponsive patient
4. Treatment of **Vfib** and **Vtach** requires alternating attempts at electrical and pharmacologic cardioversion
5. **Pulseless electrical activity** (PEA) consists of detectable cardiac electrical conduction with the absence of cardiac output
6. **Asystole** is the absence of cardiac activity

B. **Acute stroke (see Figure 7-7)**
1. Initial workup differentiates between embolic and hemorrhagic types
2. Appropriateness for anticoagulation and thrombolysis should be considered

IV. Traumatology
A. **Mechanisms of injury**
1. **Acceleration-deceleration injuries**
   a. Seen in falls, blunt trauma, and **motor vehicle accidents**
   b. Injury secondary to shearing forces in tissues and organs caused by sudden changes in momentum and sudden forces applied to tethered portions of organs (e.g., aortic arch, mesentery)
2. **Penetrating injuries**
   a. Include **gun shot wounds, stab wounds**
   b. Missile damages tissue in path of trajectory and causes indirect damage from fragmented bone and external objects

B. **Trauma assessment**
1. Patient assessment is performed in organized manner to detect all injuries and judge their severity
2. Initial assessment focuses on patient **ABCs**

 All cardiovascular emergency protocols are based on the **ABC** concept: **Airway, Breathing, Circulation.**

 Cardiac arrest lasting >10 min without cardiac output is generally considered consistent with severe brain injury or brain death.

 Do not resuscitate (DNR) status should be documented for any inpatient; documentation can be provided by a close relative or primary care provider to guide potential resuscitation attempts.

 For pulseless electrical activity, think **PEA**: **P**ulseless → **E**pinephrine and **A**tropine.

SELECTED TOPICS IN EMERGENCY MEDICINE, CRITICAL CARE, AND SURGERY

FIGURE 7-4 Treatment protocol for ventricular fibrillation or pulseless ventricular tachycardia. ABC, airway, breathing, circulation; CPR, cardiopulmonary resuscitation; IV, intravenous; Vfib, ventricular fibrillation; Vtach, ventricular tachycardia.

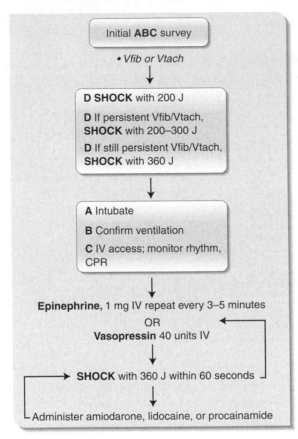

NEXT STEP Count and pair all entrance and exit gun shot wounds to suggest a number of insulting bullets and to deduce a path for each bullet.

NEXT STEP Address the ABCs and secondary survey **in order.** Do not proceed to the next step of the exam until the current segment has been addressed.

QUICK HIT Loss of consciousness is considered due to **head trauma** until ruled out.

QUICK HIT **Hypertension** with bradycardia is suggestive of increased intracranial pressure (Cushing's phenomenon).

NEXT STEP Rule out **cervical fracture** and **spinal cord injury** before performing any exam requiring head movement.

3. Secure **A**irway is established (may require intubation), oxygenation is stabilized (**B**reathing), adequate **C**irculation is confirmed, venous access is secured, and bleeding is controlled

4. Secondary assessment consists of a highly detailed exam to detect all wounds, fractures, signs of internal injury, and neurologic insult

5. Glasgow Coma Scale (GCS) and revised trauma score (RTS) are used to objectify injury severity

C. **Head trauma**

1. Head trauma may result in intracerebral or subarachnoid **hemorrhage** (see Chapter 8, Neurologic Disorders)

2. Cerebral damage may be at the point of insult (**coup**) or on the opposite side of the head (**contrecoup**)

3. H/P = evaluation should assess **level of consciousness**, sensation, motor activity, **pupil responsiveness to light** (nonresponsiveness or unequal response suggests cerebral injury), **oculocephalic reflex** (while head of unconscious patient is turned, patient's eyes normally remained fixed at a point in space [doll's eyes]; absence of this reflex in a comatose patient suggests vestibular, cranial nerve, pontine, or medullary injury), presence of skull fracture (discoloration over mastoid, blood draining from ears or nose), and intracranial pressure

4. **Radiology** = **CT** should be performed for any unconscious patient to detect intracranial hemorrhage; x-rays (anteroposterior, lateral, open-mouth odontoid) should be performed to detect skull or cervical fractures

FIGURE 7-5 Treatment protocol for pulseless electrical activity. ABC, airway, breathing, circulation; CAD, coronary artery disease; CPR, cardiopulmonary resuscitation; IV, intravenous; PE, pulmonary embolism; PTX, pneumothorax.

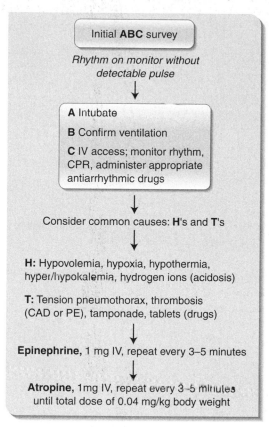

FIGURE 7-6 Treatment protocol for asystole. ABC, airway, breathing, circulation; CPR, cardiopulmonary resuscitation; IV, intravenous.

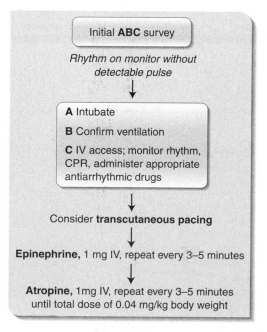

FIGURE 7-7 Treatment algorithm for suspected acute stroke. CT, computed tomography; ECG, electrocardiogram; IV, intravenous; LP, lumbar puncture; t-PA, tissue plasminogen activator.

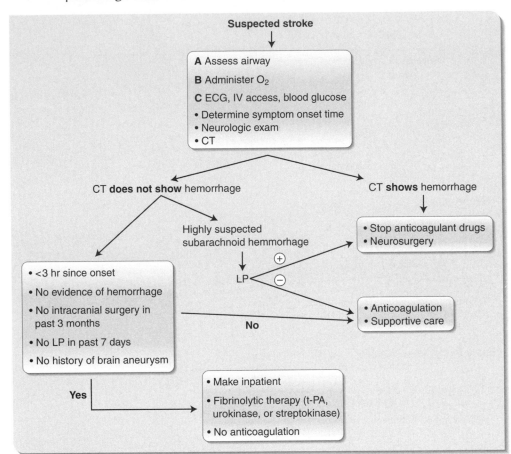

TABLE 7-4	Glasgow Coma Scale[a]	
Category	**Condition**	**Points**
Eye opening	Spontaneous	4
	To voice	3
	To pain	2
	None	1
Verbal response	Oriented	5
	Confused	4
	Inappropriate words	3
	Incomprehensible	2
	None	1
Motor response	Obeys commands	6
	Localizes pain	5
	Withdraws from pain	4
	Flexion with pain	3
	Extension with pain	2
	None	1

[a] Total score is calculated by adding component score for each category.
12+—minor brain injury with probable recovery
9–11—moderate severity requiring close observation for changes
8 or less—coma; ≤8 after 6 hours associated with 50% mortality

TABLE 7-5	Revised Trauma Score (RTS)[a]		
Coded Value[b]	Glasgow Coma Scale Score	Systolic Blood Pressure	Respiratory Rate
4	13–15	>89	10–29
3	9–12	76–89	>29
2	6–8	50–75	6–9
1	4–5	1–49	1–5
0	3	0	0

RTS, 0.9368 (GCS coded value) + 0.7326 (SBP coded value) + 0.2908 (RR coded value)

[a]RTS of 4 or greater is associated with 60% survival.
[b]Coded value is assigned to each measurement individually.
GCS, Glasgow Coma Scale; SBP, systolic blood pressure; RR, respiratory rate.

5. **Treatment** = maintain cerebral perfusion, decrease high intracranial pressure with mannitol, refer any intracranial injury to neurosurgery

D. **Spinal cord trauma** (see Chapter 8, Neurologic Disorders)
   1. Neurologic injury in any segment of spinal cord from trauma
   2. **H/P** = thorough **neurologic exam must** be performed to detect any deficits in sensation, motor activity, or autonomic function
   3. **Radiology** = x-ray should examine all cervical vertebrae and other vertebral sections of spine considered at risk for injury
   4. **Treatment** = spine must be stabilized until injury ruled out; injuries should be referred to orthopaedic surgery or neurosurgery

E. **Neck trauma**
   1. Neck is divided into **zones** based on anatomical site of injury; injury may involve trachea, esophagus, vascular structures, cervical spine, or spinal cord
   2. **H/P** = exam should focus on cervical neurologic deficits and signs of vascular damage in neck (hematoma, worsening mental status)
   3. **Radiology** = x-ray to assess cervical injury; esophagogastroduodenoscopy (EGD), angiography, and bronchoscopy used to evaluate penetrating injuries to zones I and III

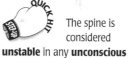 The spine is considered **unstable** in any **unconscious** patient and should not be moved until neurologic injury has been ruled out with exam and radiology.

FIGURE 7-8 Zones of the neck used to determine treatment for traumatic injury.

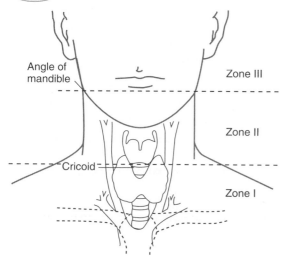

Angle of mandible

Zone III

Zone II

Cricoid

Zone I

4. **Treatment** =
   a. Trauma to **zones I or III** with stable vital signs may be treated **conservatively**
   b. Penetrating trauma to **zone II** should be **surgically explored**
   c. Intubation is frequently required because of airway occlusion

F. **Chest trauma**
   1. May result in injury to lungs, heart, or GI system
   2. Aortic rupture (due to sudden acceleration and deceleration), tension pneumothorax, hemothorax, and cardiac tamponade are potentially fatal injuries
   3. **H/P** = exam should look for signs of pneumothorax (hyperresonance, decreased breath sounds), flail chest (multiple rib fractures), **tamponade** (decreased breath sounds, jugular venous distention, and pulsus paradoxus), and aortic rupture (unstable vital signs); ECG and central venous pressure are useful in assessing cardiac function
   4. **Radiology** =
      a. CXR and neck x-rays may show pneumothorax, hemothorax, cardiac hemorrhage, aortic injury
      b. EGD and bronchoscopy are used to assess injury to esophagus and bronchi
      c. Angiography can detect vascular injury
   5. **Treatment** = urgent **thoracotomy** for thoracic cavity **hemorrhage**; **pericardiocentesis** for suspected cardiac **tamponade**; chest tube for pneumothorax or hemothorax

G. **Abdominal trauma**
   1. May cause injury to any abdominal organ or severe bleeding from the aorta, aortic branches, mesentery, spleen, or liver
   2. Penetrating trauma requires exploratory laparotomy; blunt trauma may be treated conservatively if there are no signs of an acute abdomen
   3. **H/P** =
      a. In cases where exploratory laparotomy is not automatically performed, exam must look for signs of **abdominal bleeding** (decreased blood pressure, cyanosis, anxiety, flank discoloration, severe abdominal tenderness, abdominal rigidity, shock)
      b. **Peritoneal lavage** (saline infused by catheter into abdominal cavity and then removed and examined) is useful for detecting presence of blood or fecal matter in uncertain cases
   4. **Radiology** =
      a. Abdominal radiograph may detect large abdominal collections of blood
      b. CT and is more sensitive for detecting abdominal fluid
      c. Focused abdominal sonography for trauma (**FAST**) is a quick and sensitive means of determining the presence of free abdominal fluid and solid organ injury and has become the primary test performed for evaluation of blunt abdominal trauma at most trauma centers
   5. **Treatment** =
      a. All **penetrating abdominal trauma** needs **exploratory laparotomy**
      b. Diagnosed **intra-abdominal bleeding** or visceral damage from blunt trauma requires **laparotomy** for repair
      c. **Retroperitoneal hematomas** in **upper** abdomen (pancreas, kidneys) require **laparotomy** for repair
      d. **Low retroperitoneal bleeding** should be treated with **angiography** and **embolization**

H. **Genitourinary and pelvic trauma**
   1. Injury may result from initial insult or indirectly from fracture of the pelvis

Sites of significant (>**1500 mL**) blood loss frequently not found by physical exam include blood left at the **injury scene, pleural cavity** bleeding (seen with CXR), **intra-abdominal** bleeding (seen with CT or US), **pelvic** bleeding (seen with CT), and bleeding into the **thighs** (seen on x-ray).

STEP
NEXT The **hemodynamically unstable** blunt trauma patient should be taken to the **operating room** and not to radiology.

2. **H/P =**
   a. Exam should look for blood at the **urethral meatus** or hematuria (indicative of urologic injury), "high-riding" prostate (urethral injury in men), or scrotal or penile hematoma
   b. Pelvic exam should be performed in women
   c. Patients with a **pelvis fracture** should be given a thorough **neurovascular exam**
3. **Radiology =**
   a. Intravenous pyelogram (IVP) can detect renal pelvis injury
   b. Retrograde urethrogram or cystogram can detect urethral or bladder injury
   c. X-ray can detect pelvis fracture
   d. CT can detect renal damage and pelvic blood collections
4. **Treatment =**
   a. **Penetrating** injuries need **surgical exploration**
   b. Urethral and renal pelvis injuries require cystoscopy and surgical repair; **bladder** and **renal parenchymal** injuries may be treated **nonoperatively**
   c. Pelvic fractures are repaired with intramedullary fixation

I. **Extremity trauma**
   1. Injury may involve **bones, vasculature, soft tissues,** or **nerves** in extremities
   2. **H/P =** a thorough **neurovascular exam** must be performed; gross deformities are indicative of fracture
   3. **Radiology =** x-ray detects fractures; angiography can detect vascular injury
   4. **Treatment =**
      a. Superficial or soft tissue wounds require irrigation and approximation (sutures, Steri-Strips®, dermatologic adhesive)
      b. Bone injury alone is treated with internal or external fixation
      c. Combined bone, vessel, and nerve injuries are treated by repair of fracture **followed** by vascular and neurologic repair
      d. Large wounds frequently require debridement or amputation

J. **Trauma during pregnancy**
   1. Leading cause of **nonobstetric** maternal death
   2. Anatomic differences
      a. Inferior vena cava (IVC) compression by uterus makes pregnant women more susceptible to **poor cardiac output** following injury
      b. Decreased risk of GI injury from lower abdominal trauma because of **superior displacement of bowel** by uterus (but greater risk of GI injury from upper abdominal or chest trauma)
   3. Low risk of fetal death with minor injuries (high risk in life-threatening injuries)
   4. Trauma increases the risk of **placental abruption**
   5. **H/P =** immediate assessment of cardiovascular stability, mother should be evaluated for injury **prior** to fetus, examination should be performed with mother in **left lateral decubitus position** to minimize IVC compression, obstetric assessment performed following maternal stabilization
   6. **Treatment =** needs of **mother** are **prioritized**, caesarian section should be performed for fetuses >24 weeks of gestation that are in **distress** or in any mother with **cardiovascular compromise** not responsive to early CPR, mother should be monitored for 4–48 hours (based on severity of trauma) to detect fetal distress, **RhoGAM®** should be given to any Rh⁻ mother with bleeding

A Foley catheter should **never** be placed in a patient with a **suspected urethral rupture** (e.g., blood seen at the urethral meatus) to avoid further urologic injury unless performed under cystoscopic guidance.

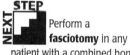
Perform a **fasciotomy** in any patient with a combined bone and neurovascular extremity injury because of the high risk of **compartment syndrome.**

V. Abuse and sexual assault

A. **Abuse**
1. Most frequently seen in children, spouses/partners (especially women), and the elderly
2. **Child** abuse
   a. **H/P** = **injury** may be **inconsistent** with **explanation** and multiple injuries may be evident; **well-defined burns** and **injuries to the back** are suggestive of abuse; depression, social withdrawal, low weight for age, or malnutrition are occasionally seen in children
   b. **Treatment** = physician has **obligation** to report any suspected cases of abuse to child protective services
   c. Suspected cases should be **well documented**
3. **Spousal/partner abuse**
   a. **H/P** = **history** may be **inconsistent** with **injury**; patients are frequently depressed; partner may be very attentive or vigilant during visit
   b. Patient should be interviewed **without** partner present
   c. **Treatment** = provide victim with information on safety plans, escape strategies, legal rights, and shelters; care should be taken not to force victim into any action
4. **Elder abuse**
   a. Occurs when elderly live with younger relatives or friends
   b. **H/P** = multiple bruises or fractures, malnutrition, depression, or **signs of neglect**
   c. **Treatment** = physician has **obligation** to report suspected cases to an official state agency

B. **Sexual assault**
1. **Nonconsensual** sexual activity with physical contact; forced intercourse is **rape**
2. Victims may be children or adults
3. **H/P** =
   a. **Detailed history** must be collected and thoroughly documented in cases where patient reports assault
   b. Exam should focus on entire body with particular attention to genitals, anus, and mouth to look for signs of assault
   c. Patients who have not admitted to being assaulted may appear depressed or very uncomfortable with examination
4. **Labs** =
   a. Collect oral, vaginal, and penile cultures to test for sexually transmitted diseases
   b. In cases of rape, all injuries must be well documented and vaginal fluid and pubic hair should be collected for evidence (i.e., rape kit)
   c. Pregnancy testing should be performed to look for incidental conception occurring during assault
5. **Treatment** = referral to **social support systems** and **counseling** is very important; appropriate treatment should be given for infections

QUICK HIT

Another healthcare worker (chaperone) must be present when a sexual examination is performed, and the patient should be made to feel as comfortable as possible with the history and physical exam.

● BASIC CRITICAL CARE

I. Issues in the intensive care unit (ICU)

A. **Role of the ICU**
1. Provides intensive nursing care for **critically ill patients**
2. Patients may require intubation, ventilation, **invasive monitoring**, **vasoactive** and antiarrhythmic medications, and close nursing supervision
B. **Pulmonary concerns**
1. **Intubation** and **ventilation** required when patient at risk for airway obstruction or needs support in breathing

2. Ventilator support is required in patients to maintain respiratory effort or in poor-oxygenation states (see Chapter 2, Pulmonary Disorders)

C. **Invasive monitoring**

1. **Arterial line** (A-line)

    a. Placed in either radial, femoral, axillary, or brachial artery

    b. Used to record more accurate blood pressure than blood pressure cuff

2. **Pulmonary artery catheter** (Swan-Ganz catheter)

    a. Catheter inserted through subclavian or jugular vein; runs through heart to pulmonary artery

    b. Measures pressures in **right atrium** and **pulmonary** artery; balloon may be inflated at catheter tip to measure wedge pressure (equivalent to **left atrium pressure**)

    c. Also may measure **cardiac output**, mixed venous O_2 saturation, systemic vascular resistance

II. Hemodynamic stability

A. **Transfusions**

1. Infusion of blood products to treat insufficient supply of a given blood component

2. ABO blood groups

    a. Blood is defined by **A** and **B** antigens and antibodies to absent antigens

    b. Blood with **both** antigens **will not have antibodies** to either antigen in plasma (i.e., AB blood type)

    c. Blood with **neither** antigen will have **antibodies to both** antigens in plasma (i.e., O blood type)

    d. Transfusions must be matched for each patient's particular ABO blood type

TABLE 7-6 Types of Blood Products Used in Transfusions

Blood Product	Definition	Indications
Whole blood	Donor blood not separated into components (full volume blood)	Rarely used except for massive transfusions for severe blood loss
Packed RBCs	RBCs separated from other donor blood components (2/3 volume of transfusion unit is RBCs)	Product of choice for treatment of low Hct due to blood loss or anemia
Autologous blood	Blood donated by patient prior to elective surgery or other treatment. Blood is frozen until needed by patient	Elective surgery or chemotherapy
FFP	Plasma from which RBCs have been separated	Warfarin overdose, clotting factor deficiency, DIC, TTP
Cryoprecipitate	Clotting factor and vWF-rich precipitate collected during thawing of FFP. Smaller volume than FFP	Same indications as FFP. Preferable to FFP in cases where large transfusion volume is unwanted
Platelets	Platelets separated from other plasma components	Thrombocytopenia not due to rapid platelet destruction
Clotting factors	Concentrations of a specific clotting factor pooled from multiple donors	Specific clotting factor deficiencies (e.g., hemophiliac)

DIC, disseminated intravascular coagulation; Hct, hematocrit; FFP, Fresh frozen plasma; RBCs, red blood cells; TTP, thrombotic thrombocytopenic purpura; vWf, von Willebrand factor.

TABLE 7-7 Vasopressors Commonly Used in the Intensive Care Unit

Drug	Mechanism	Effects	Indication
Phenylephrine	Agonist for α-adrenergic receptors ($\alpha_1 > \alpha_2$)	Vasoconstriction, reflex bradycardia	SVT, shock
Norepinephrine	Agonist primarily for α-adrenergic receptors	Vasoconstriction	Shock
Epinephrine	Agonist for both α- and β-adrenergic receptors; α effects (vasoconstriction) predominate at high doses	Increased heart rate and contractility (increased CO), vasoconstriction, bronchodilation	Bronchospasm, **anaphylactic** shock
Dopamine	Agonist for β_1-adrenergic receptors (low dose) and α adrenergic receptors (high dose); binding with dopaminergic receptors causes **renal vascular vasodilation**	Increased heart rate and contractility (increased CO), vasoconstriction (high dose only), increased renal blood flow	**Shock** (renal sparing)
Dobutamine	Agonist for β_1-adrenergic receptors	Increased heart rate and contractility (increased CO)	**CHF,** insufficient CO
Isoproterenol	Agonist for β-adrenergic receptors	Increased heart rate and contractility (increased CO), bronchodilation	Contractility stimulant in cardiac arrest

CHF, congestive heart failure; CO, cardiac output; SVT, supraventricular tachycardia.

 AB+ patients are **"universal recipients;"** they can **receive any** donor blood type because they have no antibodies to blood antigens in their plasma but can **only donate** to other **AB+** patients.

 O− patients are **"universal donors."** RBCs from these patients will not induce antibody reactions in other patients but can **only receive** blood from other **O−** donors.

 Clerical errors are the most common cause of transfusion reactions.

3. **Rh blood groups**
   a. Patient will either have Rh antigen (Rh+) or will not (Rh−)
   b. **Rh−** patients have **antibodies to Rh factor** in plasma
   c. Transfusions must be matched for each patient's Rh factor
4. **Transfusion reactions**
   a. Reaction that occurs when incompatible blood is infused into a patient
   b. Types
      (1) **Febrile nonhemolytic**—most common reaction; due to HLA antibodies; treated with acetaminophen; recurrence is uncommon
      (2) **Acute hemolytic**—due to ABO incompatibility; requires supportive care
      (3) **Delayed hemolytic**—due to Kidd or Rh antibodies; determine responsible antibody type to help prevent future reactions
      (4) **Anaphylactic**—rapid onset of shock and hypotension; due to transfused anti-IgA antibodies in patient with IgA deficiency; requires epinephrine, volume maintenance, and airway maintenance
      (5) **Urticarial**—due to plasma present in donor blood; treated with diphenhydramine
   c. **H/P** = occurs in patient receiving transfusion; pain in vein receiving transfusion, chills; flushing, pruritis; fever, jaundice
   d. **Labs** = both patient's and donor's blood should be rechecked and retyped
5. **Treatment = acetaminophen, diphenhydramine**, stop transfusion; mannitol or bicarbonate may be required in severe reactions to prevent hemolytic debris from clogging vessels
B. **Vasoactive medications**
   1. Drugs used to **maintain hemodynamic stability** by increasing blood pressure and cardiac output (i.e., pressors) or decreasing blood pressure and cardiac output (i.e., vasodilators and negative inotropic agents)
   2. Vasopressors frequently used in cases of shock and insufficient cardiac output
   3. Vasodilators reduce vascular tone; negative inotropic drugs decrease cardiac contractility (see Chapter 1, Cardiovascular Disorders)

● BASIC SURGICAL CONCERNS

Most surgical issues are discussed in the chapters concerning the appropriate systems. The following sections reflect concerns not addressed elsewhere.

I. Preoperative and postoperative issues

A. **Preoperative risk assessment**

1. In elective surgery, patient must be assessed prior to operation to determine if he/she will tolerate a procedure

2. **Cardiac risk**

   a. Cardiac function (ejection fraction, rate, rhythm), cardiac disease (congestive heart failure, coronary artery disease [CAD], recent MI), and age assessed prior to surgery

   b. Young, healthy patients may be cleared with a normal ECG by a primary care physician

   c. Other patients should be cleared by cardiologist

   d. Findings consistent with high surgical risk

      (1) **Age**—>70 years old

      (2) **Pulmonary**—Po_2 <60 mm Hg, Pco_2 >50 mm Hg, pulmonary edema

      (3) **Cardiac**—MI within past six months, nonsinus arrhythmia, pathologic Q waves on preoperative ECG, severe valvular disease, decompensated congestive heart failure with poor ejection fraction

      (4) **Renal**—BUN >50, Cr >2.6

      (5) **Surgery type**—vascular, anticipated high blood loss

   e. Patients determined to be at **high risk** for cardiac complications should **not be operated upon** until cardiac function is stabilized

   f. Minimally invasive techniques may be appropriate in high-risk patients

3. **Pulmonary concerns**

   a. **Smoking** increases risk of infection and postoperative ventilation

   b. Smoking should be stopped prior to surgery; nicotine replacement may help patients stop smoking 6–8 weeks prior to surgery

   c. Patients with chronic obstructive pulmonary disease (COPD) should be given preoperative antibiotics if showing signs of infection

   d. Patients with respiratory concerns (e.g., smokers, COPD, myasthenia gravis) should have pulmonary function tests performed to assess their respiratory capacity and to anticipate the need for lengthy ventilation and tracheostomy placement

   e. **Incentive spirometry**, deep breathing exercises, pain control, and **physical therapy** are all very important postoperatively to help prevent **atelectasis** and **pneumonia**

   f. Bronchodilators and inhaled steroids may be beneficial in postoperative patients with pre-existing disease

4. **Renal concerns**

   a. Patients with renal insufficiency may have electrolyte abnormalities, anemia, or poor immune function

   b. **Dialysis** may be required before surgery

   c. **Acetylcysteine** may be used as a renal protectant in patients with renal insufficiency who are expected to receive intraoperative contrast dye

5. **Hepatic concerns**

   a. Mortality increases with increased bilirubin, decreased albumin, prolonged prothrombin time (PT), and encephalopathy

   b. Electrolyte disorders, coagulopathy, and encephalopathy should be corrected prior to operation

6. **Diabetes mellitus (DM)**

   a. **Diabetic** patients have increased infection risk, worse wound healing, increased cardiac complication risk, and increased postoperative mortality

    b. Blood sugar levels should be well controlled via subcutaneous insulin sliding scale and frequent glucose checks

7. **Coagulation concerns**
   a. A history of **abnormal bleeding** or **easy bruising** should raise concerns for a coagulopathy (increased risk of bleeding complications intraoperatively and postoperatively)
   b. Patients taking **warfarin** prior to surgery should **stop** their warfarin use **3–4 days** before surgery
   c. Fresh frozen plasma (FFP) and vitamin K may be used for rapid reversal of warfarin therapy
   d. Patients with **recent thromboembolism** should be anticoagulated with **heparin** after stopping warfarin use until surgery and then restarted on warfarin postoperatively; heparin should be restarted 12 hours postoperatively and continued until a therapeutic INR (>2.0) is reached
   e. Patient not on prior warfarin therapy may be anticoagulated with **aspirin**, **anti-platelet drugs**, or **low molecular weight heparin** (LMWH) per surgeon's preference
   f. In general, warfarin, heparin, and LMWH are associated with a **lower risk** of postoperative **thromboembolism** than aspirin or anti-platelet medications but carry a **greater risk** of **postoperative bleeding complications**

B. **Postoperative fever**
   1. Fever develops postoperatively because of pulmonary, infectious, vascular, or pharmacological causes (Color Figure 7-1)
   2. Any postoperative fever should be evaluated with a **CXR**; **urine** and **blood cultures** should also be performed for any fever beyond the first postoperative day

C. **Wounds and healing**
   1. **Types of wounds**

> **QUICK HIT**
>
> Postoperative fevers are caused by the 5 Ws: **Wind** (pulmonary concerns), **Water** (urinary tract infection), **Walking** (deep vein thrombosis, pulmonary embolism), **Wound** (wound infection), **Wonder drugs** (medications).

TABLE 7-8 Causes of Postoperative Fever

Cause	When Seen	Diagnosis	Treatment
Atelectasis	**Initial 1–3 days** postoperatively	Time of occurrence, infiltrates on CXR	**Ambulation, incentive spirometry**
Pneumonia	**After** 3rd postoperative day	**Productive** cough, positive sputum Gram stain or culture, infiltrates or consolidation on CXR	Antibiotics, bronchoscopy
Urinary tract infection	**3–5** days postoperatively	Urine Gram stain or culture, urine nitrates, presence of **Foley catheter**	Antibiotics, remove Foley
Deep vein thrombosis	Any time postoperatively	Lower extremity warmth and tenderness; US demonstrates noncompressable vein	Anticoagulation, IVC filter
Pulmonary embolism	Any time postoperatively	Dyspnea, tachycardia, pleuritic chest pain, **increased A-a gradient, V-Q mismatch**	Anticoagulation, IVC filter
Wound infection	**5–8** days postoperatively	Red warm surgical wound, drainage from wound (possibly purulent)	Antibiotics, irrigation and drainage, surgical debridement
Medications	Any time postoperatively	Onset linked to new medication; antibiotics are frequent cause	Stop offending agent

A-a, alveolar-arterial; CXR, chest x-ray; IVC, inferior vena cava; US, ultrasound, V-Q, ventilation-perfusion.

a. **Clean**—surgical incisions through disinfected skin; no GI or respiratory entry; 1–3% infection risk

b. **Clean-contaminated**—similar to clean wounds but with GI or respiratory entry; 2–8% infection risk

c. **Contaminated**—gross contact of wound with GI or genitourinary contents; traumatic wounds; 6–15% infection risk

d. **Infected**—established infection in tissue prior to incision

2. **Wound approximation and healing**

a. **Primary intention**—low risk of infection (clean and clean-contaminated wounds or contaminated wounds with good clean-up in healthy patient); full closure of tissue and skin performed

b. **Secondary intention**—high risk for infection; wound left open and allowed to heal through epithelialization

c. **Delayed primary closure**—heavily contaminated wounds; left open for few days and cleaned prior to wound closure

d. **Skin grafts**—portion of epidermis and dermis from other body site transferred to wound that are too large to close by themselves; large deeper grafts with revascularization are called flaps

3. Closed wounds require dressings for **initial 48 hours** after closure

4. Open wounds require debridement and specialized dressings

5. Wound healing may be inhibited by malnutrition, corticosteroids, smoking, hepatic or renal failure, or DM

II. Surgical emergencies

A. **Acute abdomen**

1. **Severe abdominal pain** and rigidity lasting up to several hours that requires **prompt** treatment

TABLE 7-9 Causes of Acute Abdomen

Condition	H/P	Diagnosis	Treatment
GI strangulation (due to adhesions, hernias, tumors)	**Previous surgery,** abdominal distention, crampy pain	Abdominal radiograph shows distended loops of bowel and air-fluid levels Barium studies may locate site of obstruction	**Surgical lysis of adhesions,** hernia repair, surgical excision of tumors
Severe diverticulitis	**Left lower quadrant** pain, blood in stool	Abdominal radiograph may show free air from perforation Increased WBC	Surgical repair
Massive GI hemorrhage (perforation)	Sudden severe pain, **hematemesis, hematochezia,** hypotension	Colonoscopy or EGD visualizes lesion; technetium scan may detect smaller bleeding sources	Octreotide, **angiography with embolization,** surgical repair of detectable site of bleeding
Appendicitis	**Right lower quadrant** pain, psoas sign, rectal exam tenderness	Increased WBC Free air on abdominal radiograph if perforated	**Appendectomy**
Pancreatitis	**Back** pain, history of gallstones or alcoholism	CT shows inflamed pancreas Increased amylase and lipase	Nasogastric tube, NPO, analgesics
Ruptured ectopic pregnancy	**Amenorrhea,** lower abdominal pain, possible vaginal bleeding, or palpable pelvic mass	US **unable** to locate intrauterine pregnancy in presence of **positive urine pregnancy test**	Surgical excision

CT, computed tomography; EGD, esophagogastroduodenoscopy; GI, gastrointestinal; H/P, history and physical; NPO, nothing by mouth; US, ultrasound; WBC, white blood cell count.

TABLE 7-10 Common Types of Organ Transplantation

Type	Indications	Contraindications	Results
Heart (may be performed with lung transplant)	Severe heart disease (CAD, congenital defects, cardiomyopathy) with estimated death within 2 yr without transplant	**Pulmonary hypertension, smoking** (prior 6 months), renal insufficiency, COPD	Acute rejection common, higher mortality risk in 1st yr, 70% **5-yr** survival
Lung	**COPD** (particularly α_1-antitrypsin deficiency), primary pulmonary hypertension, **cystic fibrosis;** estimated death with 2 yr	**Smoking** (prior 6 months), poor cardiac function, renal or hepatic insufficiency	60% acute rejection, pneumonia common, **70% 1-yr** survival, **chronic rejection** common
Liver	Chronic hepatitis B or **C,** alcoholic cirrhosis, primary biliary cirrhosis, primary sclerosing cholangitis, biliary atresia, progressive Wilson's disease	**Alcoholism,** multiple **suicide** attempts (e.g., acetaminophen poisoning), liver cancer, cirrhosis from chronic hepatitis (may receive transplants from donors with hepatitis)	40% acute rejection, success correlates with patient health at time of surgery (generally 60–70% 5-yr survival)
Renal	**End-stage renal disease** requiring dialysis (glomerulonephritis, DM, polycystic kidney disease, interstitial nephritis, renal hypertension)	Stable health (dialysis is always an option for unstable patients)	Living-donor kidneys have 20% acute rejection and a half-life (time in which 1/2 of transplanted kidneys have failed) of 15–30 yr. Cadaver kidneys have 40% acute rejection and half-life of 10–15 yr
Pancreas (frequently performed with renal transplant)	**DM type I** with renal failure	Age >60 yr, CAD, PVD, obesity, **DM type II**	60–80% 1-yr survival, acute rejection common

CAD, coronary artery disease; COPD, chronic obstructive pulmonary disease; DM, diabetes mellitus; PVD, peripheral vascular disease.

2. **H/P = Abdominal pain** (severe or crampy, rapidly or gradually progressive), nausea, vomiting, possible history of recent surgery; fever, abdominal tenderness (with possible **rebound tenderness**, rigidity, **guarding**, spasm, or mass), possible hypotension; pelvic or testicular exam should be performed to rule out gynecologic or testicular condition
3. **Labs** = increased white blood cell count (WBC) in cases of infection or bowel perforation; increased amylase in pancreatitis; increased liver function tests with hepatobiliary dysfunction
4. **Radiology** = abdominal radiograph helpful to recognize bowel gas patterns, air collections, and calcifications; IVP, barium studies, or ultrasound (US) may also be helpful

TABLE 7-11 Forms of Transplant Rejection

Type	When Seen	Cause	Treatment
Hyperacute	**Initial 24 hr** after transplantation	Antidonor antibodies in recipient	**Untreatable;** should be avoided by proper cross-matching
Acute	**6 days–1 yr** after transplantation	Antidonor T cell proliferation in recipient	**Frequently reversible** through immunosuppressive agents
Chronic	**>1 yr** after transplantation	Development of multiple cellular and humoral immune reactions to donor tissue	Usually untreatable; immunosuppression may serve some role

5. **Treatment** = adequate pain control; **emergent laparotomy/laparoscopy** may be needed depending on pathology

B. **Malignant hyperthermia**

1. Rare genetic disorder in which inhalational anesthetics (especially halothane) induce hyperthermia (>40° C or 104° F)
2. **H/P** = symptoms begin after anesthesia use: rigidity, tachycardia, continually rising **body temperature**
3. Uncontrolled hyperthermia may lead to arrhythmias, disseminated intravascular coagulation (DIC), acidosis, cerebral dysfunction and electrolyte abnormalities
4. **Labs** = mixed acidosis acutely; abnormal increase in muscle contraction following in vitro treatment with halothane or caffeine (testing performed as outpatient)
5. **Treatment** = evaporative cooling (patient sprayed with water and placed in front of fans), cold inhaled O_2, cold GI lavage, cool IV fluids, **dantrolene, stop offending agent**

III. Transplantation

A. **Indications and selection**

1. Organ transplantation is considered in cases of **end-stage organ failure** that are untreatable by other means or are incompatible with survival without treatment by extraordinary means (e.g., frequent dialysis)
2. **Transplant frequency**
   a. Renal transplants are most common type
   b. Liver, pancreas, heart, lung, and cornea transplants also performed
   c. Small bowel transplant has been performed on a very limited basis with limited success
3. **Donor selection**
   a. Donors are most frequently brain-dead or living voluntary donors, without cancer, sepsis, or organ insufficiency
   b. Donors are selected based on **ABO blood group compatibility, cross-match compatibility** (presence of anti-donor antibodies on recipient T cells), and **HLA matching**

 Individuals with a specific infection (e.g., **hepatitis**) may be used as donors for patients with the same infection if no significant donor organ injury is detected.

TABLE 7-12	Immunosuppressive Drugs to Prevent Transplant Rejection		
Drug	**Indication**	**Mechanism**	**Adverse Effects**
Cyclosporine	Rejection prevention	**Helper** T cell inhibition	**Nephrotoxicity,** androgenic effects, HTN
Azathioprine	Rejection prevention	Inhibits T cell proliferation	**Leukopenia**
Tacrolimus	Rejection prevention and reversal	Inhibitor of T cell function	**Nephrotoxicity,** neurotoxicity
Corticosteroids	Rejection prevention and reversal	Inhibits **all leukocyte** activity	Cushing's syndrome, weight gain, AVN of bone
muromonab-CD3 (OKT3)	Rejection reversal and **early** rejection maintenance	Inhibitor of T cell function and depletes T cell population	Induces **one-time cytokine release** (fever, bronchospasm); limited to **short-term therapy**
Rapamycin	Rejection prevention	Helper T cell inhibition	Thrombocytopenia, hyperlipidemia
Mycophenolic acid	Rejection prevention	Inhibits T cell proliferation	**Leukopenia**
Antithymocyte globulin	Rejection reversal and **early** rejection maintenance	Depletes T cell population	Limited to **short-term therapy**

AVN, avascular necrosis; HTN, hypertension.

    c. HLA matching is **more** important for **kidney** and **pancreas** transplants and **less** important for **heart** and **liver**

  4. Transplant rejection may be hyperacute, acute, or chronic

  5. Patients must be given **immunosuppressive** agents to reduce risk of rejection

  6. Transplant patients have greater risks of **infection** (secondary to immunosuppression), **cancer** (skin, B cell lymphoma, oral squamous cell, cervical, vaginal), and infertility

B. **Graft vs. host disease**

  1. Reaction of **donor** immune cells in transplanted organ to host cells

  2. Host is immunocompromised to avoid transplant rejection and is unable to prevent attack by donor cells

  3. **Risk factors** = HLA mismatch, old age, donor-host gender disparity, **immunosuppression**

  4. **H/P** = **maculopapular rash**, abdominal pain, nausea, vomiting, diarrhea, recurrent infections, easy bleeding

  5. **Labs** = increased liver function tests, decreased immunoglobulin levels, decreased platelets; biopsy of skin or liver detects an inflammatory reaction with significant cell death

  6. **Treatment** = corticosteroids, tacrolimus, and mycophenolate are useful for decreasing graft response

  7. **Complications** = patients without an early response to therapy frequently develop **chronic** disease with skin sclerosis, hepatic insufficiency, GI ulceration, and pulmonary fibrosis

Neurologic Disorders

I. Normal neurologic and neurovascular function

A. **Cerebral vasculature (see Figure 8-1 and Table 8-1)**

1. The **Circle of Willis** is a system of collateral vessels that supplies all regions of the brain

2. Symptoms seen with a stroke may be used to determine the site of insult based on association with a particular region of the brain

B. **Neurologic organization (see Figure 8-2 and Tables 8-2, 8-3, and 8-4)**

1. Sensory and motor neurons are organized into distinct tracts in the spinal cord

2. Lesions of the spinal cord cause symptoms that are dependent upon the lesion location

3. Cranial nerves (CNs) have distinct functions within the head and neck

II. Neurologic infection

A. **Bacterial meningitis (see Table 8-5)**

1. Infection of meningeal tissue in brain or spinal cord; common bacterial agents differ, depending on patient age

2. Infection is usually caused by hematogenous spread, local extension, or cerebral spinal fluid (CSF) exposure to bacteria (e.g., neurosurgery)

3. **Risk factors** = ear infection, sinusitis, immunocompromise, neurosurgery, maternal group β streptococci infection during birth

4. **H/P =**

   a. Headache, **neck pain,** photophobia, malaise, vomiting, confusion; fever

   b. **Brudzinski's** sign (neck flexion in supine patient causes hip flexion) and **Kernig's** sign (painful knee extension occurs with hip flexion in supine patient) are not reliable tests

   c. Petechiae are seen in *Neisseria meningitidis* infection

   d. Change in mental status, seizures, decreased consciousness seen with worsening infection

   e. Symptoms in children may be nonfocal

5. **Labs** = increased white blood cell count; lumbar puncture (LP) useful for differentiating causes of meningitis from each other and from healthy patients; CSF culture may determine exact agent

6. **Radiology** = computed tomography (CT) or magnetic resonance imaging (MRI) may be helpful for ruling out other pathologies

7. **Treatment** = initially, cephalosporins (3rd generation) until specific agent is identified, then agent-specific antibiotics; close contacts of patient should be given **rifampin for prophylaxis** in cases of *Neisseria*

 First-order neurons are **preganglionic;** second-order neurons are **postganglionic.**

 UMN conditions are those that originate in the brain or first-order neurons; LMN conditions are those caused by pathology in second order neurons.

 H. influenzae has been significantly reduced as a cause of meningitis owing to childhood **vaccination.**

 Young children with meningitis frequently have **negative** Brudzinski's and Kernig's signs.

STEP NEXT Neurologic exam must be performed before LP. If there are signs of **increased ICP** (papilledema, focal neurologic deficits, pupil asymmetry), do **not** perform LP because of increased risk of uncal **herniation.**

FIGURE
8-1   Arteries of the brain including the Circle of Willis, and their anatomical relationship to selected cranial nerves. CN, cranial nerve.

A. Arteries of the base of the brain and brain stem

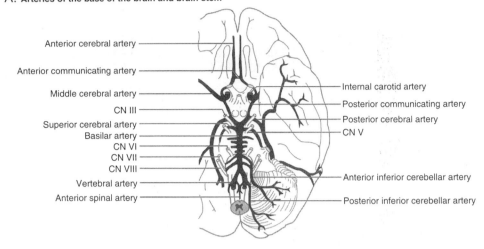

B. Arterial blood supply to the cortex

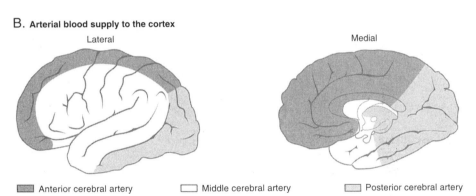

Lateral   Medial

▨ Anterior cerebral artery   ☐ Middle cerebral artery   ▨ Posterior cerebral artery

CN=cranial nerve

(Used with permission from Mehta S, Milder EA, Mirachi AJ, Milder E. *Step-Up: A High-Yield, Systems-Based Review for the USMLE Step 1.* 2nd Ed. Philadelphia: Lippincott Williams & Wilkins; 2003.)

TABLE 8-1 Regions of the Brain Supplied by Vessels in the Circle of Willis	
Artery	**Region of Brain Supplied**
Anterior cerebral artery (ACA)	Medial and superior surfaces and frontal lobes
Middle cerebral artery (MCA)	Lateral surfaces and temporal lobes
Posterior cerebral artery (PCA)	Inferior surfaces and occipital lobes
Basilar artery	Midbrain, brainstem (pons)
Anterior inferior cerebellar artery (AICA)	Brainstem (pons)
Posterior inferior cerebellar artery (PICA)	Brainstem (medulla)

FIGURE
8-2 Neuronal pathways of the spinal cord in a thoracic cross section.

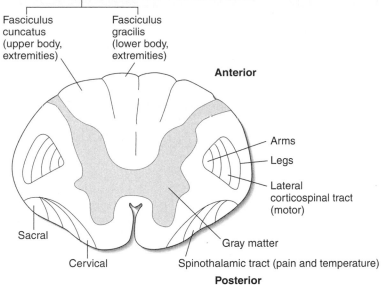

Dorsal columns
(pressure, vibration, touch, proprioception)

Fasciculus cuncatus (upper body, extremities)

Fasciculus gracilis (lower body, extremities)

Anterior

Arms
Legs
Lateral corticospinal tract (motor)

Sacral

Gray matter

Cervical

Spinothalamic tract (pain and temperature)

Posterior

(Used with permission from Le T, Amin C, Bhushan V, Choo E. *First Aid for the USMLE Step 2*, 3rd Ed. New York: McGraw-Hill; 2001.)

infection and for *H. influenzae* infection in children without prior vaccination

8. **Complications** = seizures, increased intracranial pressure (ICP), subdural effusion, or empyema, brain abscess

B. **Viral meningitis** (aseptic meningitis)
   1. Meningitis due to viral infection by enterovirus, echovirus, herpes simplex virus, lymphocytic choriomeningitis virus, mumps virus

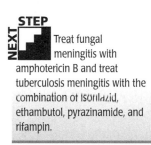

NEXT STEP Treat fungal meningitis with amphotericin B and treat tuberculosis meningitis with the combination of isoniazid, ethambutol, pyrazinamide, and rifampin.

TABLE 8-2 Sensory and Motor Tracts of the Spinal Cord

Pathway	Location	First-Order Neurons	Second-Order Neurons	Function
Dorsal columns	Posterior spinal cord	Enter at ipsilateral dorsal horn, ascend in fasciculus gracilis and cuneatus, synapse in nucleus gracilis and cuneatus	Decussate at medulla, ascend as medial lemniscus	**Two point discrimination,** sense vibration, sense **proprioception**
Spinothalamic tract	Anterior spinal cord	Originate in dorsal root ganglion, synapse in dorsolateral tract of Lissauer	Decussate in ventral white commissure, ascend in lateral spinothalamic tract	**Senses pain,** senses **temperature**
Corticospinal tract	Lateral spinal cord	Descend from internal capsule and midbrain, decussate in medullary pyramids, descend in corticospinal tract, synapse in ventral horn through interneurons	Exit cord through ventral horn	**Voluntary movement** of striated muscle

NEUROLOGIC DISORDERS

TABLE 8-3	Common Lesions of the Spinal Cord	
Condition	**Tracts Affected**	**Symptoms**
Amyotrophic lateral sclerosis (ALS)	Corticospinal tract, ventral horn	Spastic and flaccid paralysis
Poliomyelitis	Ventral horn	Flaccid paralysis
Tabes dorsalis (**tertiary syphilis**)	Dorsal columns	Impaired proprioception
Spinal artery syndrome	Corticospinal tract, spinothalamic tract, ventral horn, lateral gray matter (**dorsal columns spared**)	Bilateral loss of pain and temperature (one level below lesion), bilateral spastic paresis (below lesion), bilateral flaccid paralysis (level of lesion)
Vitamin B_{12} deficiency	Dorsal columns, corticospinal tract	Bilateral loss of vibration/discrimination and bilateral spastic paresis affecting legs before arms
Syringomyelia	Ventral horn, ventral white commissure	Bilateral loss of pain and temperature (one level below lesion), bilateral flaccid paralysis (level of lesion)
Brown-Séquard syndrome	**All** tracts on one side of cord	Ipsilateral loss of vibration and discrimination (below lesion), ipsilateral spastic paresis (below lesion), ipsilateral flaccid paralysis (level of lesion), contralateral loss of pain and temperature (below lesion)

Common arboviruses include St. Louis and California strains. Common flaviviruses include **West Nile** and Japanese strains.

In young children encephalitis may be due to **Reye's syndrome** (reaction in children with viral infection who are given ASA).

2. **H/P** = vomiting, headache, neck pain, malaise; fever; symptoms generally **milder** than for bacterial meningitis
3. **Labs** = LP helpful for diagnosis; viral culture will confirm etiology
4. **Treatment** = empiric antibiotics may be started until viral cause is confirmed; supportive care usually sufficient for confirmed viral cases

C. **Encephalitis**
1. Inflammation of brain parenchyma due to **viral** infection (varicella-zoster virus, herpes simplex virus, mumps virus, poliovirus, rhabdovirus, Coxsackie virus, arbovirus, flavivirus, measles) or immunologic response to viral infection
2. **H/P** =
   a. Malaise, headache, vomiting, neck pain, decreased consciousness; change in mental status, focal neurologic deficits (hemiparesis, pathologic reflexes, nerve palsy), fever
   b. Skin lesions seen with herpes simplex virus
   c. Parotid swelling seen with mumps
3. **Labs** =
   a. LP shows increased white blood cells (WBCs), normal glucose
   b. Culture generally not reliable
   c. Serologic testing may be useful to identify viral cause
   d. Brain biopsy may be useful but is generally impractical
4. **Radiology** = CT or MRI may show inflamed region of brain with effusion
5. **Treatment** = maintain normal ICP, supportive care; herpes simplex virus treated with acyclovir

TABLE 8-4 Cranial Nerves and Their Functions

Nerve	Type	Function/Innervation
Olfactory (CN I)	Sensory	Smell
Optic (CN II)	Sensory	Sight
Oculomotor (CN III)	Motor	Medial/superior/inferior rectus muscles, inferior oblique muscle, ciliary muscle, sphincter muscle of eye
Trochlear (CN IV)	Motor	Superior oblique muscle of eye
Trigeminal (CN V)	Both	Sensation of face; muscles of mastication
Abducens (CN VI)	Motor	Lateral rectus muscle of eye
Facial (CN VII)	Both	Taste (anterior $2/3$ of tongue); muscles of facial expression, stapedius muscle, stylohyoid muscle, digastric muscle (posterior belly); lacrimal, submandibular, sublingual glands
Vestibulocochlear (CN VIII)	Sensory	Hearing, balance
Glossopharyngeal (CN IX)	Both	Taste (posterior $1/3$ of tongue), pharyngeal sensation; stylopharyngeus muscle; parotid gland
Vagus (CN X)	Both	Sensation of trachea, esophagus, viscera; laryngeal, pharyngeal muscles; visceral autonomics
Accessory (CN XI)	Motor	Sternocleidomastoid and trapezius muscles
Hypoglossal (CN XII)	Motor	Tongue

CN, cranial nerve.

D. **Brain abscess**
1. Collection of pus in brain parenchyma resulting from extension of local bacterial infection, head wound, or hematogenous spread of bacteria
2. **H/P** = headache, nausea, vomiting, malaise; change in mental status, focal neurologic deficits, papilledema
3. **Labs** = brain biopsy or culture of abscess material performed during surgical drainage may be used to confirm bacterial identity
4. **Radiology** = CT or MRI may localize lesion
5. **Treatment** = empiric antibiotics until specific agent identified, corticosteroids, surgical drainage

TABLE 8-5 Common Causes of Meningitis by Age Group

Age	Most Common Agent	Other Common Agents
Newborn	Group β streptococci	*Escherichia coli, Listeria, Haemophilus influenzae*
1 month–2 yr old	*Streptococcus pneumoniae / Neisseria meningitidis*	Group β streptococci, *Listeria, H. influenzae*
2–18 yr old	*N. meningitidis*	*S. pneumoniae, Listeria*
18–60 yr old	*S. pneumoniae*	*N. meningitidis, Listeria*
60+ yr old	*S. pneumoniae*	*Listeria,* gram-negative rods

TABLE 8-6 CSF Findings for Different Causes of Meningitis				
Status	**WBCs**	**Pressure**	**Glucose**	**Protein**
Healthy patient	<5	50–180 mm H$_2$O	40–70 mg/dL	20–45 mg/dL
Bacterial infection	↑ (PMNs)	↑	↓	↑
Viral infection	↑ (lymphocytes)	Normal	Normal	Normal
Fungal infection or tuberculosis	↑ (lymphocytes)	↑	↓	↑

CSF, cerebral spinal fluid; PMNs, polymorphonuclear cells; WBCs, white blood cells.

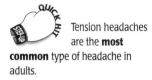

Poliomyelitis may rarely occur after **oral** polio vaccine administration, so inactivated intramuscular polio vaccine is now more commonly used.

E. **Poliomyelitis**
1. Poliovirus (an enterovirus) infection of brain and motor neurons
2. Nearly eradicated through polio vaccine given in childhood
3. **H/P** = possibly asymptomatic; headache, neck pain, vomiting, sore throat; fever, **normal sensation, muscle weakness** that may progress to paralysis in severe cases
4. **Labs** = **positive polio-specific antibody;** LP consistent with viral meningitis; viral culture helpful for diagnosis
5. **Treatment** = with supportive care, most patients recover fully; assisted respiration may be required if respiratory muscles are affected

F. **Rabies**
1. Rhabdovirus transmitted to humans by **bite of infected animal**
2. Causes severe encephalitis with neuronal degeneration and inflammation
3. **H/P** = malaise, headache, restlessness, **fear of water ingestion** (secondary to laryngeal spasm); progressive cases exhibit severe central nervous system (CNS) excitability, **foaming at mouth,** very painful laryngeal spasms, **alternating mania and stupor**
4. **Labs** =
   a. Suspected animal should be caught and tested or observed for signs of rabies
   b. If animal appears to be infected, it should be euthanized and the brain should be tested for presence of virus and **Negri bodies** (round eosinophilic inclusions in neurons)
   c. Viral testing in humans with symptoms is confirmatory of disease
5. **Treatment** = clean wound area thoroughly; administer rabies immunoglobulin and vaccine to patient if animal was infected or if rabies suspicion is high
6. **Complications = 100% mortality** without treatment

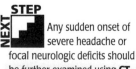

Tension headaches are the **most common** type of headache in adults.

STEP Any sudden onset of severe headache or focal neurologic deficits should be further examined using **CT without contrast** or MRI to rule out hemorrhage.

III. **Headache (see Table 8-7)**
A. Head pain that may be a primary disorder (migraine, cluster, tension) or secondary to other pathology (hemorrhage, encephalopathy, meningitis, temporal arteritis, neoplasm)
B. **Trigeminal neuralgia**
1. Head and **facial pain** in trigeminal nerve distribution possibly due to compression or irritation of trigeminal nerve root
2. **H/P** = severe pain in distributions of maxillary and mandibular branches; "trigger zone" stimulation may induce pain
3. **Radiology** = MRI may identify lesions related to nerve compression
4. **Treatment** = **carbamazepine,** baclofen, phenytoin, gabapentin, valproic acid, clonazepam, or other **anticonvulsants;** surgical decompression of nerve may be helpful

TABLE 8-7 **Primary Headache Disorders**

Variable	Migraine	Cluster	Tension
Patients	10–30 yr old, **female** > male	Young **men**	Female > male
Pathology	Poorly understood; likely due to vascular abnormalities	Poorly understood	Poorly understood
Precipitating factors	Stress, oral contraceptives, **menstruation,** foods containing tyramine or nitrates (chocolate, cheese, processed meats)	Alcohol, vasodilators	Stress, fatigue
Pain characteristics	Unilateral, throbbing	Severe, unilateral, **periorbital,** recurrent ("in clusters" over time)	**Bilateral,** tightness, occipital or neck pain
Other symptoms	**Nausea, vomiting,** preceding aura (visual abnormalities), photophobia	**Horner's syndrome** (ptosis, myosis, anhidrosis), lacrimation, nasal congestion	Anxiety
Treatment	NSAIDs, ergots, sumatriptan; prophylaxis includes tricyclic antidepressants, β-blockers, calcium channel blockers, ergots	100% O₂, ergots, sumatriptan; prophylaxis similar to that for migraines	NSAIDs, ergots, sumatriptan, relaxation exercises

NSAIDs, nonsteroidal anti-inflammatory drugs.

IV. Cerebrovascular and hemorrhagic diseases

A. **Transient ischemic attack (TIA)**
1. Acute focal neurologic deficits that last **less than 24 hours** and are due to temporarily impaired vascular supply to brain (e.g., emboli, aortic stenosis, vascular spasm)
2. **Risk factors** = hypertension (HTN), diabetes mellitus (DM), coronary artery disease, tobacco, hyperlipidemia, hypercoagulable states
3. **H/P =**
   a. Sudden appearance of focal neurologic deficits, including weakness, paresthesias, brief unilateral blindness (amaurosis fugax) or other vision abnormality, impaired coordination, vertigo
   b. Carotid bruits suggest carotid atherosclerosis
   c. Harsh systolic murmur suggests aortic stenosis
4. **Radiology** = ultrasound (US) may quantify degree of carotid or aortic stenosis; MRI or angiography may locate intracranial vascular defects
5. **Treatment =**
   a. **Carotid endarterectomy or angioplasty** performed for carotid narrowing >70%
   b. β-Blockers, valvuloplasty, or valve replacement used in treatment of aortic stenosis
   c. Anticoagulants used for arrhythmias; **aspirin (ASA)** for mild vascular stenosis
   d. Treat other underlying disorders
B. **Stroke** (cerebrovascular accident)
1. Acute focal neurologic deficit **lasting >24 hours,** due to ischemia of brain via **impaired perfusion** (ischemic stroke) or **hemorrhage** (hemorrhagic stroke)
2. Ischemic stroke may be **thrombotic** (obstruction of supplying artery by clot) or **embolic** (blockage of supplying artery by embolization of distant thrombus)

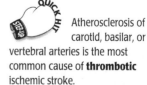

Most TIAs last <2 hours and are recurrent.

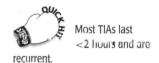

Atherosclerosis of carotid, basilar, or vertebral arteries is the most common cause of **thrombotic** ischemic stroke.

The **middle cerebral artery** is most common artery involved in **embolic ischemic** stroke. Most emboli originate in heart, aorta, carotid, or intracranial arteries.

FIGURE
8-3 Motor and sensory cortex and corresponding arterial supply.

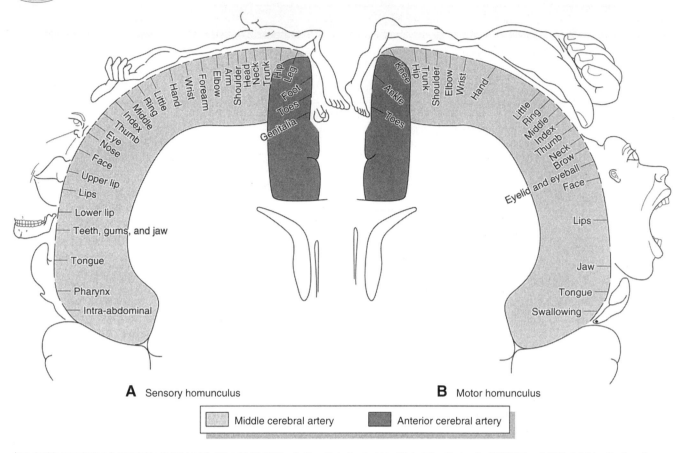

A Sensory homunculus   **B** Motor homunculus

| Middle cerebral artery | Anterior cerebral artery |

(Used with permission from Mehta S, Milder EA, Mirachi AJ, Milder E. *Step-Up to the Bedside: Clinical CaseReview for USMLE Step 1.* Philadelphia: Lippincott Williams & Wilkins; 2002.)

3. **Risk factors** = increased age, family history, obesity, DM, HTN, tobacco, atrial fibrillation (Afib)
4. Area of neurologic deficit is dependent upon location of stroke
5. **H/P** =
   a. Sudden appearance of focal neurologic deficit lasting >24 hours
   b. Constellation of symptoms depends on location of pathology
   c. Stable findings indicate stable stroke, but progressive findings indicate evolving stroke
6. **Radiology** = **CT without contrast** or MRI useful to differentiate ischemic from hemorrhagic stroke; angiography or magnetic resonance angiography (MRA) may be helpful for locating ischemic cause
7. **Electrocardiogram (ECG)** = detection of new onset arrhythmia or history of Afib seen on prior ECG may be useful in determining cause
8. **Treatment** =
   a. **Heparin** for evolving ischemic stroke (thrombotic or embolic)
   b. **ASA** or **warfarin** for prevention of additional thromboembolic events
   c. **Thrombolytic therapy** may be administered for ischemic stroke if **within 3 hours** of onset and there are no contraindications (evidence of hemorrhage on CT, recent surgery, anticoagulant use, recent hemorrhage, blood pressure >185/110 mm Hg)
   d. Physical therapy is useful in improving persistent deficits
   e. Hemorrhagic stroke requires control of ICP (e.g., mannitol, hyperventilation, anesthesia), elimination of HTN, reversal of

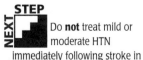
NEXT STEP Do **not** treat mild or moderate HTN immediately following stroke in order to **maintain cerebral perfusion.**

TABLE 8-8 Common Stroke Locations and Corresponding Signs and Symptoms

Location of Stroke	Signs and Symptoms
ACA	Contralateral lower extremity and trunk weakness
MCA	Contralateral face and upper extremity weakness and decreased sensation, bilateral visual abnormalities, aphasia (if dominant hemisphere), neglect and inability to perform learned actions (if nondominant hemisphere)
PCA	Contralateral visual abnormalities, blindness (if bilateral PCA involvement)
Lacunar arteries	Focal motor or sensory deficits, loss of coordination, difficulty speaking
Basilar artery	Cranial nerve abnormalities, contralateral full body weakness and decreased sensation, vertigo, loss of coordination, difficulty speaking, visual abnormalities, coma

ACA, anterior cerebral artery; MCA, middle cerebral artery; PCA, posterior cerebral artery.

anticoagulation, and possible surgical decompression for large lesions

 f. Treatment of underlying disorders is important for **prevention** of future strokes

 9. **Complications** = better prognosis for recovery in young patients with greater overall health and limited deficits; some deficits may not improve despite treatment

C. **Parenchymal hemorrhage**
 1. Bleeding within brain parenchyma due to HTN, arteriovenous malformation (AVM), or stimulant abuse
 2. **H/P** = headache, nausea, vomiting; change in mental status, motor or sensory deficits
 3. **Radiology** = CT without contrast used to localize and determine extent of bleeding
 4. **Treatment** = supportive care, maintain normal ICP, **anticonvulsants** for seizure prophylaxis; surgical decompression for large hemorrhages to reduce risk of herniation
 5. **Complications** = significant supratentorial bleeding may cause transtentorial (uncal) herniation (brainstem damage) and CSF flow obstruction (leading to hydrocephalus and brainstem compression); large hemorrhages are frequently fatal

D. **Subarachnoid hemorrhage** (SAH)
 1. Bleeding between the pia and arachnoid meningeal layers due to rupture of **arterial aneurysm** (berry aneurysm), AVM, or trauma
 2. **H/P** = **sudden severe headache,** neck pain, nausea, vomiting; fever, loss of or decreased consciousness, possible seizure, possible CN III palsy (ptosis, pupil dilation, lateral deviation of pupil)
 3. **Labs** = LP shows red blood cells, xanthochromia (yellowish discoloration of CSF), increased pressure
 4. **Radiology** = CT without contrast shows blood in the subarachnoid space; MRA or angiography can localize site of bleeding
 5. **Treatment** = prevent increase in ICP (raise head of bed, administer mannitol), treat HTN, administer anticonvulsants, perform interventional radiologic/surgical clipping or embolization of aneurysm or AVM
 6. **Complications** = recurrence of bleeding, arterial vasospasm, hydrocephalus; permanent neurologic damage or death may result

 Bleeding from parenchymal hemorrhage may extend into the subarachnoid space.

 Berry aneurysms are associated with **adult polycystic kidney disease.**

 Patients may describe the headache in SAH as the "**worst headache of my life.**"

 Patients with imminent rupture of a berry aneurysm may have multiple, though less severe, sentinel headaches in the preceding weeks.

 STEP If SAH is suspected despite a **negative** CT, perform an LP.

FIGURE 8-4 Subarachnoid hemorrhage seen on CT without contrast; blood is evident in the subarachnoid space (*white arrows*).

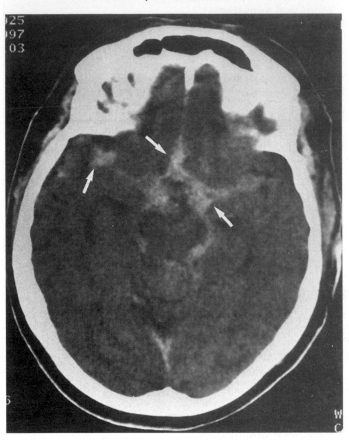

(Used with permission from Daffner RH. *Clinical Radiology: The Essentials.* 2nd Ed. Philadelphia: Lippincott Williams & Wilkins; 1999.)

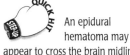
The most common cause of epidural hematoma is damage to the **middle meningeal artery** from blunt trauma.

An epidural hematoma may appear to cross the brain midline on CT; subdurals do not.

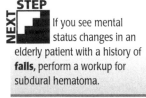
If you see mental status changes in an elderly patient with a history of **falls,** perform a workup for subdural hematoma.

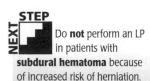
Do **not** perform an LP in patients with **subdural hematoma** because of increased risk of herniation.

E. **Epidural hematoma**
  1. Collection of blood between dura and skull due to arterial hemorrhage
  2. **H/P** = initial **"lucid interval"** between start of bleeding and onset of symptoms for a few hours or less with no change in consciousness; headache and decreased consciousness, hemiparesis, pupil abnormalities (blown pupil) may appear after lucid interval
  3. **Radiology** = CT without contrast shows **convex** hyperdensity compressing brain at site of injury, adjacent skull fracture may be apparent in traumatic cases
  4. **Treatment** = **emergent** drainage of hematoma either under radiographic guidance or by surgical burr hole
  5. **Complications** = permanent neurologic injury or death usually results without prompt treatment
F. **Subdural hematoma**
  1. Collection of blood between the dura and arachnoid meningeal layers due to rupture of bridging veins following trauma
  2. **H/P** =
     a. **Slowly progressive** headache (days to weeks); change in mental status, contralateral hemiparesis, increased deep tendon reflexes (DTRs)
     b. Large hematomas may cause transtentorial herniation with decreased consciousness and pupil abnormalities
  3. **Radiology** = CT without contrast shows **concave** hyperdensity compressing brain that does **not** cross midline
  4. **Treatment** = surgical drainage or supportive therapy

FIGURE 8-5 **A.** Epidural hematoma: note **convex** hyperdensity due to blood (*white arrows*). **B.** Subdural hematoma: note **faint concave** hyperdensity due to blood (*white arrows*).

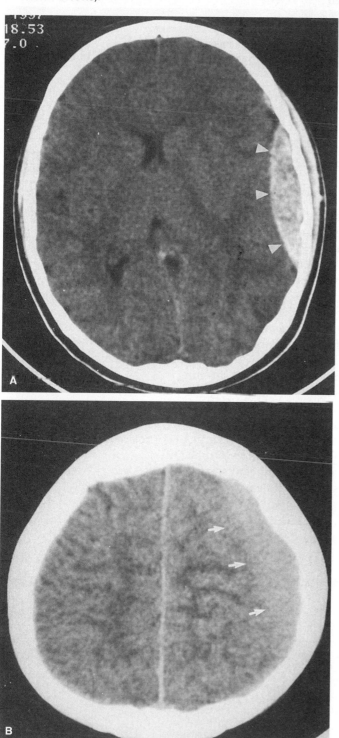

(Used with permission from Daffner RH. *Clinical Radiology: The Essentials.* 2nd Ed. Philadelphia: Lippincott Williams & Wilkins; 1999.)

TABLE 8-9	Common Classifications of Aphasias		
Type	**Area Injured**	**H/P**	**Treatment**
Broca's (expressive)	Inferior frontal gyrus	Few words, difficulty producing words **(nonfluent); good comprehension;** face and arm hemiparesis, loss of oral coordination	Speech therapy
Wernicke's (receptive)	Posterior superior temporal gyrus, inferior parietal lobe	Word substitutions, meaningless words, meaningless phrases (**poor comprehension,** "word salad")	Speech therapy
H/P, history and physical.			

G. Aphasias
1. Disorders in speech due to injury of specific regions of the brain following stroke or hemorrhage
2. **Broca's and Wernicke's aphasias are the most common types of aphasia although other types exist**
H. **Normal pressure hydrocephalus**
1. Collection of excess CSF in cerebral ventricles and spinal thecal sac; may follow **SAH**
2. **H/P** = cognitive impairment, incontinence, gait abnormalities
3. **Radiology** = CT shows enlarged cerebral ventricles with little cortical atrophy
4. **Treatment** = ventriculoperitoneal shunting

V. Seizure disorders
A. **Causes of seizures**
1. Due to excessive synchronized discharge of cortical neurons in a limited (focal) or generalized distribution of the brain
2. **Epilepsy** is condition of **recurrent** seizures
3. Common causes of seizures vary with age

TABLE 8-10	Common Causes of Seizures by Age Group
Age Group	**Causes**
Infant	Infection Metabolic defects Perinatal injury
Children	Idiopathic Infection Fever Trauma
Adult	Idiopathic Drug withdrawal Trauma Neoplasm
Elderly	Stroke Metabolic defects Neoplasm Drug withdrawal Trauma

TABLE 8-11 Types of Seizures

Type	Involvement	H/P	EEG	Treatment
Simple partial	Focal cortical region of brain	**Focal** sensory (paresthesias, hallucinations) or motor (repetitive or purposeless movement) deficit; **no loss of consciousness**	Distinct focal conductive abnormality	Phenytoin, carbamazepine; surgery may be helpful
Complex partial	Focal region of **temporal** or medial frontal lobes	**Hallucinations** (auditory, visual, olfactory), **automatisms** (repeated coordinated movement), déjà vu, impaired consciousness, postictal confusion	Focal abnormalities in temporal lobe	Phenytoin, carbamazepine; surgery may be helpful
Generalized tonic-clonic	Bilateral cerebral cortex	Loss of consciousness, **tonic** (sustained) contraction of extremities and back (approx. 30 sec), **clonic** (repetitive) muscle contraction and relaxation (approx. 1 min), incontinence, delayed return of consciousness, significant postictal confusion, possible focal neurologic deficit lasting several days after seizure (Todd's paralysis)	**Generalized** electrical abnormalities	Phenytoin, carbamazepine, valproic acid; surgery may be helpful
Absence	Bilateral cerebral cortex	**Brief** (few seconds) episodes of **impaired consciousness,** normal muscle tone, possible eye blinking, no postictal confusion; more common in **children**	Generalized 3-cycle-per-second **spike and wave pattern**	Ethosuximide, valproic acid

EEG, electroencephalogram; H/P, history and physical.

B. **Types of seizures**
1. Classified according to electrical activity and extent of brain involvement
2. Electroencephalogram (EEG) used to measure cortical neuron activity and differentiate types of seizures
3. Anticonvulsants are the mainstay of therapy
C. **Status epilepticus**
1. **Repetitive seizures** without any period of regained consciousness
2. Due to withdrawal of anticonvulsants, alcohol withdrawal, trauma, pre-existing seizure disorder, metabolic abnormalities
3. **H/P** = uninterrupted seizures lasting >**20 minutes** (frequently several hours) **without** return to normal consciousness
4. **Labs** = complete blood count (CBC), glucose, electrolytes, toxicology, liver function tests (LFTs), blood urea nitrogen (BUN), and creatinine may be useful to determine underlying cause
5. **EEG** = shows prolonged abnormal electrical activity

Generalized seizures involve **the entire cortex.** Partial seizures involve **focal** neurologic deficits and may progress to **secondary** generalization (as distinguished from primary generalized seizures).

STEP Delay CT and EEG during status epilepticus until patient is stabilized.

TABLE 8-12	Anticonvulsant Medications Used in Epilepsy Treatment		
Drug	**Mechanism**	**Indications**	**Adverse Effects**
Phenytoin	Stabilizes neuronal membranes by decreasing Na⁺ passage, suppresses neuronal firing	**Partial and tonic-clonic** seizures, **status epilepticus**	Nausea, vomiting, gingival hyperplasia, anemia, confusion, **birth defects,** interactions with other P450-metabolized drugs
Carbamazepine	Inhibits action potentials by blocking Na⁺ channels	Partial and tonic-clonic seizures	Vertigo, drowsiness, blurred vision, nausea, vomiting, hepatotoxicity
Valproic acid	Reduces electrical propagation through enhanced GABA activity	Tonic-clonic and absence seizures	Hepatotoxicity, nausea, vomiting, drowsiness, tremor
Ethosuximide	Reduces electrical propagation in the brain	**Absence** seizures	Nausea, vomiting, drowsiness, inability to concentrate
Gabapentin	GABA analogue	Partial and tonic-clonic seizures	Drowsiness
Lamotrigine	Blocks Na⁺ channels, inhibits glutamate and aspartate release	Partial and tonic-clonic seizures	Drowsiness, rash
Benzodiazepines (diazepam, etc.)	Suppresses electrical propagation	**Status epilepticus**	Drowsiness
Barbiturates (phenobarbital, pentobarbital)	Suppresses electrical propagation, increases seizure threshold	Status epilepticus not responding to benzodiazepines	Drowsiness, general cognitive depression, vertigo, nausea, vomiting, rebound seizures

GABA, γ-aminobutyric acid.

6. **Treatment =**
   a. Maintain airway, breathing, circulation (ABCs)
   b. **IV benzodiazepines** used to end seizure activity, phenytoin given to prevent recurrence
   c. Refractive seizure activity may be treated with phenobarbital or pentobarbital
   d. Treat underlying disorder
7. **Complications =** >20% mortality if not controlled promptly

VI. Degenerative neurologic disorders

A. **Parkinson's disease**
   1. Idiopathic dopamine depletion and loss of dopaminergic striated neurons in the substantia nigra, leading to abnormal cholinergic input to cortex
   2. Similar syndrome may be induced by MPTP intoxication
   3. **H/P = resting tremor** ("pill rolling" tremor of hands), decreased or slowed voluntary movement (bradykinesia), mask-like facies, **shuffling gait,** involuntary acceleration of gait following initiation, **"cogwheel"** rigidity (increased tone of agonist and antagonist muscles), memory loss, difficulty initiating movement, postural instability
   4. **Treatment =**
      a. Dopaminergic agonists (levodopa, carbidopa, bromocriptine, amantadine), anticholinergic agents (benztropine)
      b. Pallidotomy or thalamotomy may be helpful in severe refractory cases
      c. Deep brain electrical stimulation may be helpful

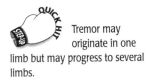

Tremor may originate in one limb but may progress to several limbs.

TABLE 8-13 Medications Used in Treatment of Parkinson's Disease

Drug	Mechanism	Indications	Adverse Effects
Levodopa	Dopamine precursor	Initial therapy	Nausea, vomiting, anorexia, tachycardia, hallucinations, mood changes
Carbidopa	Dopamine decarboxylase inhibitor that reduces levodopa metabolism	Combined with levodopa to augment effects	Reduces adverse effects of levodopa by allowing smaller dosage
Bromocriptine	Dopamine receptor agonist	Increases response to levodopa in patients with declining response	Hallucinations, confusion, nausea, hypotension, cardiotoxicity
Amantadine	Increases synthesis, release, or re-uptake of dopamine	More effective against rigidity and bradykinesia	Agitation, hallucinations
Antimuscarinic agents (e.g., benztropine)	Block cholinergic transmission	Adjuvant therapy	Mood changes, dry mouth, visual abnormalities, confusion, hallucinations, urinary retention

NEUROLOGIC DISORDERS

B. **Amyotrophic lateral sclerosis** (ALS)
1. Progressive loss of upper motor neurons (UMNs) and lower motor neurons (LMNs) in brain and spinal cord, involving degeneration of anterior horn cells
2. **H/P** = asymmetric **progressive weakness** in face (tongue, dysphagia) and limbs with **normal sensation and cognition;** increase or decrease in DTRs, spasticity, positive Babinski sign, flaccid paralysis, and fasciculations seen in limbs
3. **Labs** = blood tests used to rule out other pathologies
4. **Electromyogram (EMG)** = demonstrates denervation and fibrillation in >2 regions
5. **Radiology** = CT or MRI may be helpful to rule out neurologic lesions
6. **Treatment** = riluzole may slow progression; supportive care
7. **Complications** = half of patients die within three years of diagnosis secondary to respiratory failure

C. **Huntington's disease**
1. Autosomal dominant disease due to multiple CAG repeats on chromosome 4; higher numbers of CAG repeats lead to earlier onset of disease
2. Characteristic signs include movement and mental dysfunction starting in middle age
3. **H/P** = progressive, rapid irregular involuntary movement of extremities (**chorea**), dementia (e.g., irritability, antisocial behavior)
4. **Labs** = genetic analysis will detect chromosome 4 abnormality
5. **Radiology** = CT or MRI shows caudate nucleus and putamen atrophy
6. **Treatment** = dopamine antagonists may improve symptoms; genetic screening may be used in asymptomatic family members with proper counseling
7. **Complications** = usually fatal in <20 years from diagnosis

D. **Alzheimer's disease**
1. Slowly progressive dementia due to neurofibrillary tangles, neuritic plaques, amyloid deposition, and neuronal atrophy; **most common** cause of dementia

 Signs of **UMN** disease include spasticity, increased DTRs, positive Babinski sign. Signs of **LMN** disease include flaccid paralysis, decreased DTRs, fasciculations, negative Babinski sign.

 Clinical diagnosis of ALS requires signs of disease in three extremities or two extremities plus the face.

 Huntington's disease has **100%** genetic penetrance but does not become symptomatic until **middle age.**

STEP **NEXT** In elderly patients with **greater than mild** memory loss or dementia, Alzheimer's disease should be suspected.

STEP **NEXT** Distinguish dementia due to Alzheimer's disease from that due to multiple cortical infarcts with MRI. Multiple small lesions or infarcts will be apparent on MRI when there is a **vascular** cause.

STEP **NEXT** Highly suspect multiple sclerosis in a **young woman** with a confusing constellation of neurologic symptoms. Perform MRI to look for white matter lesions and LP to look for oligoclonal bands.

Lambert-Eaton syndrome is a paraneoplastic disorder (e.g., **small cell lung cancer**) with similar presentation to myasthenia gravis. It occurs because of antibodies to presynaptic Ca^{2+} channels, and is treated with immunosuppressive agents and plasmapheresis.

2. **Risk factors** = increased age, family history, Down's syndrome; female > male
3. **H/P** = progressive **short-term memory loss,** depression, **confusion,** inability to complete complex movements or tasks; severe cases have personality changes and delusions
4. **Labs** = nondiagnostic, but may be used to rule out other causes of dementia
5. **Radiology** = CT or MRI shows **cortical atrophy**
6. **Treatment** = cholinergic stimulants (donepezil, tacrine) may slow progression; occupational therapy helpful to prolong independence
7. **Complications** = death frequently occurs within 10 years of onset secondary to infection or aspiration

E. **Multiple sclerosis (**MS)
1. Progressive demyelinating disease of brain and spinal cord with possible autoimmune etiology
2. Most patients are **women** 20–40 years old
3. **H/P** =
   a. **Variable** initial presentation with multiple neurologic complaints (vertigo, vision abnormalities, paresthesias, weakness, urinary retention) that are difficult to explain through one cause
   b. Symptoms may progress slowly with several remissions and become worse during stressful events (infection, childbirth, trauma, heat)
   c. Late symptoms and signs include worsening vision, poor movement control, difficulty speaking (dysarthria), sensory abnormalities, postural and positional instabilities (cerebellar signs), spasticity, increased DTRs, and positive Babinski sign
4. **Labs** = LP shows CSF with increased protein, mildly increased WBCs, **oligoclonal bands,** increased IgG
5. **Radiology** = MRI shows multiple asymmetric **white matter lesions**
6. **Treatment** = corticosteroids and counseling the patient to avoid stress may help decrease length of exacerbations; interferon-β and copolymer 1 decrease frequency of exacerbations; supportive care
7. **Complications** = progressive neurologic abnormalities with residual deficits; many patients become chronically disabled

F. **Syringomyelia**
1. Post-traumatic cystic degeneration of spinal cord due to unknown mechanism
2. Syrinx cavity (centralized channel within spinal cord) expands and compresses adjacent neural tissue
3. **H/P** = symptoms and signs depend upon relation of nerve roots to cavity
   a. **Local to cavity**—loss of pain and temperature sensation, flaccid paralysis, decreased DTRs, fasciculations
   b. **Below cavity**—loss of proprioception and vibration sense, spasticity, increased DTRs
4. **Radiology** = MRI shows syrinx expansion
5. **Treatment** = surgical decompression; shunting may be needed for recurrent cases; supportive care

VII. **Peripheral neurologic and neuromuscular disorders**
A. **Myasthenia gravis**
1. Autoimmune disorder characterized by antibodies that bind to acetylcholine (ACh) receptors at neuromuscular junction and block normal neuromuscular transmission
2. Often associated with thymoma and thyrotoxicosis
3. Most common in **young adult women**

4. **H/P = periodic weakness** and muscle fatigue that worsens through day; ptosis, diplopia (double vision), dysphasia; severe cases may have dyspnea

5. **Labs = positive ACh receptor antibodies;** when edrophonium (anticholinesterase agent) is administered, symptoms improve

6. **Treatment** = anticholinesterase agents (neostigmine, pyridostigmine), thymectomy, immunosuppressive agents (prednisone, azathioprine), plasmapheresis, IV immunoglobulin for refractive cases

B. **Guillain-Barré syndrome**

1. Autoimmune demyelinating disorder of peripheral nerves associated with recent **viral infection,** surgery, or vaccination (rare)

2. **H/P =**
   a. Rapidly progressive **bilateral weakness** initially in distal extremities in **"stocking-glove"** distribution and extending proximally with **decreased sensation** and possible absent DTRs
   b. Recent history of viral infection/vaccination/surgery
   c. Blood pressure, heart rate, or core temperature may be labile
   d. Severe cases may include respiratory muscle weakness

3. **Labs** = LP shows increased protein with normal pressure and glucose

4. **EMG** = consistent with widespread demyelination

5. **Treatment** = self-resolving within 1 month; plasmapheresis or IV immunoglobulin may accelerate resolution; patients must be watched for signs of **respiratory failure**

6. **Complications** = respiratory failure requires intubation and ventilation; most patients recover fully

C. **Reflex sympathetic dystrophy** (RSD)

1. **Chronic pain** syndrome that occurs after trauma due to abnormal neurologic reorganization at site of injury (pain fibers may become "wired" into sympathetic neuronal pathways)

2. **H/P = hypersensitive** and painful limb following recovery from injury, edema, atrophy, abnormal tone and increased sweating at involved site; occasional cyanosis or increased hair growth at injury site

3. **Radiology** = bone scan may show decreased perfusion of injured site

4. **Treatment =**
   a. Selected nerve blocks with sensation testing may help differentiate RSD from other neuropathies
   b. Physical therapy, transcutaneous electrical nerve stimulation (TENS), regional nerve block, and corticosteroids have been suggested as initial therapies
   c. Sypathectomy may be used in refractory cases

D. **Hyperkinetic disorders (see Table 8-14)**

1. Abnormal involuntary movement associated with specific neurologic diseases or other causes

2. Described by pattern of movements

VIII. Neoplasms

A. **Primary CNS neoplasms**

1. Brain tumors that are not due to distant metastases; more common in young and middle-aged adults

2. Tumors in **adults** tend to be **above** the tentorium (fold of dural meninges that separates cerebellum below from cortex above)

3. Tumors in **children** tend to be **below** the tentorium

4. Symptoms result from focal compression (i.e., mass effect) of tumor (hydrocephalus, increased ICP, venous obstruction)

5. **H/P** = headache, vomiting, lethargy; focal neurologic abnormalities, change in mental status, possible seizures; blown pupil seen if herniation occurs

Edrophonium is a short-acting agent, making it ideal for myasthenia gravis testing (Tensilon test) but ineffective for therapy.

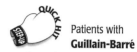
Patients with **Guillain-Barré** syndrome have sensory impairment, while patients with **ALS** retain sensation.

Glioblastoma multiforme is the most common primary brain tumor in **adults. Medulloblastoma** is the most common brain tumor in **children.**

TABLE 8-14 Common Hyperkinetic Disorders

Disorder	Movement	Associated Diseases	Treatment
Benign essential tremor	**Fixed oscillation** of hands or head	Idiopathic	β-Blockers, primidone, clonazepam
Chorea	Rapid **flinching** distal limb and facial movements	**Hyperthyroidism,** stroke, **Huntington's disease,** SLE, levodopa use, rheumatic heart disease	Treat the underlying disorder
Athetosis	**Snake-like** movement in extremities	**Cerebral palsy,** encephalopathy, Huntington's disease, Wilson's disease	Treat underlying disorder
Dystonia	Slow **writhing** proximal limb and trunk contractions	Wilson's disease, **Parkinson's disease,** Huntington's disease, encephalitis, neuroleptic use (**tardive dyskinesia**)	Carbidopa, levodopa, botulinum toxin, treat underlying disorder
Hemiballismus	**Flinging** of proximal extremities	Stroke (subthalamic nucleus)	Haloperidol
Tics	**Repetitive** brief involuntary movement (blinking, grimacing) or sound (grunting, sniffing, throat clearing)	**Tourette's syndrome,** obsessive-compulsive disorder, attention deficit hyperactivity disorder	Clonidine, haloperidol, methylphenidate, dextroamphetamine

SLE, systemic lupus erythematosus.

Metastatic brain tumors are **more common** than primary tumors.

Most metastases to the brain are **supratentorial.**

6. **Labs** = biopsy under CT guidance of detected lesion used for diagnosis
7. **Radiology** = CT with contrast or MRI detects lesion
8. **Treatment** = surgical resection (if possible), radiation, chemotherapy; corticosteroids may decrease cerebral edema, anticonvulsants used for seizure prophylaxis

B. **Metastatic CNS neoplasms**
1. Tumors that have metastasized to brain from distant site; lung, breast, kidney, gastrointestinal (GI) tract, melanoma are most common primary tumors

TABLE 8-15 Primary Central Nervous System Neoplasms

Tumor	Location	H/P	Treatment	Prognosis
Meningioma	Dura mater	Headache, seizures, focal neurologic deficits	Surgical resection, radiation	Good
Astrocytoma	Cortex	Headache, gradual increase in ICP, facial sensory and motor deficits	Surgical resection, radiation	50% 2-yr survival
Glioblastoma multiforme (high-grade astrocytoma)	Cortex	Headache, rapid increase in ICP, facial sensory and motor deficits	Surgical resection, radiation, chemotherapy	Poor; 10% 2-yr survival
CNS lymphoma	Meninges or cortex (immunocompromised patients)	Headache, seizures, focal neurologic deficits	Corticosteroids, radiation, chemotherapy	Variable
Medulloblastoma	4th cerebral ventricle	Hydrocephalus, increased ICP	Surgical resection, radiation, chemotherapy	Poor

CNS, central nervous system; H/P, history and physical; ICP, intracranial pressure.

2. **H/P** = symptoms similar to presentation for primary tumors; headache, vomiting, lethargy; focal neurologic abnormalities, change in mental status, seizures

3. **Labs** = biopsy confirms origin of tumor

4. **Radiology** = CT with contrast or MRI detects lesions

5. **Treatment** = treat original tumor; surgical resection for single metastasis, palliative radiation

6. **Complications** = poor prognosis

C. **Neurofibromatosis type 1 (von Recklinghausen's disease)**

1. Autosomal dominant disorder (NF1 gene on chromosome 17) with multiple neurologic tumor and dermatologic manifestations

2. Neurofibromatosis type 2 is a rare autosomal dominant disorder linked to chromosome 22, characterized by the development of bilateral **acoustic neuromas**

3. At least two of the following required for diagnosis:

   a. >5 **café-au-lait macules** >15 mm diameter

   b. >1 **neurofibromas** or one plexiform neurofibroma (tumors with mix of Schwann cells, fibroblasts, and mast cells)

   c. Axillary or inguinal freckling

   d. Optic glioma (tumor of optic nerve)

   e. >1 iris hamartomas (**Lisch nodules**)

   f. Bone lesions (cortical thinning of long bones, sphenoid dysplasia)

   g. 1st-degree relative with neurofibromatosis type 1

4. **H/P** =

   a. Initial signs are freckling, **café-au-lait spots, Lisch nodules, neurofibromas,** and **bone abnormalities** evident in first few years of life

   b. Severe functional limitations in movement and gait may be seen due to nonunion of bone fragments (pseudoarthrosis) and fractures during development

   c. Short stature and scoliosis may be evident

   d. Visual abnormalities may result from compression of optic nerve by glioma

5. **Labs** = genetic testing detects abnormal gene

6. **Radiology** = MRI shows multiple areas of increased signal intensity in brain and increased brain volume

7. **Treatment** = therapy directed at maintaining function and treating complications

8. **Complications** = increased risk of malignant CNS tumors, developmental delays, mental retardation, peripheral neuropathy, pheochromocytoma, vision abnormalities, severe bone abnormalities, seizures

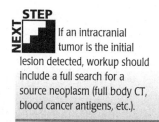

NEXT STEP If an intracranial tumor is the initial lesion detected, workup should include a full search for a source neoplasm (full body CT, blood cancer antigens, etc.).

IX. Sleep and loss of consciousness

A. **Sleep**

1. **Normal sleep cycles**

   a. Stage 1 sleep is light sleep with fast θ waves on EEG

   b. Stage 2 sleep is intermediate sleep with sleep spindles and k-complexes on EEG

   c. Stages 3 and 4 sleep are deep sleep with δ waves on EEG

   d. Rapid eye movement (REM) sleep occurs every 90–120 minutes and is characterized by rapid eye movements, dreams, and low-voltage, high-frequency EEG pattern

2. **Sleep apnea**

   a. Hypoventilation during sleep secondary to pulmonary obstruction or decreased neurologic respiratory drive (see Chapter 2, Pulmonary Disorders)

Most of sleep is spent in stage 2.
Benzodiazepines increase stage 2 sleep and decrease stages 3 and 4, and do not reproduce normal sleep architecture.

3. **Narcolepsy**
   a. Sudden onset of sleep with decreased latency until REM occurs
   b. **H/P** = sudden loss of muscle tone (cataplexy), vivid dreams, sleep paralysis; **hypersomnia** (sudden occurrence of sleep) may occur suddenly during the daytime
   c. **Treatment** = methylphenidate or pemoline help prevent hypersomnia, tricyclic antidepressants may help prevent cataplexy

B. **Syncope**
   1. Acute transient loss of consciousness frequently related to inadequate blood supply to the brain
   2. Common causes include **cardiac dysfunction** (aortic stenosis, bradycardia, decreased stroke volume), vasovagal response, hypotension, **hypoglycemia,** seizures, cerebrovascular ischemia
   3. **H/P** = lightheadedness, nausea, and weakness preceding loss of consciousness (i.e., fainting); few generalized spasms may be observed; **patient quickly regains consciousness (**though seizure patients may display postictal sleepiness**)**
   4. **Labs** = glucose levels should be measured; **orthostatics** or tilt testing (patient response is measured with rapid posture changes) with or without β-blocker infusion can help diagnose cardiovascular cause
   5. **EEG** = useful for detecting epileptic causes
   6. **Radiology** = MRI, MRA, or angiography may detect vascular abnormalities
   7. **Treatment** = treat underlying cause

C. **Coma**
   1. Condition in which patient is **unresponsive to stimuli** and **unable to communicate;** associated with bilateral cortical or brainstem reticular activating system dysfunction
   2. May be due to cerebral hemorrhage, tumor, abscess, sedating drugs (alcohol, benzodiazepines, narcotics), hypoglycemia, metabolic dysfunction, hypothermia, hepatorenal failure, or psychogenic causes
   3. **H/P** = patient unresponsive to stimuli; pertinent history and physical exam helpful for determining cause
   4. **Labs** = CBC, electrolytes, BUN and creatinine, glucose, LFTs, coagulation factors, toxicology, or arterial blood gas are helpful for diagnosis
   5. **Radiology** = CT or MRI may detect intracranial cause (hemorrhage, tumor)
   6. **Treatment** = maintain airway, breathing, and circulation (ABCs); prevent increase in ICP (hyperventilation, mannitol, elevate head); treat underlying cause

X. **Pediatric neurologic issues**
   A. **Febrile seizures**
      1. Childhood seizures between 6 months–6 years old associated with **fever**
      2. **H/P** = fever > 102° F (38.9 °C) with rapid rise in temperature; tonic-clonic seizure lasting <15 minutes; atypical seizures may occur at lower temperature and may last longer
      3. **Labs** = LP should be performed if meningitis suspected
      4. **EEG** = usually normal unless atypical seizure
      5. **Treatment** = **acetaminophen** as antipyretic; atypical seizures should receive more in-depth workup including blood labs, EEG, and MRI
      6. **Complications** =
         a. 50% of patients have recurrent febrile seizures but little increase in lifetime risk of epilepsy

A patient in a **persistent vegetative state** has normal sleep cycles, an inability to perceive and interact with the environment, and preserved autonomic function for >**1 month.** Recovery is unlikely if these symptoms last >**3 months.**

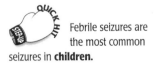
Febrile seizures are the most common seizures in **children.**

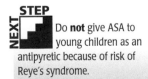
Do **not** give ASA to young children as an antipyretic because of risk of Reye's syndrome.

FIGURE 8-6 Approach to the patient in a coma.

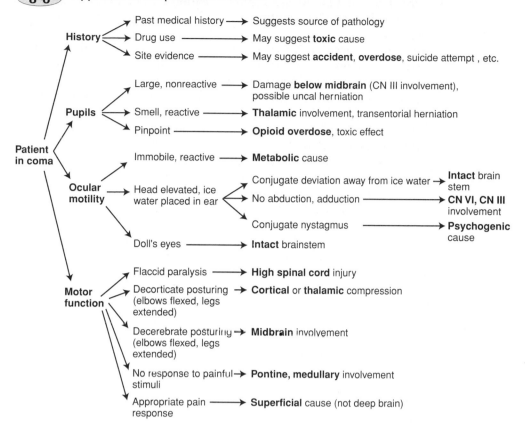

B. **Childhood hydrocephalus**
1. Hydrocephalus in children due to either obstruction of CSF circulation in 4th cerebral ventricle (**noncommunicating**) or dysfunction of subarachnoid cisterns or arachnoid villi (**communicating**)
2. **H/P = increased head growth,** bulging fontanelles, and dilated scalp veins in infants; lethargy, vomiting, poor appetite, irritability, headache, poor skull suture fusion in older children
3. **Radiology** = US, CT, or MRI will show expanded ventricles
4. **Treatment** = acetazolamide or furosemide may be used to temporarily relieve symptoms; surgical shunting usually required for most cases
5. **Complications** = increased risk of bacterial infection with shunting
C. **Tay-Sachs disease**
1. Autosomal recessive disorder due to absence of hexosaminidase A (enzyme required for lipid ganglioside metabolism)
2. **Risk factors = Ashkenazi Jews,** French Canadians
3. **H/P** = poor development, decreased alertness, hyperacute hearing; **cherry-red spots** on **retina** on fundoscopic exam, progressive paralysis, vision loss, change in mental status
4. **Labs** = decreased hexosaminidase A activity
5. **Treatment** = supportive care; genetic screening may aid parents with future childbearing decisions
6. **Complications** = death within first few years of life

Arnold-Chiari malformation type II and Dandy-Walker malformations are anatomic defects of the skull and ventricular system associated with hydrocephalus in children.

b. **Atypical** febrile seizures more likely to recur, occur over longer periods of time, and carry an increased risk of epilepsy

D. **Neural tube disorders**
1. Failure of neural tube closure during gestation leading to spectrum of defects involving CNS formation
2. Types of defects
   a. **Spina bifida occulta**—most benign type; defect in **closure of dorsal vertebral arches** above spinal cord (usually lumbosacral junction)
   b. **Meningocele**—larger defect with herniation of meninges through dorsal vertebral defect; soft mass may form in midline superficial to defect
   c. **Myelomeningocele**—severe defect with herniation of meninges and spinal cord through defect; frequent neurologic deficits including bowel and bladder incontinence, flaccid paralysis, poor sensation, LMN signs, hydrocephalus
   d. **Anencephaly**—severe disorder with failure of cranial neural tube to close; absence of forebrain, meninges, and portions of skull; death occurs within days of birth
3. **Risk factors** = anticonvulsant use or **poor folate intake** during pregnancy (both result in low maternal serum folate)
4. **H/P** =
   a. Symptom severity depends on severity of defect; patients with spina bifida may have tuft of hair over defect and may be asymptomatic
   b. More severe cases of spina bifida may include delayed motor and mental development
   c. More severe neural tube defects have more severe neurologic and developmental abnormalities
5. **Labs** = increased amniotic α-**fetoprotein, acetylcholinesterase** during gestation
6. **Radiology** = US during pregnancy may detect defects
7. **Treatment** =
   a. Surgical repair of all but mild defects needed
   b. Shunting frequently needed for meningocele and myelomeningocele to resolve hydrocephalus
   c. Physical therapy needed for gait abnormalities for patients capable of walking (spina bifida)
   d. Appropriate supportive care for children with more severe neurologic deficits and those involving the genitourinary system
   e. Pregnant women and women trying to conceive should be given folate supplementation to reduce risk of defects
8. **Complications** = increased risk of urinary tract infection and CNS infection; hydrocephalus in severe defects; children with severe defects may require lifelong care

E. **Cerebral palsy (CP)**
1. Disorders of motor function resulting from CNS damage within the first years of life; most cases are due to **perinatal complications**
2. **Risk factors** = prematurity, intrauterine growth restriction, **birth trauma,** neonatal seizures or cerebral hemorrhage, **perinatal asphyxia**
3. Types
   a. **Spastic**—spastic paresis of multiple limbs
   b. **Nonspastic**—choreoathetoid (see hyperkinetic disorders in this chapter), dystonic, or ataxic movement disorder
4. **H/P** =
   a. Patients with spastic CP have multiple limbs with increased tone, increased DTRs, weakness, gait abnormalities, and frequent mental retardation
   b. Patients with nonspastic CP have choreoathetoid, dystonic, or ataxic movements that worsen with stress as well as having difficulty speaking (dysarthria)

Spastic CP is due to damage of **pyramidal** tracts. **Nonspastic** CP is due to **extrapyramidal** pathology.

c. Both types of CP may have hyperactivity, seizures, or limb contractures

d. Some patients may exhibit symptoms of both types

5. **Treatment** =

a. Pharmacologic therapy (botulinum toxin, dantrolene, baclofen, benzodiazepines), physical therapy, bracing, and surgery may be used to alleviate contractures and improve function

b. Speech therapy is useful for dysarthria

c. Special education is needed for patients with mental retardation

F. **Retinoblastoma**

1. Malignant tumor of retina in children and the most common **intraocular tumor** in children

2. Some cases have genetic link that increases risk of tumor for both eyes

3. **H/P** = rarely, patients experience decrease in vision or eye inflammation; ophthalmologic exam may detect poor red-light reflex in affected eye (**leukocoria**) or white retinal mass (Color Figure 8-1)

4. **Labs** = mutation of RB1 gene apparent on genetic testing

5. **Radiology** = US and CT detect size and extent of tumor; finding of calcified mass with normal globe size on CT is needed before initiation of therapy can begin

6. **Treatment** =

a. Enucleation performed for large tumors with no vision potential

b. Radiation may be used for bilateral tumors or tumors near optic nerve

c. Cryotherapy or laser photocoagulation used for smaller tumors

d. Chemotherapy used for metastases or vision salvage

7. **Complications** = good prognosis if metastasis has not occurred; risk of vision loss is high if tumor is adjacent to cornea

XI. Ophthalmology

A. **Normal eye function**

1. Retinal artery and vein are vasculature for the retina; vascular pathology affects vision (e.g., occlusion, DM retinopathy)

2. Nerves

a. Optic nerve (CN II) responsible for vision

b. Trochlear nerve (CN IV) controls superior oblique muscle (downward medial gaze, inward eye rotation)

c. Abducens nerve (CN VI) controls lateral rectus muscle (abduction)

d. Oculomotor nerve (CN III) controls all other eye muscles

e. Medial longitudinal fasciculus (MLF) maintains conjugate gaze when one eye abducts

f. Specific distortions in vision result from neuronal injury depending on site of insult

B. **Common vision abnormalities (see Table 8-17)**

1. Types of visual irregularity are due to abnormal eye shape, gaze alignment, or eye focal orientation

2. Usually correctable through **lenses,** visual training, or surgery

C. **Eye inflammation and infection**

1. **Conjunctivitis**

a. Inflammation of eye mucosa secondary to bacterial or viral infection or allergic reaction

b. **H/P** = mildly painful eye, **inflamed conjunctiva,** possible lymphadenopathy, pruritic eye when due to allergy; purulent discharge seen with bacterial infection

c. **Labs** = Gram stain and culture of discharge may indicate bacterial cause

d. **Treatment** = self-limited; topical sulfonamides reduce duration of bacterial infection; antihistamines improve symptoms due to allergic

Conjunctivitis facts:

- Adenovirus is the most common cause

- Typically highly contagious and may be spread by contact with towels or linens or by close contact

- May be caused by *N. gonorrhoeae* and *Chlamydia trachomatis* after sexual contact

- May occur in the perinatal period if mother is infected with *N. gonorrhoeae* or *C. trachomatis.*

TABLE 8-16 Common Pupil and Gaze Abnormalities

Abnormality	Presentation	Cause
Argyll-Robertson pupil	Accommodation to near objects, nonreactive to light	Syphilis, SLE, DM
Marcus Gunn pupil	Light in affected pupil causes minimal bilateral constriction, light in normal pupil causes normal bilateral constriction	Afferent nerve defect
Horner's syndrome	Ptosis, miosis, anhidrosis	Sympathetic trunk lesion (e.g., Pancoast tumor)
Adie's pupil	Nonreactive dilated pupil	Abnormal innervation of iris
MLF syndrome	With lateral gaze there is absent contralateral eye adduction	Intracranial lesion, MS

DM, diabetes mellitus; MLF, medial longitudinal fasciculus; MS, multiple sclerosis; SLE, systemic lupus erythematosus.

reaction; fastidious handwashing decreases community spread of infection

2. **Uveitis**
   a. Inflammation of iris, choroids, and ciliary bodies due to infectious (viral, syphilis), autoimmune (ankylosing spondylitis, **juvenile rheumatoid arthritis**), or inflammatory (ulcerative colitis, **Crohn's** disease) conditions
   b. **H/P** =
      (1) **Anterior uveitis**—pain and photophobia; slit lamp exam shows inflammation of eye and keratin deposits on cornea
      (2) **Posterior uveitis**—mild vision abnormalities; slit lamp exam shows eye inflammation and retinal lesions

FIGURE 8-7 Visual field defects resulting from neuronal injury.

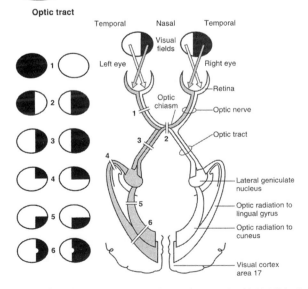

(Used with permission from Mehta S, Milder EA, Mirachi AJ, Milder E. *Step-Up: A High-Yield, Systems-Based Review for the USMLE Step 1.* 2nd Ed. Philadelphia: Lippincott Williams & Wilkins; 2003.)

TABLE 8-17 Common Vision Abnormalities

Disorder	Cause	H/P	Treatment
Myopia	Refracting power of eye is too great causing image focal point to be anterior to retina	Blurred vision, vision quality worsens as objects move farther away	Corrective lenses, laser correction
Hyperopia	Refracting power of eye is insufficient causing image focal point to be posterior to retina	Blurred vision, vision quality worsens as objects move closer	Corrective lenses, laser correction
Astigmatism	Asymmetrical cornea surface causing inconsistent refraction of light	Blurred vision	Corrective lenses
Strabismus	Deviation of eye unable to be overcome by normal motor control	Gaze for each eye is in different directions, double vision, progressive blindness	Vision training, surgery frequently required to achieve bilateral alignment
Amblyopia ("lazy eye")	Developmental defect in neural pathways of eye	Poor visual acuity, spatial differentiation in affected eye	Vision training, levodopa, carbidopa

H/P, history and physical.

    c. **Treatment** = topical or systemic corticosteroids; treat underlying condition

D. **Cataracts**
   1. **Clouding** of lens leading to progressive vision loss
   2. May be due to trauma (caustic substances), DM, corticosteroid use, **age,** or tobacco use
   3. **H/P** = progressive hazy and blurred vision occurring over months to years; exam reveals opacity of lenses and decreased red reflex
   4. **Treatment** = lens replacement surgery

E. **Glaucoma**
   1. Increased intraocular pressure (IOP) leading to loss of vision
   2. **Open angle glaucoma**
     a. **Gradual** bilateral increase in IOP
     b. **Risk factors** = increased age, African American, DM, myopia, family history
     c. **H/P** = initially asymptomatic; gradual loss of vision (from **peripheral to central**), halos seen around lights, headache, and poor adaptation to changes in light; **cupping** of optic disc seen on fundoscopic examination
     d. **Labs** = IOP testing (tonometry) shows increased pressure over several tests performed at 2–4 week intervals
     e. **Treatment** =
       (1) Topical β-blockers (e.g., timolol) decrease aqueous humor production; pilocarpine increases aqueous humor removal
       (2) Laser surgery improves aqueous humor drainage in refractory cases
       (3) Prevention is important for all at-risk patients, who should receive **regular ophthalmologic exams**
     f. **Complications** = progressive, permanent vision loss
   3. **Closed angle glaucoma**
     a. **Acute** increase in IOP secondary to narrowing of anterior chamber angle and obstructed drainage of aqueous humor from eye
     b. **Risk factors** = increased age, Asian, hyperopia, dilated pupils (e.g., low-light environments, optometry exam dilation)

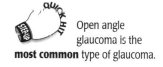

Open angle glaucoma is the **most common** type of glaucoma.

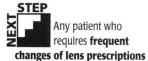

STEP
Any patient who requires **frequent changes of lens prescriptions** should be suspected for having glaucoma and pressure testing should be performed.

Closed angle glaucoma is usually **unilateral.**

STEP
NEXT **Never** induce additional pupil dilation during exam of patient with suspected closed angle glaucoma because it will acutely worsen the condition.

Macular degeneration is the most common cause of **bilateral** vision loss in the elderly.

c. **H/P** = severe eye pain, blurred vision, halos seen around lights, nausea, and vomiting; eye is inflamed and **hard** with a **dilated** and nonreactive pupil

d. **Labs** = tonometry demonstrates increased IOP

e. **Treatment** =

    (1) Acetazolamide decreases pressure; pilocarpine administered after pressure is lowered to reduce obstruction

    (2) Laser iridotomy should be performed to prevent recurrence (frequently performed on unaffected eye as prophylaxis)

f. **Complications** = rapid permanent vision loss

F. **Macular degeneration**

1. Atrophic (slow) or exudative (rapid) degeneration of retina, leading to **retinal fibrosis** and **permanent vision loss**

2. **Risk factors** = Caucasian, tobacco, family history; female > male

3. **H/P** = painless, gradual loss of vision **(central to peripheral)**; retinal pigmentation and hemorrhage in macular region and possible retinal detachment seen on fundoscopic examination

4. **Radiology** = fluorescein angiography may show neovascular membranes and retina

5. **Treatment** = laser photocoagulation may delay progression

6. **Complications** = treatment effectiveness is limited; gradual progression to severe vision loss

G. **Retinal detachment**

1. Separating of retina from adjacent epithelium, leading to acute vision loss

2. **Risk factors** = trauma, cataract surgery, myopia

3. **H/P** = painless acute loss of vision **("window shade pulled over eye")**; gray retina floating in vitreous humor seen on fundoscopic examination

4. **Treatment** = laser photocoagulation or cryotherapy to halt tear progression and reattach retina (may not fully restore loss of vision)

H. **Retinal vessel occlusion**

1. Occlusion of retinal artery or vein resulting in sudden loss of vision

2. Most commonly due to atherosclerosis, DM, HTN, **thromboembolic disease (Color Figures 8-2, 8-3, and 8-4)**

3. **H/P** = acute painless loss of vision (more sudden in arterial occlusion); fundoscopic examination shows **cherry-red spot** in fovea and poor arterial filling in arterial occlusion and **cotton wool spots,** edema, **retinal hemorrhages,** and dilated veins in venous occlusion

4. **Treatment** =

    a. Thrombolysis of arterial occlusion should be performed within 8 hours of onset

    b. Acetazolamide and O_2 administration also used to decrease congestion and increase perfusion for arterial occlusion

    c. Laser photocoagulation may be useful for venous occlusion

5. **Complications** = without prompt treatment, permanent vision loss results

XII. Audiovestibular disorders

A. **Otitis media**

1. Infection of middle ear caused by *Streptococcus pneumoniae, Haemophilus influenzae, Moraxella catarrhalis, Streptococcus pyogenes,* or viruses

2. Increased risk in children secondary to shorter and more horizontal ear canal than in adults, pacifier use, hypertrophic tonsillar tissue

3. **H/P** = ear pain, decreased hearing; fever, **bulging** tympanic membrane with **decreased mobility,** poor light reflex; possible bloody discharge with perforation

4. **Treatment** =

    a. Initially observation and supportive care

      b. For unresolved cases amoxicillin for 10 days; resistant strains may require trimethoprim-sulfamethoxazole (TMP-SMX)

      c. Recurrent cases may require surgical placement of tympanic tubes to assist in middle ear drainage

   5. **Complications** = mastoiditis, meningitis, hearing loss, sigmoid sinus thrombosis, or brain abscess may occur in untreated cases

B. **Otitis externa ("swimmer's ear")**

   1. Infection of outer ear canal most commonly by *Escherichia coli, Pseudomonas,* or *Proteus;* frequently associated with water in ears (e.g., swimming)

   2. **H/P** = painful, swollen ear with possible white discharge; **ear canal** is red and **swollen,** tenderness of pinna

   3. **Treatment** = topical polymyxin, neomycin, and hydrocortisone; oral cephalosporins or ciprofloxacin may be used for *Pseudomonas* infection or infection that spreads to involved skull; topical drying agents after H_2O exposure to prevent recurrent infection

C. **Benign paroxysmal positional vertigo** (BPPV)

   1. Vertigo (abnormal feeling of rotational movement leading to poor balance and coordination) caused by a dislodged otolith in the inner ear that interferes with semicircular canal stabilization

   2. **H/P** =

      a. Brief episodic vertigo that may be brought on by certain head movements accompanied by nausea, vomiting

      b. Nystagmus may be seen during episodes

      c. **Dix-Hallpike maneuver** (moving from sitting to supine while quickly turning head to side) induces symptoms and confirms diagnosis

   3. **Labs** = normal thyroid-stimulating hormone (TSH) level rules out thyroid pathology

   4. **Radiology** = CT or MRI can rule out intracranial lesion

   5. **Treatment** = physical maneuvers designed to free otolith from semicircular canal can alleviate recurrent episodes

D. **Ménière's disease** (endolymphatic hydrops)

   1. Vertigo caused by distension of endolymphatic compartment of inner ear

   2. **H/P** = acute vertigo lasting **several hours,** nausea, vomiting, decreased hearing, feeling of ear fullness, tinnitus (ringing in ears)

   3. **Labs** = audiometry shows **low-frequency hearing loss**

   4. **Treatment** = anticholinergics and antihistamines improve exacerbations; salt restriction and acetazolamide may reduce frequency of episodes; surgical decompression needed in refractory cases

   5. **Complications** = progressive hearing loss

E. **Acoustic neuroma (Schwannoma)**

   1. Benign tumor of Schwann cells of CN VIII that may lead to hearing loss secondary to nerve compression

   2. **H/P** = hearing loss, dizziness, tinnitus; unilateral facial palsy, decreased sensation may be seen on examination

   3. **Labs** = audiometry shows sensorineural hearing loss

   4. **Radiology** = MRI can localize tumor

   5. **Treatment** = surgical excision

   6. **Complications** = large tumors may compress cerebellum or brain stem

- Conductive hearing loss:
  - Pathology occurs along conductive pathway from outer ear to inner ear
  - Audiometry shows **preserved air** conduction, but consistently low hearing threshold (negative Rinne test)
- Sensorineural hearing loss:
  - Pathology in neural pathways from ear to brain
  - Audiometry shows both **impaired bone** and **air conduction** (asymmetric Weber test, positive Rinne test)

Musculoskeletal Disorders

I. Common adult orthopaedic conditions

A. Carpal tunnel syndrome

1. Syndrome resulting from the **median** nerve being compressed at the wrist
2. **Risk factors** =
   a. **Pregnancy,** rheumatoid arthritis (RA), diabetes mellitus (DM), acromegaly, hypothyroidism, obesity, **overuse** (activities requiring significant wrist motion including typing, piano playing, writing, etc.)
   b. Most common in 30–55 year olds; female > male
3. **H/P** =
   a. Wrist pain that radiates up arm and worsens with hand flexion and grasping, decreased hand strength, numbness in thumb and index and middle fingers, decreased two-point discrimination except on the radial side of the palm
   b. Positive **Tinel's** sign (tapping palmaris longus tendon elicits wrist tingling and pain) and **Phalen's** sign (placing dorsal side of hands together and flexing wrists 90° causes the onset of symptoms within a minute)
   c. Thenar muscle atrophy is seen in long-term cases
4. **Electromyogram (EMG)** = can be used in addition to nerve conduction studies to evaluate nerve compromise
5. **Treatment** = wrist splints, **activity modification,** nonsteroidal anti-inflammatory drugs (NSAIDs), corticosteroid injections, surgical diversion of the transverse carpal ligament

B. Dislocations

1. **Shoulder**
   a. Most commonly **anterior** (posteriorly directed force on distal humerus or forearm during abduction causes cantilever effect that drives humeral head forward and tears anterior shoulder capsule)
   b. **Posterior** dislocations most frequently occur following **seizures** and **electrical shock** (strong contraction in internally rotated, adducted arm causes humeral head dislocation)
   c. **Treatment** = closed reduction, sling; chronic dislocations may require surgery to improve joint stability
   d. **Complications** = axillary artery and nerve injury, increased risk of future dislocations
2. **Hip**
   a. Most commonly **posterior** via a posteriorly directed force on an internally rotated, flexed, and adducted hip (e.g., dash board injury)
   b. **Treatment** = closed reduction, bracing, abduction pillow

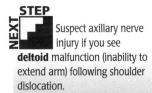

NEXT STEP
Suspect axillary nerve injury if you see **deltoid** malfunction (inability to extend arm) following shoulder dislocation.

FIGURE 9-1 Tendonous and neurovascular structures superficial and deep to the transverse carpal ligament in the wrist.

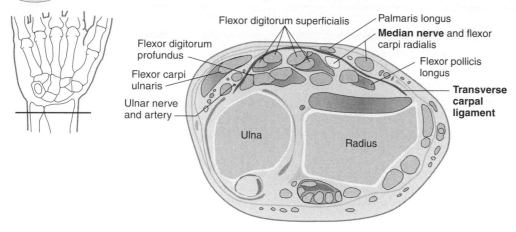

(Modified from Moore KL. *Clinically Oriented Anatomy.* 3rd Ed. Baltimore: Williams & Wilkins; 1992.)

C. **Fractures (see Table 9-1)**
   1. Fractures are associated with a particular mechanism of injury and carry different options depending on location
D. **Sprains**
   1. Common in the ankle and knee
   2. Injuries to **ligaments** and surrounding soft tissues in a joint; structures may be partially or completely torn at ligament-bone interface or within ligament substance
   3. **H/P** — pain in involved joint with weight bearing or movement
   4. **Treatment** = **RICE**: **R**est, **I**cing, and **C**ompression of swelling, **E**levation of joint; analgesics
E. **Ligament tears**
   1. Occur from excessive stress on joints
   2. **H/P** = pain and swelling that worsens with joint stress
   3. **Radiology** = magnetic resonance imaging (MRI) may confirm tear
   4. **Treatment** = initially as for sprains; may require surgical repair
F. **Meniscus tears (knee)**
   1. Result from repetitive microtrauma and degeneration
   2. Frequently associated with anterior cruciate ligament (**ACL**) injury (especially from blunt trauma or sports injuries)
   3. **H/P** = vague pain inside knee joint; clicking or locking of joint
   4. **Radiology** = MRI may detect tear
   5. **Treatment** = NSAIDs, physical therapy, arthroscopic repair
   6. **Complications** = arthroscopic debridement may predispose knee to developing osteoarthritis
G. **Compartment syndrome**
   1. Trauma (surgical or accidental) in extremities leads to reperfusion injury and swelling of fascial compartments; **intracompartmental swelling** may cause compression of **neurovascular** structures leading to **ischemia**
   2. Most common in **lower leg** (e.g., tibial fracture) and forearm
   3. **H/P** = **6 Ps** are signs of progression (**Pain, Pallor, Poikilothermia, Pulselessness, Paresthesia, Paralysis**); compartment pain with passive stretching is best screening test
   4. **Labs** = elevated pressure seen in compartment pressure measurement (needle inserted into compartment and manometry)
   5. **Treatment** = **emergent fasciotomy** for pressures >30 mmHg or for pressures within 20 mmHg of diastolic blood pressure

NEXT STEP An **open** fracture (fracture penetrates skin and is exposed to outside environment) requires thorough **irrigation** in the operating room to reduce the risk of **infection.**

CT is generally more useful in the diagnosis of **bone** pathology, while **MRI** is more useful in **soft tissue** injuries.

A medially directed blow to the lateral side of the knee (valgus stress) may cause the **unhappy triad: medial meniscus** tear, **medial collateral ligament** (MCL) tear, and **ACL** tear.

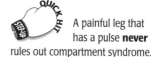

A painful leg that has a pulse **never** rules out compartment syndrome.

TABLE 9-1 **Common Fractures, Their Mechanism of Injury, and Appropriate Treatment**

Type	Bones Involved	H/P	Treatment	Clinical Pearls
Colles	Distal radius	**Fall on outstretched hand,** forearm dorsally displaced and angulated (forearm profile looks like a **dinner fork**)	Closed reduction Long arm cast Possible surgery	Most common wrist fracture
Scaphoid	Scaphoid	"Snuffbox" tenderness, fall on radially deviated outstretched hand	Thumb spica cast Possible surgery	Increased risk of AVN; **not seen on x-ray for 1–2 weeks after injury;** most common carpal fracture
Boxer's	5th-metacarpal neck	Punching hard object or surface with a strong force applied to 5th metacarpal	Closed reduction Ulnar gutter splint Surgical pinning	Beware the "fight bite"—open wounds from teeth will need surgical exploration to rule out tendon involvement
Humerus	Humerus	Trauma (motor vehicle accident, blunt trauma, etc.)	Closed reduction Splint Possible surgery	If you see wrist drop or weakened thumb abduction, think radial nerve injury
Monteggia	Dislocation of radial head and ulnar diaphyseal fracture	Defense against blunt trauma (e.g., nightstick injury)	Closed reduction of radial head Surgical repair of ulna	
Galeazzi	DRUJ dislocation and radial diaphyseal fracture	Trauma (direct blow or fall)	Surgical repair Cast forearm in supination to maintain reduction of DRUJ	
Hip	Femoral head or neck	Fall, motor vehicle accident, trauma Injured leg is shortened and externally rotated Frequently occurs from strong axial force (e.g., fall or knee hitting a car dashboard)	Surgical repair May require joint replacement	Increased risk for **AVN** and DVT Particularly dangerous in elderly Anticoagulate
Femur	Femoral diaphysis	Trauma	Surgical repair	Increased risk of fat embolization
Tibial	Tibia	Trauma	Cast Surgical repair	
Ankle	Medial, lateral, and/or posterior malleoli	Trauma, excessive twist of ankle (most commonly supination and external rotation	Cast Possible surgical repair	
Rib	Nonfloating ribs	Trauma, pain worse during deep breathing	Pain control Possible splinting	
Pelvic	Pelvis	Big trauma	Surgical repair	**High risk of major blood loss**

AVN, avascular necrosis; DRUJ, distal radial-ulnar joint; DVT, deep venous thrombosis; H/P, history and physical.

FIGURE
9-2 Differential diagnosis for back pain.

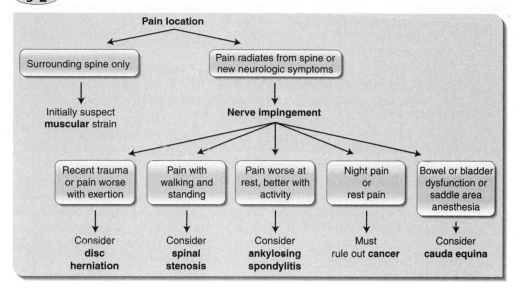

II. Spine

A. **Back pain**
   1. Back pain may be due to musculoskeletal, neurologic, neoplastic, infectious, or rheumatic causes
   2. **Treatment** = NSAIDs, physical therapy, or rest for muscular injuries

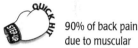
90% of back pain due to muscular injury resolves within six weeks regardless of treatment.

B. **Degenerative disc disease**
   1. Vertebral disc is composed of a dense annulus fibrosus and a gelatinous nucleus pulposus
   2. Degenerative changes in disc lead to **herniation** (most frequently posterior or posterior lateral) of nucleus pulposus and **nerve impingement**
   3. Herniation is most common in the lumbosacral region (L4–L5, L5–S1 discs) but may also be cervical
   4. **H/P** = pain extending from nerve root **along path of compressed nerve,** characteristic sensory and motor deficits depending on nerve root involved; pain worsens with straight leg raises or Valsalva maneuver
   5. **Radiology** = MRI confirms diagnosis; computed tomography (CT) is helpful for analysis of bone structure
   6. **Treatment** = disease may be self-limited; NSAIDs, activity modification, epidural injection of anti-inflammatory agents, or surgical decompression may be used depending on duration and severity of symptoms

C. **Spinal stenosis**
   1. Generalized narrowing of bony spaces in the spine secondary to arthritic changes causes nerve compression
   2. Most common in middle-aged and **older** adults
   3. **H/P** = radiating pain that is worse with walking and standing
   4. **Radiology** = CT or x-ray confirms diagnosis; MRI may also be helpful to rule out herniation
   5. **Treatment** = analgesics (NSAIDs), physical therapy, epidural injections, surgical decompression

D. **Cauda equina syndrome**
   1. Cauda equina is extension of the dural-arachnoid sac beyond the inferior tip of the spinal cord that contains nerves
   2. Trauma can damage nerves running in the sac; neoplasms may cause nerve compression

TABLE 9-2	H/P for Compression of Specific Cervical and Lumbosacral Nerve Roots		
Nerve Root	**Reflex**	**Motor Deficit**	**Sensory Deficit**
C5	Biceps	Deltoid, biceps	Shoulder
C6	Brachioradialis	Biceps, wrist extensors	Lateral forearm
C7	Triceps	Triceps, wrist flexors, finger extensors	Posterior forearm
C8	None	Finger flexors	4th and 5th fingers, medial forearm
L4	Patellar	Tibialis anterior (foot dorsiflexion)	Medial leg
L5	None	Extensor hallucis longus (1st-toe dorsiflexion)	Medial forefoot and leg
S1	Achilles	Peroneus longus and brevis (foot eversion)	Lateral foot
H/P, history and physical.			

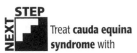
STEP
NEXT
Treat **cauda equina syndrome** with **immediate** surgical decompression because it can quickly result in permanent neurologic injury.

3. **H/P = urinary retention** following trauma, change in bowel habits; anesthesia in perineal region **(saddle anesthesia),** decreased rectal tone or bulbocavernosus reflex

4. **Treatment = emergency** surgical decompression of cauda equina, corticosteroids commonly given despite poor evidence of effectiveness, radiation used in cases of neoplasm

FIGURE 9-3 MRI of lumbar spine demonstrating herniation of L5-S1 disc (*arrows*) and compression of spinal cord.

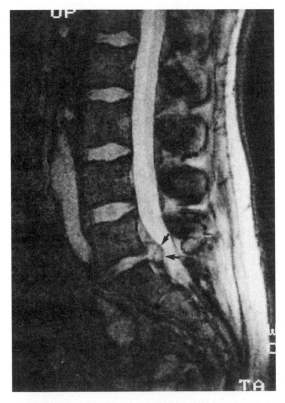

(With permission from Daffner RH. *Clinical Radiology: The Essentials.* 2nd Ed. Philadelphia: Lippincott Williams & Wilkins; 1999.)

FIGURE
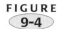
9-4 Diagram of brachial plexus anatomy. (Asset provided by Anatomical Chart Company.)

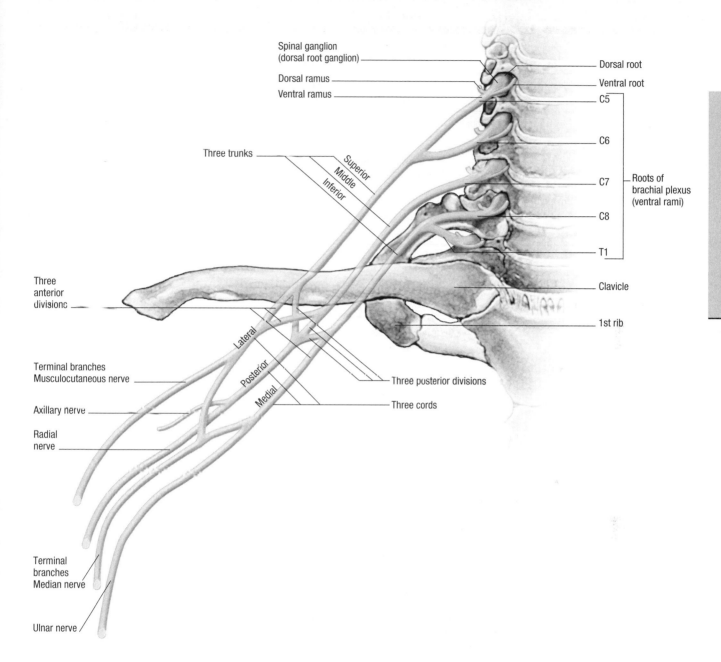

Spinal ganglion
(dorsal root ganglion)

Dorsal ramus

Ventral ramus

Three trunks

Superior
Middle
Inferior

Three
anterior
divisions

Lateral

Posterior

Medial

Terminal branches
Musculocutaneous nerve

Axillary nerve

Radial
nerve

Terminal
branches
Median nerve

Ulnar nerve

Dorsal root

Ventral root

C5

C6

C7 — Roots of
brachial plexus
(ventral rami)

C8

T1

Clavicle

1st rib

Three posterior divisions

Three cords

E. **Brachial plexus (see Table 9-3)**
1. The brachial plexus is composed of nerve roots C5–T1 and innervates the upper extremity
2. Brachial plexus disorders are related to specific mechanisms of injury

III. Metabolic bone diseases
A. **Osteoporosis**
1. Substantial osteopenia (decreased bone density) but normal mineralization in existing bone stock
2. Results from decreased bone formation or increased resorption of bone
3. Peak bone mass occurs at 20–25 years of age
4. **Risk factors** = inadequate dietary calcium during young adulthood, smoking, excessive alcohol consumption, sedentary lifestyle, decreased

TABLE 9-3 **Common Brachial Plexus Disorders**

Condition	Site of Injury	Cause of Injury	Clinical Features
Erb-Duchenne palsy	Superior trunk	Hyperadduction of arm causing widening of the humeral-glenoid gap (e.g., **birth**)	**Waiter's tip** (arm extended and adducted with pronated forearm)
Claw hand	Ulnar nerve	Epiphyseal separation of medial epicondyle of humerus	Weak finger adduction, poor 4th- and 5th-finger flexion
Wrist drop	Posterior cord/radial nerve	Mid-humerus fracture causes nerve impingement or tear	Inability to extend fingers, loss of sensation from dorsal hand
Deltoid paralysis	Axillary nerve	**Anterior shoulder dislocation** causes axillary nerve impingement or stretching	Poor shoulder function
Klumpke's palsy	Posterior/medial cords	Hyperabduction of arm places excess tension on lower cords and nearby sympathetic chain	**Claw hand,** poor wrist and hand function, association with Horner's syndrome

Osteoporosis is **less** likely to occur in **obese** people because the increased load placed on bones helps to prevent osteopenia.

Hormone and electrolyte levels will be normal for age in osteoporosis unless there is an underlying **endocrine** disorder.

X-rays will only show changes in osteoporotic bone after significant bone loss.

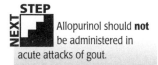

Allopurinol should **not** be administered in acute attacks of gout.

estrogen (e.g., postmenopausal), long-term steroid use, hyperparathyroidism, hyperthyroidism; typical patients are thin, white, postmenopausal women
5. **H/P** = usually asymptomatic until fractures (e.g., Colles, femoral neck, and vertebral) and neurovascular impingement occur
6. **Radiology** = decreased bone density evident on dual-energy x-ray absorptiometry (DEXA), x-ray, and CT
7. **Treatment** =
   a. Prevention is key, with exercise and sufficient calcium and vitamin D in diet (especially prior to the peak bone density age of 35 years old) important for maintaining bone stock
   b. Bisphosphonates decrease osteoclast activity (less bone resorption), increase bone density, and decrease fracture risk
   c. Hormone replacement therapy has been recommended in the past, but recent studies have shown that it may carry other risks (breast cancer, etc.)

B. **Gout**
1. Peripheral mono-arthritis due to deposition of **sodium urate crystals** in joints
2. **Risk factors** = renal disease, male gender, urate underexcretion, diuretic use, cyclosporine use, cancer, hemoglobinopathies, excessive alcohol consumption
3. **H/P** =
   a. **Sudden severe pain** and **swelling** in one joint that frequently starts at night
   b. 1st metatarsophalangeal joint most commonly affected (**podagra**); ankle, knee, and foot joints also common sites
   c. Possible concurrent fever, chills, or malaise
4. **Labs** = serum uric acid may be normal or increased; joint aspiration shows **needle-shaped, negatively birefringent crystals** and several leukocytes (Color Figure 9-1)
5. **Radiology** = x-ray may show punched-out bone lesions in chronic cases
6. **Treatment** =
   a. NSAIDs (especially indomethacin), colchicine, corticosteroids
   b. Decreasing alcohol and diuretic use, avoidance of foods high in purines (e.g., red meats, fish) helps prevent exacerbations
   c. Probenecid (inhibits kidney uric acid resorption) or allopurinol (inhibits uric acid formation) used in cases of chronic gout to prevent flare-ups

7. **Complications** = long-standing disease leads to chronic tophaceous gout with formation of nodular tophi (large deposits of crystals in soft tissues), leading to permanent deformity

C. **Pseudogout** (calcium pyrophosphate dihydrate deposition disease, or CPPD)
1. Calcium pyrophosphate dehydrate crystal deposition in joints
2. Familial condition associated with other endocrine diseases (e.g., DM, hyperparathyroidism)
3. **H/P** = similar presentation to gout but **less severe symptoms; knee** and **wrist** most commonly initially affected joints
4. **Labs** = joint aspiration shows **positively birefringent, rhomboid crystals (Color Figure 9-2)**
5. **Radiology** = x-ray may show chondrocalcinosis (calcification of articular cartilage in joints)
6. **Treatment** = NSAIDs, colchicine

D. **Paget's disease of bone**
1. Overactive osteoclasts and osteoblasts leading to excessive bone turnover and disorganized bony architecture
2. **H/P** = possibly asymptomatic or deep bone pain, increased incidence of fractures; **tibial bowing,** kyphosis, **increased cranial diameter,** deafness (due to changes in auditory ossicles)
3. **Labs** = increased alkaline phosphatase; increased urine hydroxyproline; normal calcium and phosphorus
4. **Radiology** = x-rays may demonstrate osteolytic lesions and expanded hyperdense bone
5. **Treatment** = bisphosphonates, calcitonin

E. **Osteogenesis imperfecta**
1. Defective production of collagen due to genetic disorder
2. Diagnosis primarily made during childhood
3. **H/P** = frequent **fractures** from **minimal** trauma, **blue sclera,** skin and teeth deformities, possible deafness, joint hypermobility (may resemble child abuse)
4. **Treatment** = activity restriction, surgical correction of bony misalignment

F. **Osteopetrosis**
1. Increased bone density due to impaired osteoclast activity
2. **H/P** = increased incidence of fractures, possible blindness or deafness, variable neurologic symptoms (due to bony compression of nerves)
3. **Labs** = decreased hemoglobin, decreased hematocrit (Hct) (via narrowing of marrow cavities), increased acid phosphatase, increased creatine phosphokinase (CPK)
4. **Radiology** = general increased bone density seen on x-ray including thickening of cranium and vertebrae
5. **Treatment** = transfusion of marrow components necessary for osteoclast production

IV. Infection
A. **Septic joint and septic arthritis**
1. Most commonly occurs through hematogenous spread of bacteria or direct inoculation (e.g., open fracture)
2. Most commonly due to *Staphylococcus aureus;* consider *Neisseria gonorrhoeae* in sexually active patients (may also have tenosynovitis)
3. Consider gram-negative rods in patients with DM, cancer, or other underlying illnesses
4. Preexisting arthritis increases risk
5. **H/P** = sudden onset joint pain or several days of migratory polyarthralgias; warm, red, tender, swollen joint; possible overlying skin lesions

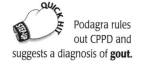
Podagra rules out CPPD and suggests a diagnosis of **gout.**

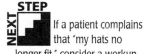
If a patient complains that "my hats no longer fit," consider a workup for Paget's disease or osteopetrosis.

MUSCULOSKELETAL DISORDERS

MUSCULOSKELETAL DISORDERS

TABLE 9-4	Findings in Aspirated Joint Fluid for Common Inflammatory Joint Conditions	
Conditions	**Joint Aspiration Leukocytes**	**Histology**
Osteoarthritis, trauma	<2,000 per mm³	May see signs of hemarthrosis (bleeding into joint) for trauma; otherwise negative
Inflammatory arthropathies (e.g., rheumatoid arthritis, gout, pseudogout)	5,000–50,000 per mm³	Needle-shaped, negatively birefringent crystals for **gout** Positively birefringent rhomboid crystals for **pseudogout**
Septic joint	>**50,000** per mm³	Many **WBCs**; infrequently see bacteria

WBC, white blood cells.

While **Salmonella** should be considered in patients with sickle cell disease and **Pseudomonas** should be considered in intravenous drug abusers, **S. aureus** is still the **most common** cause of osteomyelitis in these patients.

6. **Labs** = joint aspiration shows **numerous white blood cells (WBCs)** (lower for *N. gonorrhoeae* than *S. aureus*) and decreased glucose; positive cultures (frequent false negatives for *N. gonorrhoeae*)
7. **Treatment** = for *N. gonorrhoeae,* use IV ceftriaxone and doxycycline for possible *Chlamydia* co-infection; for *S. aureus* use penicillinase-resistant penicillin; for gram-negative bacteria use aminoglycosides

B. **Osteomyelitis**
1. **Bone infection** via hematogenous spread or local extension
2. *S. aureus* and *Pseudomonas* most common causes; consider *Salmonella* in **sickle cell** patients
3. **H/P** = bone pain, tenderness, fever, chills; possible skin involvement with a draining sinus
4. **Labs** = increased WBCs; increased erythrocyte sedimentation rate (ESR); cultures needed to define appropriate antibiotic therapy
5. **Radiology** = x-rays are **not** helpful initially and only show signs of infection after 10 days; bone scan will show increased uptake after 72 hours
6. **Treatment** = must irrigate and **debride** infected tissue; IV antibiotics for 4–6 weeks

C. **Lyme disease**
1. Caused by *Borrelia burgdorferi;* the organism is most commonly delivered through the bite of the *Ixodes* tick
2. **H/P** =
   a. Chills, fatigue, arthralgias, headache; **erythema chronicum migrans** (bullseye rash), fever (Color Figure 9-3)
   b. Later symptoms include **myocarditis weeks to months** after infection, cardiac arrhythmias, heart block, **Bell's palsy,** sensory-motor neuropathies, aseptic meningitis, or meningoencephalitis
   c. After a **few months to years** later chronic synovitis, **monoarthritis or oligoarthritis,** subacute encephalopathy, or polyneuropathy may develop
3. **Labs** = positive immunologic assays (frequent false-negatives); joint aspiration is not helpful
4. **Treatment** = doxycycline, amoxicillin

V. Osteoarthritis
A. **Degenerative joint disease**
1. Chronic, noninflammatory joint degeneration involving **articular cartilage deterioration** and osteophyte formation
2. Most commonly affects weight-bearing joints; also affects distal interphalangeal (DIP) joints and proximal interphalangeal (PIP) joints; can cause spinal stenosis in vertebral bodies
3. **Risk factors** = family history, obesity, previous joint trauma
4. **H/P** = joint crepitus, insidious onset of joint stiffness and pain that **worsens with activity and weight-bearing** and is relieved by rest, no systemic symptoms; patients have decreased range of motion, bony protuberances in DIP **(Heberden nodes)** and PIP **(Bouchard nodes)** joints
5. **Labs** = normal ESR; less than 2,000 leukocytes on joint aspiration
6. **Radiology** = x-ray demonstrates osteophyte formation, joint space narrowing, increased subchondral bone density
7. **Treatment** = rest, heat, analgesics (NSAIDs), weight loss, physical therapy, corticosteroid injections, joint replacement in advanced cases

VI. Rheumatologic diseases
A. **Rheumatoid arthritis (RA)**
1. Chronic inflammatory disorder with infiltration of synovial joints by inflammatory cells
2. **Synovial hypertrophy** with granulation tissue formation on articular cartilage **(pannus formation)** results from joint inflammation
3. Most commonly seen in middle-aged women; increased frequency in people with HLA-DR4 serotype
4. **PIP** and metacarpophalangeal (**MCP**) usually first joints involved; **symmetric polyarthropathy** involving ankles, knees, shoulders, hips, elbows, and spine develops

- **Osteoarthritis:** typically **asymmetrical** and may only affect one joint; DIP joints are frequently involved.
- **RA:** affects joints on both sides of the body in a **symmetrical** distribution; DIP joints are spared.

FIGURE 9-5 Osteoarthritis in a right hip joint; synovial cysts (*black arrows*) and osteophytes (*white arrow*) are evident.

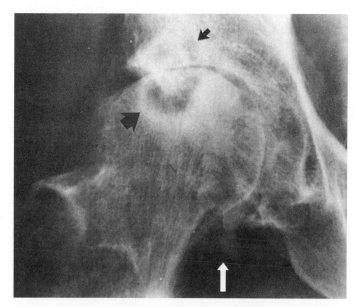

(Modified with permission from Daffner RH. *Clinical Radiology: The Essentials.* 2nd Ed. Philadelphia: Lippincott Williams & Wilkins; 1999.)

5. **H/P** =
   a. Malaise, weight loss, insidious onset of **morning stiffness with pain,** decreased mobility
   b. Warm joints, joint swelling, fevers, ulnar deviation of fingers; MCP hypertrophy, **swan neck deformities** (flexed DIP plus hyperextended PIP), **boutonniere deformities** (flexed PIP), subcutaneous nodules, pleuritis, pericarditis, scleritis, chorea
6. **Labs** =
   a. Rheumatoid factor (RF) positive in 75% of patients but not specific for the disease
   b. Positive antinuclear antibodies (ANA) in <50% of patients (see Table 9-5)
   c. Increased ESR, increased IgG, and IgM
   d. Joint aspiration shows 5,000–50,000 leukocytes
7. **Radiology** = x-rays may demonstrate soft tissue swellings, joint space narrowing, marginal bony erosions, or subluxation
8. **Treatment** =
   a. Initially NSAIDs, physical therapy, and corticosteroids as needed
   b. Methotrexate is a second-line agent
   c. Gold, hydroxychloroquine sulfate, and azathioprine may be used in severe cases

B. **Juvenile rheumatoid arthritis (JRA)**
   1. Nonmigratory monoarthropathy or polyarthropathy in **children** lasting more than 3 months; resolves before puberty in 95% of patients
   2. Characteristics of JRA vary with the subtype described
   3. **Labs** = no good diagnostic test; RF-positive in only 15% of patients; ESR may be normal
   4. **Radiology** = x-ray findings of arthritic process in child may be helpful in making diagnosis
   5. **Treatment** =
      a. NSAIDs, physical therapy, corticosteroids
      b. Methotrexate is a second-line drug
      c. Regular ophthalmologic exams
      d. 50% patients with systemic form and almost all with pauciarticular form have resolution of symptoms before 10 years old

FIGURE
9-6 Variants of juvenile rheumatoid arthritis (JRA).

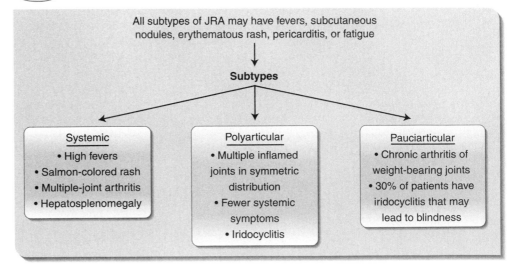

All subtypes of JRA may have fevers, subcutaneous nodules, erythematous rash, pericarditis, or fatigue

↓

Subtypes

Systemic
- High fevers
- Salmon-colored rash
- Multiple-joint arthritis
- Hepatosplenomegaly

Polyarticular
- Multiple inflamed joints in symmetric distribution
- Fewer systemic symptoms
- Iridocyclitis

Pauciarticular
- Chronic arthritis of weight-bearing joints
- 30% of patients have iridocyclitis that may lead to blindness

FIGURE

9-7 MD SOAP CHAIR mnemonic for symptoms of systemic lupus erythematosus. BUN, blood urea nitrogen; MCPs, metacarpophalangeal joints, PIPs, proximal interphalangeal joints.

Malar (butterfly) rash
Discoid (patchy) rash

Serositis (pleuritis, pneumonitis, pleural effusion)
Oral ulcers
Arthritis (symmetric, PIPs, MCPs, wrists, knees, feet)
Photosensitivity

Central nervous system (psychosis, seizures, stroke, neuropathy)
Heart and hemotologic issues (pericarditis, myocarditis, arrythmias, Libman-Sacks endocarditis, chronic anemia, autoimmune hemolytic anemia, leukopenia, thrombocytopenia, thrombus formation, Raynaud's phenomenon)

Anti-nuclear antibodies (ANA) increased
Immunologic issues (anti-double-stranded DNA [dsDNA] and anti-Smith [Sm] antibodies)

Renal issues (immune complex glomerulonephritis, interstitial nephritis, proteinuria, increased BUN, increased serum creatine)

6. **Complications** = increased risk of **blindness** in polyarticular and pauciarticular forms; one third of patients with systemic form, few with pauciarticular form, and most with polyarticular form have chronic arthritis

C. **Systemic lupus erythematosus (SLE)**
  1. Multisystem autoimmune disorder involving a variety of autoantibodies
  2. Antibody-mediated cellular attack occurs with deposition of antigen-antibody complexes in affected tissues
  3. **Risk factors** = young women, African American
  4. Hydralazine, procainamide, isoniazid, methyldopa, quinidine, chlorpromazine can cause similar symptoms that resolve when the **drug is discontinued**
  5. **H/P** =
    a. Think **MD SOAP CHAIR**
    b. May also experience fevers, malaise, weight loss, abdominal pain, vomiting, conjunctivitis, blindness
    c. Any combination of symptoms is possible and may change during the course of the disease
  6. **Labs** =
    a. Positive ANA in 95% of patients
    b. Anti-dsDNA antibodies in 60% of patients but not found in other rheumatologic disorders
    c. Presence of anti-Sm antibodies is very specific for disease
    d. Anti-histone antibodies may be seen for drug-induced lupus-like symptoms
    e. Patients frequently have a **false-positive test** for **syphilis**
  7. **Treatment** = avoidance of sun, NSAIDs, corticosteroids for immunosupression, other immunosuppressant drugs in cases resistant to corticosteroids, anticoagulation
  8. **Complications** = lupus anticoagulant and anticardiolipin antibodies increase the risks of miscarriage and fetal death; patient death results from progressive impairment of lung, heart, brain, and kidney function

D. **Polymyositis and dermatomyositis**
  1. Progressive systemic diseases with skeletal muscle inflammation; one third of patients with polymyositis also have dermatomyositis

TABLE 9-5 Immunologic Markers Found in Rheumatic Diseases

Disease	Immunologic Markers
Systemic lupus erythematosus (SLE)	ANA (95% of patients) Anti-dsDNA antibodies (60% of patients) Anti-Sm antibodies False-positive RPR (syphilis test)
Drug-induced lupus	Anti-histone antibodies
Rheumatoid arthritis (RA)	RF (75% of patients) ANA (<50% of patients) HLA-DR4 common
Polymyositis/dermatomyositis	ANA Anti-Jo-1 antibodies
Ankylosing spondylitis	HLA-B27 (90% of patients)
Psoriatic arthritis	Possible HLA-B27
Scleroderma	Anti-scl-70 ANA
CREST syndrome	Anti-centromere antibodies
Mixed connective tissue disease (MCTD)	Anti-RNP ANA
Sjögren's syndrome	Anti-Ro (anti-SSA) ANA Anti-LA (anti-SSB) ANA

ANA, antinuclear antibodies; CREST, calcinosis, Raynaud's, esophageal dysmotility, sclerodactyly, and telangiectasias; RF, rheumatoid factor; RPR, rapid plasma reagin.

2. **Risk factors** = more common in women, African Americans, elderly
3. **H/P** =
    a. Symmetric progressive **proximal** muscle weakness (occurs in **legs first**), muscle atrophy in later stages of disease
    b. Cutaneous manifestations of dermatomyositis are a **red heliotropic rash** on the face, upper extremities, chest, or back, violet discoloration of eyelids, or scaly patches over hand joints
    c. Patients with lung involvement have dyspnea and poor oxygenation saturation
4. **Labs** =
    a. Increased creatinine, aldolase, creatine phosphokinase (CPK), AST, ALT, and LDH
    b. ANA frequently positive
    c. Anti-Jo-1 antibodies in patients with interstitial lung disease (see Table 9-5)
    d. Muscle biopsy shows inflammatory cells and muscle degeneration, inflammatory cells **within** muscle fascicles in **polymyositis** and **surrounding** muscle fascicles in **dermatomyositis**
5. **EMG** = spontaneous fibrillations
6. **Treatment** = high-dose corticosteroids for 4–6 weeks followed by tapered dosing
7. **Complications** = possible conduction defects, myocarditis, interstitial lung disease
E. **Polymyalgia rheumatica** (PMR)
    1. Rheumatic disease frequently associated with **temporal arteritis;** most common in elderly women (see Chapter 1, Cardiovascular Disorders)

2. **H/P** = pain and stiffness in shoulder and pelvic girdle, difficulty raising arms and getting out of bed, malaise, unexplained weight loss; fever, minimal joint swelling

3. **Labs** = decreased Hct, **markedly increased ESR,** negative RF

4. **Treatment** = low-dose corticosteroids followed by tapered dosing

F. **Fibromyalgia**

1. Disease causing **chronic pain** in muscles and tendons

2. Unknown etiology but frequently associated with **depression,** anxiety, and irritable bowel disease

3. Possible predisposition with hypothyroidism, RA, sleep apnea; more common in women, 20–50 years old

4. **H/P** = myalgias and weakness without inflammation; "trigger points" on exam (specific locations that when stimulated reproduce pain symptoms)

5. **Treatment** = stretching, antidepressants (tricyclic antidepressants [TCAs], selective serotonin reuptake inhibitors [SSRIs]), patient education, physical therapy modalities

G. **Ankylosing spondylitis**

1. Chronic inflammatory disease of the **spine** and pelvis that results in eventual bone fusion

2. **Risk factors** = 20–40 years old, male > female, white > African American

3. **H/P** =

a. Hip and low back pain that is **worse in the morning** and **following inactivity; pain improves over course of day**

b. Possible limited range of motion in spine, hip, or chest

c. Painful kyphosis that is relieved by bending forward

d. Possible self-limited anterior uveitis

4. **Labs** = positive HLA-B27 in 90% of patients, increased or normal ESR, negative RF, negative ANA (see Table 9-5)

5. **Radiology** = x-ray shows **bamboo spine** (multiple vertebral fusions)

6. **Treatment** = physical therapy, NSAIDs; exercise helps to prevent or delay permanent deformities

H. **Psoriatic arthritis**

1. Arthritis that develops in approximately 1% of patients with **psoriasis**

2. **H/P** = may be asymmetrical arthritis involving few joints or may be similar to presentation of RA

3. **Labs** = negative RF and ANA, possible positive HLA-B27 (see Table 9-5)

4. **Radiology** = x-rays show findings similar to RA; highly destructive lesions of DIP and PIP joints ("pencil in cup" deformities)

5. **Treatment** = NSAIDs, methotrexate, sulfasalazine

I. **Scleroderma**

1. Chronic multisystem sclerosis with accumulation of connective tissue, skin thickening, and visceral involvement

2. **H/P** = **Raynaud's phenomenon** (blue distal extremities due to arteriolar spasm), **skin thickening, esophageal dysmotility,** intestinal hypomotility

3. **Labs** = positive anti-scl-70 ANA (see Table 9-5)

4. **CREST syndrome** is variant with **C**alcinosis, **R**aynaud's phenomenon, **E**sophageal dysmotility, **S**clerodactyly, and **T**elangiectasias

a. Skin thickening limited to distal extremities and face

b. Labs show anti-centromere antibodies (see Table 9-5)

c. Better prognosis than scleroderma

5. **Treatment** = supportive care, angiotensin-converting enzyme (ACE) inhibitors for malignant renal hypertension, calcium channel blockers to relieve Raynaud symptoms

6. **Complications** = pulmonary fibrosis, acute renal failure due to malignant renal hypertension

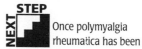

Weakness is a symptom of **polymyositis** but not of polymyalgia rheumatica.

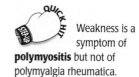

Once polymyalgia rheumatica has been diagnosed, the patient should automatically be worked up for **temporal arteritis.**

MUSCULOSKELETAL DISORDERS

J. **Mixed connective tissue disease** (MCTD)
1. Overlapping features of SLE, scleroderma, and polymyositis
2. May progress to a single diagnosis
3. **H/P** = possible Raynaud's phenomenon, polyarthralgias, arthritis, swollen hands, proximal muscle weakness, esophageal hypomotility, or pulmonary abnormalities
4. **Labs** = positive anti-ribonucleoprotein (RNP) ANA (see Table 9-5)
5. **Treatment** = corticosteroids, supportive measures

K. **Sjögren's syndrome**
1. Autoimmune disorder with lymphocytic infiltration of exocrine glands
2. May be seen in association with RA, SLE, or primary biliary cirrhosis
3. **H/P** = **dry eyes, dry mouth,** enlarged parotid glands, possible symmetrical arthritis associated with other autoimmune conditions
4. **Labs** = positive anti-Ro (anti-SSA) and anti-LA (anti-SSB) ANA (see Table 9-5)
5. **Treatment** = supportive care

Sicca syndrome is Sjögren's syndrome **without** a secondary autoimmune association.

VII. Neoplasms
A. **Osteosarcoma**
1. Most common **primary** malignant bone tumor; more common in adolescents, male > female
2. Most frequently involves distal femur, proximal tibia, or proximal humerus
3. **Risk factors** = Paget's disease of bone, p53 genetic mutations, familial retinoblastoma, radiation exposure, bone infarcts
4. **H/P** = deep bony pain, later development of palpable bony mass
5. **Radiology** = x-ray shows bone lesion with a **sunburst** pattern and **Codman's triangle** (periosteal new bone formation at the diaphyseal end of the lesion); MRI useful for determining extent of lesion
6. **Treatment** = surgical excision, chemotherapy
7. **Complications** = 60% five-year survival rate

B. **Bone metastases**
1. Most common bone tumors in adults
2. Can result from nearly any primary tumor
3. **H/P** = presence of primary form of cancer; deep bone pain, possible palpable bone mass
4. **Radiology** = lesions may be evident on bone scan or x-ray
5. **Treatment** = follows that for primary tumor

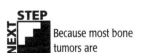
STEP
NEXT
Because most bone tumors are **metastases** and not primary tumors, any patient with a new bone tumor should undergo a full work up to look for a tumor source.

C. **Ewing sarcoma**
1. Highly malignant cartilage tumor occurring in diaphysis of long bones; most common in **children,** 5–15 years old
2. **H/P** = bony pain, tissue swelling
3. **Radiology** = x-ray may detect large destructive lesions with significant periosteal reaction
4. **Treatment** = radiation, adjuvant chemotherapy
5. **Complications** = 60% survival rate when both radiation and chemotherapy are used

D. **Osteochondroma**
1. Most common **benign** bone tumor in metaphysis of long bones; more common in patients <25 years old, male > female
2. Typically occurs in lower femur or upper tibia
3. **H/P** = nontender, palpable mass
4. **Treatment** = none necessary unless causing soft tissue irritation or neurovascular compromise or if continued growth occurs (surgical excision indicated)
5. **Complications** = rare (1%) transformation into chondrosarcoma

FIGURE
9-8   Osteosarcoma in left proximal femur; note the dense sunburst pattern of the
        lesion (*solid black arrows*) and presence of Codman's triangle (*open arrow*).

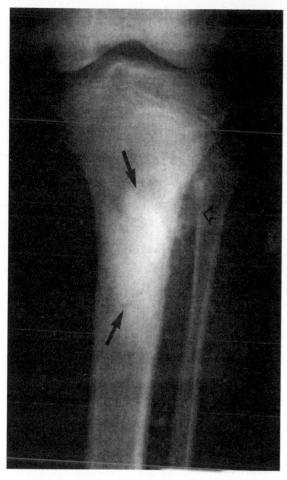

(With permission from Daffner RH. *Clinical Radiology: The Essentials.* 2nd Ed. Philadelphia: Lippincott Williams &
Wilkins; 1999.)

VIII. Pediatric orthopaedics

A. **Developmental dysplasia of the hip (DDH)**
   1. Varying displacement of proximal femur from acetabulum
   2. Occurs due to poor development of acetabulum *in utero*
   3. **Risk factors** = female > male, first-born children, babies delivered in
      breech presentation, oligohydramnios
   4. **H/P** =
      a. Children have delayed walking or abnormal gait if diagnosis not made
         early
      b. Positive **Barlow's** and **Ortolani's** maneuvers (provocation of hip
         dislocation or reduction)
      c. Knees at unequal heights when hips and knees flexed **(Galeazzi's sign)**
      d. Positive Trendelenburg sign (sagging of opposite hip)
      e. Asymmetric skin folds
   5. **Radiology** = x-rays are not helpful in making a diagnosis until after four
      months of age
   6. **Treatment = Pavlik harness;** best results occur with early treatment;
      surgery may be required in progressed cases
B. **Slipped capital femoral epiphysis** (SCFE)
   1. Separation through growth plate of femoral epiphysis from metaphysis
   2. **Risk factors = adolescent, obese,** African American

    3. **H/P** = thigh and knee pain; limp, limited internal rotation and abduction of the hip, hip flexion produces obligatory external hip rotation

    4. **Radiology** = x-rays indicate posterior and medial displacement of the femoral head from the femoral metaphysis

    5. **Treatment** = surgical pinning, weight-bearing restrictions following repair, closed reduction may help avoid surgery in acute cases

    6. **Complications** = increased risk of avascular necrosis (AVN) and premature osteoarthritis if treatment is not performed early

C. **Rickets**

    1. **Impaired calcification** of bone in children due to **vitamin D deficiency;** coexistent calcium and phosphorus deficiencies

    2. Called **osteomalacia** in adults

    3. Results from lack of sunlight and/or poor diet

    4. Epiphyseal cartilage becomes hypertrophic without calcification

    5. **H/P** = bone pain, delayed walking; **bowed legs,** kyphoscoliosis, proximal limb weakness, decreased height, softened skull bones; fractures that result from minimal trauma in adults

    6. **Labs** = decreased 25-hydroxyvitamin D_3 and 1,25-dihydroxycholecalciferol, increased parathyroid hormone, decreased phosphorus, calcium may be decreased or normal, increased alkaline phosphatase in adults

    7. **Radiology** = x-rays will demonstrate skeletal abnormalities (e.g., bowed-legs, kyphoscoliosis)

    8. **Treatment** = vitamin D, calcium, phosphorus; physical therapy is useful for gait training

D. **Osteochondritis**

    1. Inflammation of bone-cartilage interface

    2. Specifically referred to as **Osgood-Schlatter disease** when the **tibial tubercle** is involved (common in boys during growth spurt)

    3. **H/P** = pain at involved site that worsens with activity

    4. **Treatment** = activity restraint

E. **Clavicular fracture**

    1. **Most common** fracture in children (e.g., birth trauma, falls)

    2. **Treatment** = sling

F. **Nursemaid's elbow**

    1. Radial head subluxation that occurs via pulling and lifting on the hand (e.g., yanking the child out of danger by his or her arm)

    2. **H/P** = child with painful arm who will not bend elbow

    3. **Treatment** = manual reduction via supination of the arm with flexion of the elbow from 0° to 90° of flexion

G. **Legg-Calvé-Perthes disease**

    1. AVN of capital femoral epiphysis most common between 3–12 years old

    2. **H/P** = gradual progressive limp, insidious onset of pain, decreased range of motion

    3. **Treatment** = containment of hip within acetabulum via bracing or surgical means (acetabular modification)

    4. **Complications** = increased risk of hip complications in adulthood including osteoarthritis, progressive AVN, and need for early arthroplasty

H. **Club foot**

    1. Inversion of foot, plantar flexion of ankle, adduction of forefoot, and internal rotation of tibia

    2. **H/P** = child that is slow to walk, limp; obvious defect on exam

    3. **Treatment** = **serial casting** of foot in correct position; surgery required in long-standing cases

I. **Scoliosis**
1. Medial-lateral spiral **curvature** of the spine that does not passively correct to a normal alignment
2. Curvature progresses until skeletal maturity
3. Initially mainly a **cosmetic** issue; progressive curvature interferes with activities
4. Severe cases result in decreased pulmonary function
5. **H/P** = asymmetry of back musculature and palpable curve of the spine that are augmented when patient bends at the waist
6. **Treatment** = bracing for moderate curves in young patients; surgery for more severe curves or curves in older patients
7. **Complications** = severe curves may cause restrictive respiratory disease by limiting lung expansion

J. **Duchenne muscular dystrophy**
1. X-linked disorder resulting from deficiency of **dystrophin** (subsarcolemmal cytoskeletal protein)
2. **Most common** lethal muscular dystrophy
3. Onset at 2–6 years old
4. **H/P** = progressive clumsiness, easy fatigability, **difficulty standing up and walking,** waddling gait, positive **Gower's maneuver** (must push on thighs with hands to stand up); weakness occurs in proximal muscles before distal muscles; **pseudohypertrophy** occurs in calf muscles due to fatty infiltration
5. **Labs** = increased CPK; muscle biopsy shows muscle fiber degeneration and fibrosis and basophilic fibers; immunostaining for dystrophin (**absent** in disease) is diagnostic
6. **EMG** = polyphasic potentials and increased fiber recruitment
7. **Treatment** = physical therapy, tendon release of contractures as necessary
8. **Complications** = progressive cardiac issues, scoliosis, and flexion contractures; death commonly occurs by 20 years old owing to respiratory issues

Dermatology

I. Infections

A. Cellulitis

1. Acute skin infection most frequently due to *Staphylococcus aureus* or **group A streptococci**
2. **Risk factors = intravenous drug use, diabetes mellitus (DM),** immunocompromise, penetration of skin (e.g., surgery, trauma)
3. **H/P = erythematous, warm,** swollen, and painful skin, chills; fever, lymphadenopathy; skin findings may be near wound (Color Figure 10-1)
4. **Labs** = increased white blood count (WBC); wound culture may help identify pathogen
5. **Treatment** = oral cephalosporins or penicillinase-resistant β-lactams for 7 to 10 days; IV antibiotics for severe cases or bacteremia
6. **Complications** = necrotizing fasciitis

B. Skin abscess

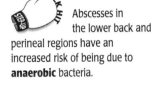

Abscesses in the lower back and perineal regions have an increased risk of being due to **anaerobic** bacteria.

1. **Subcutaneous** collection of pus most commonly due to staphylococcal bacteria
2. May occur as collection of multiple infected hair follicles (carbuncle)
3. **Hidradenitis suppurativa**
   a. Chronic follicular occlusion and **apocrine** inflammation resulting in recurrent abscesses in the axilla, groin, and perineum
   b. Chronic infection leads to scarring
   c. May require both antibiotics and surgical excision for treatment
4. **H/P** = erythematous, fluctuant, and localized swelling in skin; tender on palpation; pain frequently relieved by rupture of abscess
5. **Treatment = incision and drainage** with healing by secondary intention; antibiotics administered for facial abscesses
6. **Complications** = large, eroding facial abscess may cause cavernous sinus thrombosis

C. Necrotizing fasciitis

1. Quickly spreading group A streptococcal infection of **fascial planes**
2. **H/P** = erythematous, warm, and swollen skin; **loss of sensation** in involved tissue, crepitus in infected skin, purple discoloration
3. **Treatment** = surgical débridement, incision and drainage, IV antibiotics
4. **Complications** = sepsis, gangrene, high mortality (1/3 patients)

D. Gangrene

1. Tissue necrosis due to **poor vascular supply** or severe infection (occasionally *Clostridium* sp.)
2. **H/P** = prior skin infection or penetrating wound, severe pain in skin; fever, hypotension, skin crepitus, **rotten-smelling skin**
3. **Radiology** = subcutaneous air
4. **Treatment** = incision and drainage, débridement, antibiotics

E. **Impetigo**
1. **Contagious** skin infection that is most common in **children** caused by *S. aureus* or **group A streptococci**
2. **H/P** = facial pruritus; **yellow crusted lesions** around mucocutaneous surfaces; erythematous vesicles (blisters) seen in staphylococcal infection; erythematous pustules on face and extremities with streptococcal infections (Color Figure 10-2)
3. **Treatment** = wash all affected areas; erythromycin, cephalosporins, or topical antibiotics; unaffected family members should not share towels or clothing to prevent spread until cure achieved

F. **Acne vulgaris**
1. Inflammation of hair follicles and sebaceous glands associated with *Propionibacterium acnes,* adolescence, androgens, and obstruction of pores by exfoliated skin or personal care products
2. **H/P** =
   a. Most frequently occurs in **adolescents**
   b. Erythematous pustules predominantly on face, neck, chest, and back
   c. Cystic lesions may form in severe cases
3. **Treatment** =
   a. Benzoyl peroxide helps prevent follicular obstruction by decreasing oiliness of skin
   b. Antibiotics (oral or topical) may inhibit bacterial growth
   c. Topical or oral **vitamin A analogues** decrease sebaceous gland activity
   d. Oral contraceptives may be useful in women with excess androgen production
4. **Complications** = cystic acne may result in permanent scarring; oral vitamin A analogues may cause birth defects or hepatotoxicity (require periodic liver function tests and mandatory contraceptive use for women)

G. **Herpes simplex (HSV)**
1. Recurrent viral infection of mucocutaneous surfaces due to herpes simplex virus 1 or 2 (HSV-1, HSV-2)
2. HSV transmitted through contact with **oral** or **genital fluids**
3. **HSV-1** causes primarily **oral** disease; **HSV-2** causes primarily **genital** disease
4. After primary infection, viral genetic material remains in sensory ganglia; stress will cause reactivation of disease in distribution of involved nerves
5. **H/P** = small painful vesicles around mouth (HSV-1) or genitals (HSV-2) lasting several days; primary infection usually presents with more severe symptoms and a flu-like illness (Color Figure 10-3)
6. **Labs** = Tzanck smear of lesions shows multinucleated giant cells; viral culture confirms diagnosis
7. **Treatment** = incurable, so treatment should be directed at minimizing symptoms and exacerbations; acyclovir shortens duration of recurrences and may decrease number of recurrences in patients with frequent eruptions
8. **Complications** =
   a. Contagious whenever vesicles present
   b. Transmission from **infected mother to newborn** may cause severe disseminated disease with severe neurologic involvement
   c. Rarely, mother-to-newborn transmission may occur in absence of visible vesicles

H. **Varicella**
1. Infection by varicella-zoster virus (i.e., herpes zoster) that may present as primary disease (chickenpox) or recurrent disease (shingles) (Color Figure 10-4)
2. Chickenpox and shingles have different presentations despite being caused by the same viral infection

There is no proven association between acne vulgaris and certain types of food.

Acne usually decreases in severity as adolescence ends. **Corticosteroid use** and **androgen** production disorders are common causes of outbreaks in adulthood.

Check varicella immunity status (received vaccine or had chickenpox as child) in all **pregnant** women; **varicella immune globulin** should be given to all nonimmune pregnant women who contract the disease.

DERMATOLOGY

TABLE 10-1 **Characteristics or Primary (Chickenpox) and Recurrent (Shingles) Varicella**

Varicella Condition	Chickenpox (Primary)	Shingles (Recurrent)
Patients affected	More common in **children**	Patient with prior history of varicella-zoster infection
Timing of presentation	Symptoms 2+ weeks after infection occurs; symptoms of headache, malaise, myalgias, and fever precede development of lesions by < 3 days	Myalgias, fever, malaise preceding lesions by approximately 3 days
Type of lesion	Small red macules that evolve into papules and then vesicles that eventually become crusted	Small red macules that evolve into papules and then vesicles that eventually become crusted
Distribution of lesions	**Wide** distribution	Limited to single or few distinct **dermatomes**
Course of disease	Lesions may develop up to 1 week and resolve a few days after appearing	Lesions may exist for multiple weeks and may be **painful**
Treatment	Antipruritics aid symptoms; acyclovir used in severe cases or in immunocompromised patients	Analgesics, possible corticosteroids; acyclovir used in immunocompromised patients and trigeminal nerve distribution
Complications	More severe course in older and pregnant patients (increased risk of varicella pneumonia); may have severe consequences if passed from **infected mother to unborn fetus**	Postinfectious neuralgia (long-lasting pain at site of eruption), trigeminal neuropathy

I. **Warts**
   1. Benign epithelial tumors due to local infection by one of many types of **human papillomavirus** (HPV)
   2. **H/P** = well-defined lesions of thickened epithelium, may appear flat (plantar warts) or raised; occasional tenderness to palpation
   3. **Treatment** = occasionally self-limited; chemical, laser, or cryotherapy may be required for removal
   4. **Complications** = some forms of HPV that cause genital warts are associated with cervical cancer (see Chapter 11, Gynecologic Disorders)

J. **Molluscum contagiosum**
   1. Viral skin infection most frequently seen in children and in patients positive for HIV
   2. **H/P** =
      a. Painless, **shiny papules** with **central umbilication** (<5 mm diameter)
      b. In children found on face, back, chest, and extremities; in adults found in perineal region
   3. **Labs** = Giemsa and Wright's stains on histology show large inclusion bodies
   4. **Treatment** = chemical, laser, or cryotherapy for removal

K. **Fungal infections**
   1. Cutaneous fungal infections typically characteristic for a specific body region (Color Figure 10-5)
   2. Frequently associated with **warm or moist environments,** obesity, DM, or recent antibiotic use

TABLE 10-2 Common Cutaneous Fungal Infections

Condition	Fungus	Lesions	Diagnosis	Treatment
Tinea versicolor	*Malassezia furfur*	Small scaly macules most frequently on chest and back	KOH prep shows short hyphae, Wood's lamp exam shows extent of disease	Topical antifungal agent for several weeks or oral ketoconazole for 1–5 days
Tinea not due to *M. furfur* Described by location: corporis (body), cruris (groin), pedis (feet), unguium (nail beds), capitis (scalp)	• *Microsporum* • *Trichophyton* • *Epidermophyton*	Pruritic, erythematous, scaly plaques with central clearing	KOH prep shows hyphae	• Topical antifungal agent for multiple weeks • Oral antifungal agent for resistant cases
Intertrigo	*Candida albicans*	Pruritic, painful, erythematous plaques with pustules most commonly in skin creases	KOH prep shows pseudohyphae	• Topical antifungal agent • Topical corticosteroid

KOH, potassium hydroxide.

L. **Scabies**
1. Cutaneous infestation by *Sarcoptes scabiei* mite
2. **Risk factors = crowded living conditions,** poor hygiene
3. **H/P** = severe pruritus at site of involvement (most commonly extremities) that worsens after a hot bath; **mite burrows** with nearby papules may be seen on close examination of skin
4. **Labs** = mites and eggs may be seen in skin scrapings under microscope
5. **Treatment** =
   a. Permethrin cream or oral ivermectin; diphenhydramine to relieve pruritus
   b. All clothing, towels, and linens must be washed in hot water
6. **Complications = infection of close contacts** common

II. Inflammatory skin conditions
A. **Hypersensitivity reactions in skin**
1. Allergic reaction seen in skin due to cutaneous **contact** or **ingestion** of a given allergen (e.g., drugs)
2. Mechanism of reaction
   a. **Type I**—due to mast cell degranulation; light diffuse rash (urticaria) appears soon after exposure and lasts only several hours
   b. **Type IV**—due to lymphocyte activity; measles-like (morbilliform) rash appears several days after second exposure to allergen (mechanism for most allergic contact dermatitis)
3. **H/P** =
   a. Pruritus, erythematous rash in distinct patterns (lines, shapes) in contact dermatitis
   b. Ingestion of an allergen (food, drug reaction) may cause rash in a characteristic location or in a poorly defined area
   c. History of drug ingestion, contact with allergen, or previous reaction is helpful for diagnosis (Color Figure 10-6)
4. **Treatment** =
   a. Stop offending agent or remove contact with allergen
   b. Mild cases may be treated with topical corticosteroids and antihistamines
   c. Oral corticosteroids may be required in worse cases

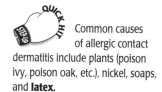

Common causes of allergic contact dermatitis include plants (poison ivy, poison oak, etc.), nickel, soaps, and **latex.**

STEP Use the pattern of a rash to distinguish between an **outside** cause (**defined** shape) from an **internal** cause (**nondefined** distribution) of rash.

Penicillins, sulfonamides, NSAIDs, oral contraceptives, and anticonvulsants are agents most frequently associated with erythema multiforme.

HSV and *Mycoplasma pneumoniae* are common infectious causes of erythema multiforme.

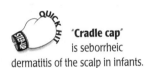

'Cradle cap' is seborrheic dermatitis of the scalp in infants.

20% of patients with psoriasis also have **psoriatic arthritis** (see Chapter 9, Musculoskeletal Disorders).

B. **Erythema multiforme**
   1. More serious cutaneous hypersensitivity reaction due to **drugs, infection,** or vaccination
   2. **H/P** = malaise, myalgias; macules (small nonpalpable lesions), plaques (large nonpalpable lesions), or vesicles on extremities (especially palms, soles); **target lesions** (erythematous center surrounded by pale inner ring and erythematous outer ring) may be evident
   3. **Labs** = increased eosinophils; skin biopsy shows increased lymphocytes and necrotic keratinocytes
   4. **Treatment** = may be self-limited; stop offending agent; corticosteroids, analgesics

C. **Stevens-Johnson syndrome**
   1. **Severe** form of erythema multiforme involving mucous membranes, and severe plaque formation
   2. **Skin sloughing** may be evident; high risk of dehydration
   3. **Treatment** = **stop offending agent;** corticosteroids, analgesics, IV fluids; frequently treated in burn unit

D. **Toxic epidermal necrosis** (TEN)
   1. Most severe form of hypersensitivity reaction with **significant skin sloughing** and **full-thickness epidermal necrosis (Color Figure 10-7)**
   2. **Labs** = decreased WBC, decreased hemoglobin, decreased hematocrit, increased ALT, increased AST
   3. **Treatment** =
      a. **Stop offending agent**
      b. Treat patient in **burn center,** IV hydration, **surgical débridement,** corticosteroids, intravenous immune globulin
      c. Acyclovir may be useful in cases due to HSV

E. **Seborrheic dermatitis**
   1. Chronic hyperproliferation of epidermis most commonly on **scalp** or face
   2. Most common in adolescents and infants
   3. **H/P** = pruritus; erythematous **plaques with yellow, greasy scales**
   4. **Treatment** = shampoo containing selenium, tar, or ketoconazole; 1% hydrocortisone cream may be used intermittently on face
   5. **Complications** = frequent recurrence

F. **Atopic dermatitis** (i.e., eczema)
   1. Chronic inflammatory skin rash characterized by **dry skin patches** with papules
   2. Both **infantile** (resolves with initial years of life) and **adult** (recurrent) forms
   3. **Risk factors** = **asthma,** allergic rhinitis, family history
   4. **H/P** = pruritic lesions; erythematous patches of dry skin on flexor surfaces, dorsum of hands and feet, chest, back, or face; lesions more commonly on face and scalp in infants (Color Figure 10-8)
   5. **Treatment** = moisturizing creams or topical corticosteroids; severe cases may be treated with oral corticosteroids and antihistamines

G. **Psoriasis**
   1. Inflammatory skin disorder characterized by epidermal hyperproliferation
   2. **H/P** = possible pruritus; well-defined **red plaques** with **silvery scales** on **extensor surfaces** (especially knees and elbows) that bleed easily with scale removal (Auspitz sign), pitted nails, lifting of nails (Color Figure 10-9)
   3. **Labs** = negative for rheumatoid factor; skin biopsy shows thickened epidermis, absent granular cell layer, and nucleated cells in stratum corneum; possible increased uric acid, increased erythrocyte sedimentation rate (ESR)
   4. **Treatment** = topical corticosteroids, tar, retinoids, or antifungal agents; phototherapy, methotrexate, cyclosporine, or immune modulators may be used in severe disease

COLOR PLATES

Positron emission tomography (PET scan) using N-13 ammonia to examine perfusion and Fl-18 flurodeoxyglucose to examine metabolism in a patient with perfusion-metabolism mismatch (open arrows) and tissue with impaired function due to scarring (closed arrows).

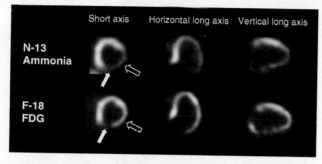

(Used with permission from Topol EJ. *Textbook of Cardiovascular Medicine,* 2ⁿᵈ ed. Philadelphia: Lippincott Williams & Wilkins, 2002, Figure 55.8.)

Paired gram-positive cocci seen in sputum consistent with *S. pneumoniae* pneumonia.

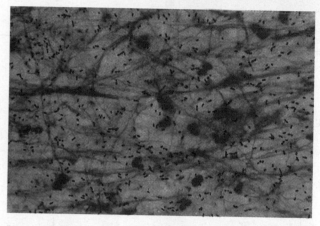

(Used with permission from McClatchey KD. *Clinical Laboratory Medicine,* 2ⁿᵈ ed. Philadelphia: Lippincott Williams & Wilkins, 2002. Figure 51.3.)

Numerous acid-fast bacilli seen in pulmonary histologic section consistent with *Mycobacterium tuberculosis* infection.

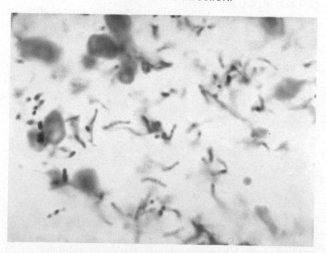

(Used with permission from Rubin E, Farber JL. *Pathology,* 3ʳᵈ ed. Philadelphia: Lippincott Williams & Wilkins, 1999, Figure 9-46.)

Giardiasis; several trophozoites are seen with characteristic pear shape and paired nuclei resembling owls' eyes.

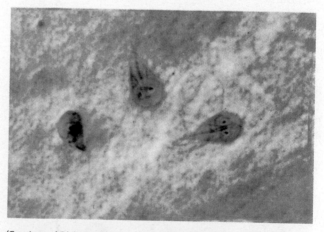

(Courtesy of Dickson Despommier, Ph.D., Department of Parasitology, Columbia Presbyterian Medical Center, New York, NY. Used with permission from Fenoglio-Preiser CM, Lantz PE, Listrom MB, Davis M, Rilke FO. *Gastrointestinal Pathology. An Atlas and Text.* 2ⁿᵈ ed. Philadelphia: Lippincott Williams & Wilkins, 1999, Fig. 9-126.)

COLOR FIGURE 3-2 Jaundice in a patient with hyperbilirubinemia; note the yellow sclera and skin compared to the normal hue of the examiner's hand.

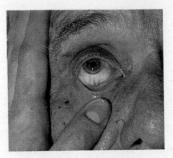

(Used with permission from Bickley LS, Szilagyi P. *Bate's Guide to Physical Examination and History Taking,* 8th ed. Philadelphia: Lippincott Williams & Wilkins, 2003, Table 4-2.)

COLOR FIGURE 4-1 Autosomal dominant polycystic kidney disease; note enlargement of the kidney with many cysts of various sizes.

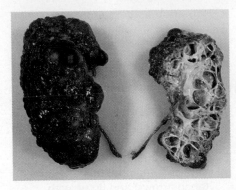

(Used with permission from Rubin E, Farber JL. *Pathology,* 3rd ed. Philadelphia: Lippincott Williams & Wilkins, 1999, Fig. 16-10.)

COLOR FIGURE 6-1 Microangiopathic hemolytic anemia demonstrating multiple schistocytes (fragmented RBCs).

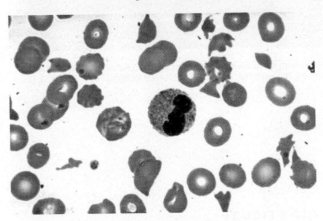

(Used with permission from Rubin E, Farber JL. *Pathology,* 3rd ed. Philadelphia: Lippincott Williams & Wilkins, 1999, Figure 20-31.)

COLOR FIGURE 6-2 Hereditary spherocytosis; blood smear shows numerous spherocytes with decreased diameter, increased staining, and absence of central pallor.

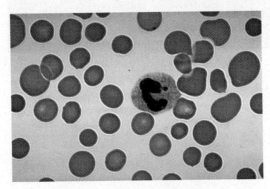

(Used with permission from Rubin E, Farber JL. *Pathology,* 3rd ed. Philadelphia: Lippincott Williams & Wilkins, 1999, Figure 20-27.)

COLOR FIGURE 6-3 Microcytic hypochromic RBCs characteristic of iron deficiency anemia.

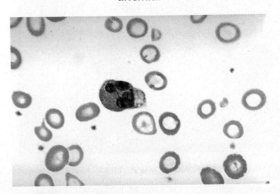

(Used with permission from Rubin E, Farber JL. *Pathology,* 3rd ed. Philadelphia: Lippincott Williams & Wilkins, 1999, Figure 20-22.)

COLOR FIGURE 6-4 Lead poisoning anemia; note the hypochromic RBCs and basophilic stippling seen in some cells.

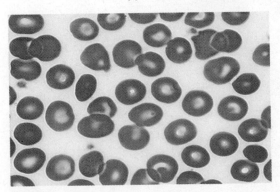

(Used with permission from Anderson SC, Poulsen KB. *Anderson's Atlas of Hematology.* Philadelphia: Lippincott Williams & Wilkins, 2003, Figure IIA2-18.)

COLOR FIGURE 6-5 Blood smear in a patient with sideroblastic anemia; note several red blood cells surrounded by rings of iron granules (ring sideroblasts).

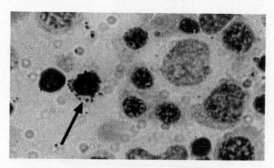

(Used with permission from Handin RI, Lux SE, Stossel TP. *Blood: Principles and Practice of Hematology,* 2nd ed. Philadelphia: Lippincott Williams & Wilkins, 2003, Color Figure 3-6D.)

COLOR FIGURE 6-7 α-thalassemia, Hemoglobin H type; note hypochromic RBCs and occasional target cells.

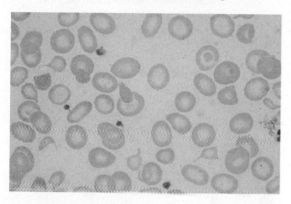

(Used with permission from Anderson SC, Poulsen KB. *Anderson's Atlas of Hematology.* Philadelphia: Lippincott Williams & Wilkins, 2003, Figure IIA2-2.)

COLOR FIGURE 6-9 RBC (arrow) demonstrating signs of *Plasmodium* infection (malaria); note enlarged size, intracellular ring signifying Plasmodium infiltration, and eosinophilic Schuffner's granules.

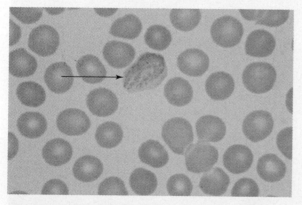

(Used with permission from Anderson SC, Poulsen KB. *Anderson's Atlas of Hematology.* Philadelphia: Lippincott Williams & Wilkins, 2003, Figure IA1-49.)

COLOR FIGURE 6-6 Anemia due to vitamin B12 deficiency; note the macrocytic RBCs and presence of a hypersegmented neutrophil.

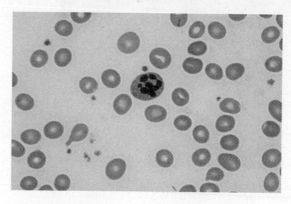

(Used with permission from Anderson SC, Poulsen KB. *Anderson's Atlas of Hematology.* Philadelphia: Lippincott Williams & Wilkins, 2003. Figure IIA3-3.)

COLOR FIGURE 6-8 Sickle cell anemia; note multiple sickle cells and occasional target cells.

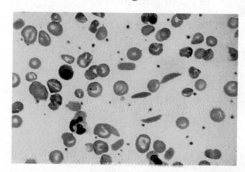

(Used with permission from Rubin E, Farber JL. *Pathology,* 3rd ed. Philadelphia: Lippincott Williams & Wilkins, 1999, Figure 20-26.)

COLOR FIGURE 6-10 Hodgkin's disease; histologic section of lymph node demonstrates pathognomonic binucleated Reed-Sternberg cells that resemble owls' eyes.

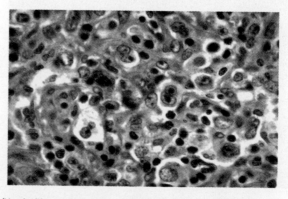

(Used with permission from Rubin E, Farber JL. *Pathology,* 3rd ed. Philadelphia: Lippincott Williams & Wilkins, 1999, Figure 20-72.)

Color Plate 3

COLOR FIGURE 6-11 Acute lymphocytic leukemia; note lymphoblasts with irregular nuclei and prominent nucleoli.

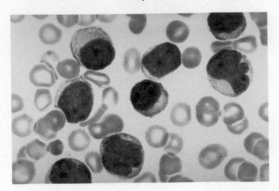

(Used with permission from Rubin E, Farber JL. *Pathology*, 3rd ed. Philadelphia: Lippincott Williams & Wilkins, 1999, Figure 20-59.)

COLOR FIGURE 6-12 Acute myelogenous leukemia (AML) with monocytic differentiation; note the prominent waxy nucleoli, large size of blasts, and presence of Auer rods.

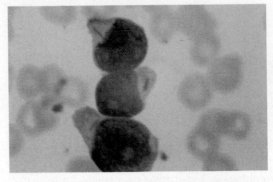

(Used with permission from Handin RI, Lux SE, Stossel TP. *Blood: Principles and Practice of Hematology,* 2nd ed. Philadelphia: Lippincott Williams & Wilkins, 2003, Color Fig. 15-1A.)

COLOR FIGURE 6-13 Chronic lymphocytic leukemia; note small lymphocytes of comparable size to nearby RBCs and presence of smudge cells (fragile lymphocytes disrupted during smear preparation) in upper portion of image.

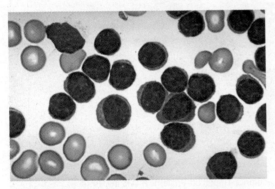

(Used with permission from Rubin E, Farber JL. *Pathology*, 3rd ed. Philadelphia: Lippincott Williams & Wilkins, 1999, Figure 20-57.)

COLOR FIGURE 7-1 Gram stain for a patient with staphylococcal bacteremia; note organization of bacteria in grape-like clusters.

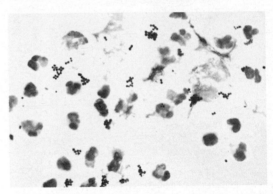

(Used with permission from McClatchey KD. *Clinical Laboratory Medicine,* 2nd ed. Philadelphia: Lippincott Williams & Wilkins, 2002, Figure 51-1.)

COLOR FIGURE 8-1 Leucokoria in a child with a left-eye retinoblastoma.

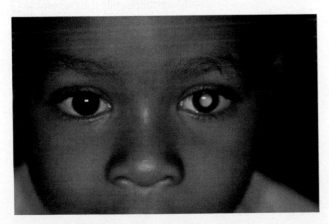

(Used with permission from Rubin E, Farber JL. *Pathology*, 3rd ed. Philadelphia: Lippincott Williams & Wilkins, 1999, Figure 29-23A.)

COLOR FIGURE 8-2 Diabetic retinopathy; note yellowish lipid exudates and multiple small retinal hemorrhages.

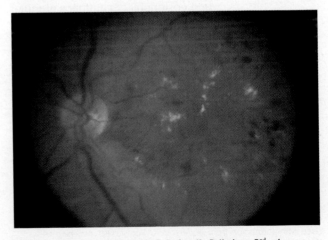

(Used with permission from Rubin E, Farber JL. *Pathology*, 3rd ed. Philadelphia: Lippincott Williams & Wilkins, 1999, Figure 29-11A.)

COLOR FIGURE 8-3 Retinal artery occlusion; note generalized retinal edema and presence of cherry-red spot.

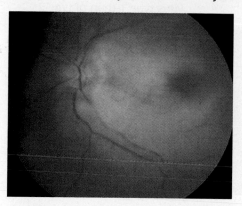

(Used with permission from Gold DH, Weingeist TA. *Color Atlas of the Eye in Systemic Disease.* Philadelphia: Lippincott Williams & Wilkins, 2001, Figure 75-2.)

COLOR FIGURE 8-4 Retinal vein occlusion; note edematous retina, retinal hemorrhages, cotton wool spots, and venous dilation.

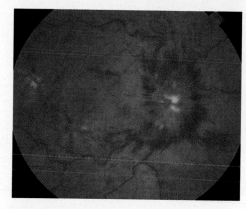

(Used with permission from Gold DH, Weingeist TA. *Color Atlas of the Eye in Systemic Disease.* Philadelphia: Lippincott Williams & Wilkins, 2001, Figure 29-1.)

COLOR FIGURE 9-1 Synovial aspirate from patient with gout; note needle-shaped negatively birefringent sodium urate crystals that are visible under polarized light microscopy.

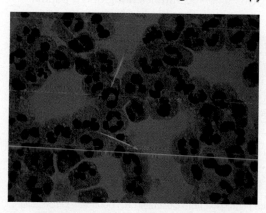

(Used with permission from McClatchey KD. *Clinical Laboratory Medicine,* 2nd ed. Philadelphia: Lippincott Williams & Wilkins, 2002, Figure 27-17.)

COLOR FIGURE 9-2 Synovial aspirate from patient with calcium pyrophosphate dehydrate deposition disease; under polarized light microscopy rhomboid-shaped calcium pyrophosphate dehydrate crystals appear positively birefringent.

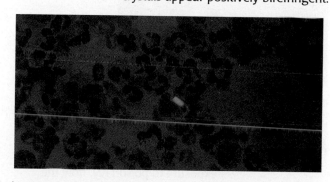

(Used with permission from McClatchey KD. *Clinical Laboratory Medicine,* 2nd ed. Philadelphia: Lippincott Williams & Wilkins, 2002, Figure 27-22.)

COLOR FIGURE 9-3 Patient with Lyme disease exhibiting erythema chronicum migrans (bull's eye rash).

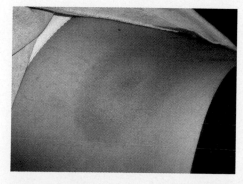

(Used with permission from Goodheart HP. *Goodheart's Photoguide of Common Skin Disorders,* 2nd ed. Philadelphia: Lippincott Williams & Wilkins, 2003, Figure 7-19.)

COLOR FIGURE 10-1 Cellulitis of the right pretibial region; note the erythematous, swollen skin with mild desquamation.

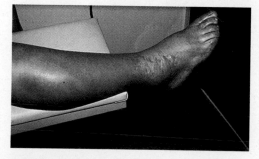

(Used with permission from Goodheart HP. *Goodheart's Photoguide of Common Skin Disorders,* 2nd ed. Philadelphia: Lippincott Williams & Wilkins, 2003, Figure 2-69.)

COLOR FIGURE 10-2 Impetigo involving left nostril due to *S. aureus* infection; note presence of greasy yellow scales within lesion.

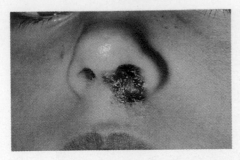

(Used with permission from Smeltzer SC, Bare BG. *Textbook of Medical-Surgical Nursing,* 9th ed. Philadelphia: Lippincott Williams & Wilkins, 2000, Figure 52-1.)

COLOR FIGURE 10-4 Chicken pox in a child due to varicella zoster infection; while the small crusted vesicles are distributed across the body in the childhood form, reactivated infection in adults (shingles) occurs in a single dermatome.

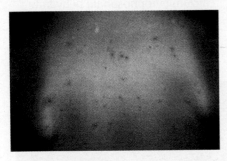

(Used with permission from Goodheart HP. *Goodheart's Photoguide of Common Skin Disorders,* 2nd ed. Philadelphia: Lippincott Williams & Wilkins, 2003, Figure 8-2.)

COLOR FIGURE 10-6 Allergic contact dermatitis due to exposure to poison ivy; note the linearity of the rash consistent with an outside-of-body cause.

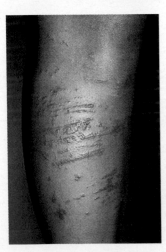

(Used with permission from Goodheart HP. *Goodheart's Photoguide of Common Skin Disorders,* 2nd ed. Philadelphia: Lippincott Williams & Wilkins, 2003, Figure 2-48.)

COLOR FIGURE 10-3 Herpes simplex; these perioral vesicles are more indicative of infection with herpes simplex virus type 1 than of type 2.

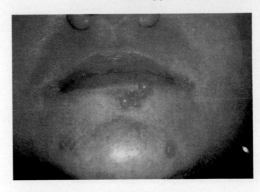

(Used with permission from Weber J, Kelley J. *Health Assessment in Nursing,* 2nd ed. Philadelphia: Lippincott Williams & Wilkins, 2003, Display 13-1a.)

COLOR FIGURE 10-5 Tinea corporis; fungal infection of skin characterized by scaly rash on the body with central clearing and a papular border.

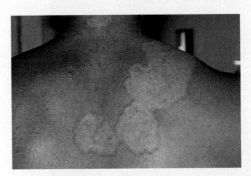

(Used with permission from Goodheart HP. *Goodheart's Photoguide of Common Skin Disorders,* 2nd ed. Philadelphia: Lippincott Williams & Wilkins, 2003, Figure 4-12.)

COLOR FIGURE
10-7

Toxic epidermal necrolysis (TEN). This severe dermatologic condition begins as a generalized erythematous rash that progresses into widespread desquamation and erosion formation.

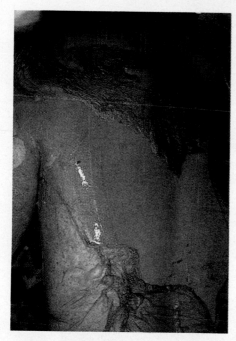

(Used with permission from Elder D, Elenitsas R, Johnson B Jr., et al. *Synopsis and Atlas of Lever's Histopathology of the Skin*. Philadelphia: Lippincott Williams & Wilkins, 1999, Clin. Fig. IVC2.c.)

COLOR FIGURE
10-9

Red plaques with silver scales on extensor forearm surface of a patient with psoriasis; similar lesions may also be seen on the extensor surfaces of the knee.

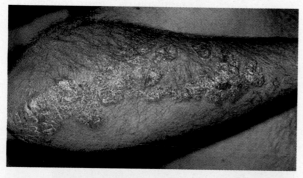

(Used with permission from Goodheart HP. *Goodheart's Photoguide of Common Skin Disorders*, 2nd ed. Philadelphia: Lippincott Williams & Wilkins, 2003, Figure 2-23.)

COLOR FIGURE
10-8

Adult atrophic dermatitis (eczema) characterized by erythematous patches of dry skin.

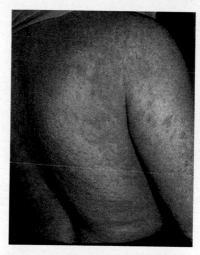

(Used with permission from Goodheart HP. *Goodheart's Photoguide of Common Skin Disorders*, 2nd ed. Philadelphia: Lippincott Williams & Wilkins, 2003, Figure 2-8.)

COLOR FIGURE
10-10

Pityriasis rosea; these scaled papules fan out across the chest or back to give the overall appearance of a Christmas tree pattern.

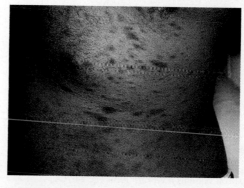

(Used with permission from Goodheart HP. *Goodheart's Photoguide of Common Skin Disorders*, 2nd ed. Philadelphia: Lippincott Williams & Wilkins, 2003, Figure 4-4.)

COLOR FIGURE
10-11

Pemphigus vulgaris. Fragile bullae develop which rupture easily leading to widespread erosions and desquamation.

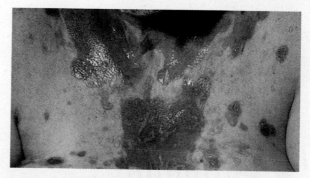

(Used with permission from Elder D, Elenitsas R, Johnson B Jr., et al. *Synopsis and Atlas of Lever's Histopathology of the Skin*. Philadelphia: Lippincott Williams & Wilkins, 1999, Clin. Fig. IVD3.b.)

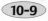
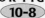

Color Plate 7

COLOR FIGURE 10-12 Bullous pemphigoid. Multiple large bullae form on an erythematous base leading to severe erosions.

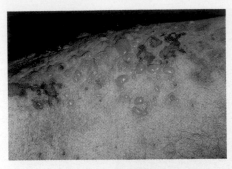

(Used with permission from Elder D, Elenitsas R, Johnson B Jr., et al. *Synopsis and Atlas of Lever's Histopathology of the Skin.* Philadelphia: Lippincott Williams & Wilkins, 1999, Clin. Fig. IVE3.)

COLOR FIGURE 10-13 Actinic keratosis; these lesions are superficial papules covered by dry scales and are a result of sun exposure.

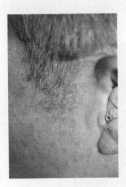

(Used with permission from Sauer GC. *Manual of Skin Diseases,* 5th ed. Philadelphia: JB Lippincott, 1985, Table 4-4.)

COLOR FIGURE 10-14 Squamous cell carcinoma with erythematous base and ulceration.

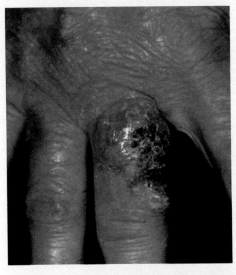

(Used with permission from Rubin E, Farber JL. *Pathology,* 3rd ed. Philadelphia: Lippincott Williams & Wilkins, 1999, Fig. 24-76A.)

COLOR FIGURE 10-15 Basal cell carcinoma; note the pearly appearance of a papule with central ulceration.

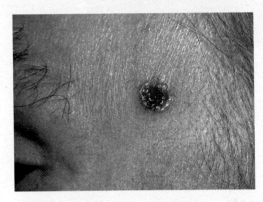

(Used with permission from Goodheart HP. *Goodheart's Photoguide of Common Skin Disorders,* 2nd ed. Philadelphia: Lippincott Williams & Wilkins, 2003, Figure 22-17.)

COLOR FIGURE 10-16 Melanoma, superficial spreading type; note the ABCDs of the lesion—asymmetry, irregular border, inconsistent color, and large diameter (>20 mm).

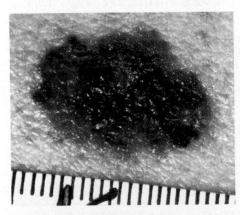

(Used with permission from Rubin E, Farber JL. *Pathology,* 3rd ed. Philadelphia: Lippincott Williams & Wilkins, 1999, Figure 24-51.)

COLOR FIGURE 10-17 Melanocytic nevus; unlike melanoma, this lesion is near symmetrical, has better border regularity, is a more consistent color, and is a smaller diameter.

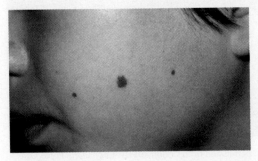

(Used with permission from Goodheart HP. *Goodheart's Photoguide of Common Skin Disorders,* 2nd ed. Philadelphia: Lippincott Williams & Wilkins, 2003, Figure 21-1.)

H. **Pityriasis rosea**
  1. Mild inflammatory skin disorder in children with possible viral association characterized by papular lesions
  2. **H/P =**
     a. Pruritus; oval erythematous papules covered with white scale located primarily on chest, back, and extremities
     b. Rash begins with appearance of **"herald patch"** (single round lesion up to 5 cm in diameter) a few days before generalized eruption (Color Figure 10-10)
  3. **Treatment** = self-limited; topical steroids, phototherapy, or erythromycin may decrease duration of exacerbation

I. **Erythema nodosum**
  1. Inflammation of **subcutaneous fat** resulting in painful erythematous pretibial nodules
  2. Due to delayed immunologic reaction to infection, collagen-vascular diseases, inflammatory bowel disease, or drugs
  3. **H/P** = malaise, arthralgias; tender erythematous **pretibial nodules**, fever
  4. **Labs** = possible positive antistreptolysin O titer (when associated with streptococcal infection), increased ESR; skin biopsy may show fatty inflammation
  5. **Treatment** = self-limited; non-steroidal anti-inflammatory drugs (NSAIDs), potassium iodide, corticosteroids

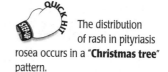

The distribution of rash in pityriasis rosea occurs in a **"Christmas tree"** pattern.

III. Bullous diseases

A. **Pemphigus vulgaris**
  1. Autoimmune disorder characterized by autoantibodies to adhesion molecules in epidermis
  2. Patients usually 30–40 years old
  3. **H/P = painful, fragile blisters** in oropharynx and on chest, face, and perineal region; blisters rupture easily and erosions are common (Color Figure 10-11)
  4. **Labs** = skin biopsy shows separating of epidermal cells (**acantholysis**) with intact basement membrane; immunofluorescence demonstrates anti-epidermal antibodies
  5. **Treatment** = corticosteroids, azathioprine, or cyclophosphamide
  6. **Complications** = sepsis, high mortality without treatment

B. **Bullous pemphigoid**
  1. Autoimmune disorder characterized by autoantibodies to epidermal basement membrane
  2. Most patients >60 years old
  3. **H/P = widespread blistering** (especially on flexor surfaces and perineal region), pruritus; erosions may form with blister rupture (Color Figure 10-12)
  4. **Labs** = immunofluorescence shows **anti-basement membrane** antibodies
  5. **Treatment** = oral or topical corticosteroids or azathioprine

C. **Porphyria cutanea tarda**
  1. Disease resulting from deficiency of hepatic uroporphyrinogen decarboxylase, an enzyme involved in heme metabolism
  2. **Risk factors** = alcoholism, hepatitis C, iron overload, estrogen use, smoking
  3. **H/P** = chronic blistering on sun-exposed skin, ruptured blisters heal poorly and result in erosions and hyperpigmented skin
  4. **Labs** = decreased uroporphyrinogen decarboxylase, increased porphyrins in serum, urine, and feces
  5. **Treatment** = periodic phlebotomy, chloroquine

NEXT STEP Even when actinic keratosis is the suspected diagnosis, biopsy a lesion to rule out squamous cell cancer.

Use of a good **sunscreen** (SPF 15 or greater) is important in the prevention of skin cancer associated with sun exposure.

Basal cell carcinoma is the **most common** type of skin cancer.

Shave biopsy should **never** be used to study a suspicious lesion because it does not provide enough tissue for clear diagnosis and cannot be used to measure lesion depth.

Nevi should be followed to look for the ABCDEs of melanoma—**A**symmetry, **B**order (irregular), **C**olor (variable), **D**iameter (large), and **E**nlargement.

The most important prognostic factor for melanoma is **thickness of lesion** (>0.76 mm associated with increased risk of metastasis).

IV. Neoplasms

A. Actinic keratosis
1. **Precancerous** skin lesion that may progress to squamous cell cancer
2. **Risk factors** = sun exposure
3. **H/P** = erythematous **papule** with rough, **yellow-brown scales** <5 mm in diameter; lesions found in **sun-exposed** areas (Color Figure 10-13)
4. **Labs** = biopsy shows dysplasia of epithelium (deeper epithelial cells show variations in shape and nuclei with increased staining)
5. **Treatment** = topical 5-flurouracil, cryotherapy
6. **Complications** = 0.1% per year risk of progression to **squamous cell carcinoma** (**60%** of squamous cell carcinomas arise from **actinic keratosis**)

B. Squamous cell carcinoma
1. Skin cancer involving **squamous** cells of epithelium
2. **Risk factors** = **sun exposure** (particularly **UVB** radiation), actinic keratosis, arsenic exposure, fair complexion, radiation
3. **H/P** = painless erythematous papule with scaling in sun-exposed area; progressive lesions may bleed, ulcerate, or be painful (Color Figure 10-14)
4. **Labs** = biopsy shows anaplastic epidermal cells extending to dermis
5. **Treatment** = surgical excision; Mohs' excision (serial shallow excisions with histological analysis performed to minimize cosmetic damage) may be performed for lesions on face; radiation may be helpful in large lesions
6. **Complications** = progresses slowly but may be large lesion by time of diagnosis if located in poorly visualized region (back, scalp); 5 to 10% of cases metastasize

C. Basal cell carcinoma
1. Skin cancer arising in **basal** epidermal cells
2. **Risk factors** = sun exposure
3. **H/P** = **pearly papule** with fine vascular markings (**telangiectasias**) (Color Figure 10-15)
4. **Labs** = biopsy shows basophilic-staining basal epidermal cells arranged in palisades
5. **Treatment** = surgical excision, Mohs' excision, radiation, or cryotherapy
6. **Complications** = lesions metastasize in <0.1% of cases

D. Melanoma
1. Malignant melanocyte tumor that spreads rapidly
2. **Risk factors** = sun exposure, fair complexion, family history, numerous nevi (moles)
3. Types
   a. **Superficial spreading**—most common type; grows laterally before invasive growth occurs
   b. **Nodular**—only grows vertically and becomes invasive rapidly; difficult to detect
   c. **Acral lentiginous**—involves palms, soles, and nail beds
   d. **Lentigo maligna**—long-lasting in situ stage prior to vertical growth
4. **H/P** =
   a. **Painless** pigmented lesion with recent changes in appearance
   b. Lesions have irregular borders, multiple colors, and may be large or rapidly growing (Color Figure 10-16)
   c. In contrast, melanocytic nevi are more symmetrical, have more regular borders, are homogenously colored, and remain relatively the same size over time (Color Figure 10-17)
5. **Labs** = biopsy shows atypical melanocytes and possible invasion into dermis
6. **Treatment** = surgical excision; chemotherapy if metastatic
7. **Complications** = aggressive cancer; lesions may be metastatic by time of discovery (most commonly lung, brain, and gastrointestinal tract)

TABLE 10-3	Common Types of Skin Grafts and Tissue Flaps Used in Wound Repair		
Type	**Description**	**Common Donor Sites**	**Indications**
Split-thickness graft	Skin graft composed of epidermis and part of dermis	Abdomen, thighs, buttocks	Skin replacement in wounds; useful to cover extensive surface area (contracts over time)
Full-thickness graft	Skin graft composed of epidermis and full dermis	Above ears (for face), forearm, groin	Defects on face, hands
Composite graft	Skin grafts that also contain other tissues (cartilage, nail bed, fat)	Fingertip, ear, etc	Site-specific anatomical reconstruction
Skin flap	Skin and subcutaneous tissue with attached vascular supply	Forehead, groin, deltopectoral region, thighs	Large defects with good vascular supply requiring padding
Muscle flap	Transferred muscle that either includes skin (myocutaneous flap) or requires additional skin graft	Tensor fascia lata, gluteal muscles, sartorius, rectus abdominus, latissimus dorsi	Areas requiring increased vascularized tissue, exposed bone, severe radiation injury

DERMATOLOGY

V. Plastic surgery

A. Grafts and flaps

1. Transfer of skin and soft tissues from one location of body to another for use in wound repair
2. Skin grafts may be autografts (from healthy tissue on same patient), allografts (donor tissue from another individual), or xenografts (donor tissue from another species)
3. Flaps may be **rotational** or **transpositional** (left partially attached to donor site and rotated or stretched to cover wound) or **free flaps** (flap completely removed from donor site and transferred in whole to wound)

B. Reconstructive surgery

1. Repair of soft tissue defects due to surgery, congenital anomalies, or wounds
2. Multiple types of tissue are used to recreate normal anatomy (skin, muscle, bone, cartilage, vessels, nerves)
3. **Types**
   a. Maxillofacial—cleft lip repair, cleft palate repair, facial trauma
   b. Breast—reconstruction following mastectomy with muscle flaps or implants
   c. Genitourinary—repair of epispadias, hypospadias, or genital agenesis
   d. Soft tissues—following sarcoma excision or for filling defects

C. Cosmetic surgery

1. Surgical alteration of appearance
2. May be performed to remove anatomical anomalies or results of massive weight loss, surgery, or injury (e.g., gynecomastia, postmastectomy, excessive skin, difficulty breathing)
3. More often used to combat effects of **aging** or to **modify** physical appearance
4. Types
   a. Facial—face-lift, brow-lift, blepharoplasty (repair of baggy eyelids), rhinoplasty
   b. Skin—removal of scarring, spider veins, age wrinkles (dermabrasion, laser treatment, chemical peel)
   c. Breast—augmentation, reduction (may be helpful to reduce back strain)
   d. Fatty tissue reduction—abdominoplasty, liposuction
5. **Psychiatric** issues must be considered, especially in patients who repeatedly request "upgrades"

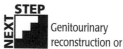

NEXT STEP Genitourinary reconstruction or gender reassignment requires a careful preoperative evaluation to determine true gender of patient, genetic causes, realistic outcomes, expectations, and psychiatric issues.

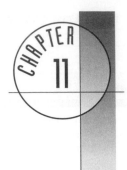

Gynecologic and Breast Disorders

The mean age of menarche is 13 years old in the United States and tends to occur earlier in African Americans than in Caucasians.

Precocious puberty in boys occurs before 9 years of age and is most commonly due to adrenal hyperplasia.

Central nervous system (CNS) lesions or **trauma** are a cause of isosexual precocious puberty in approximately 10% of cases.

I. Menstrual physiology

A. **Gynecologic development (see Tables 11-1 and 11-2 and Figure 11-1)**
1. Reproductive changes driven by follicle-stimulating hormone (FSH) and luteinizing hormone (LH) levels
2. Secondary sexual characteristics are due to androgens
3. Tanner stages describe breast and pubic hair development during puberty

B. **Precocious puberty**
1. Development of pubertal changes in **girls** before **8** years old
2. Most cases are **idiopathic**
3. Types
   a. **Heterosexual**
      (1) Virilization of girls or feminization of boys
      (2) In girls most commonly due to congenital adrenal hyperplasia, exposure to exogenous androgens, or androgen-secreting neoplasm
   b. **Isosexual**
      (1) Premature sexual development appropriate for gender
      (2) May be complete (all sexual characteristics develop prematurely) or incomplete (only one sexual characteristic develops prematurely)
4. **H/P** =
   a. Complete isosexual—normal pubertal changes take place but at **earlier-than-normal age**
   b. Incomplete isosexual—premature breast budding **(thelarche),** axillary hair growth **(adrenarche),** or pubic hair growth **(pubarche)** may take place
5. **Labs =**
   a. Increased LH release following administration of gonadotropin-releasing hormone (GnRH) suggests pituitary gland activation
   b. Increased estrogen suggests exogenous hormone production (neoplasm)
   c. Increased thyroid-stimulating hormone (TSH) with low thyroxine (T_4) and triiodothyronine (T_3) suggest precocious puberty in response to chronic hypothyroidism
6. **Radiology** = MRI or CT with contrast may detect cerebral or adrenal lesions
7. **Treatment =**
   a. **GnRH analogues** are useful for LH and FSH suppression in **idiopathic** and pituitary gland hyperactivity pathologies
   b. Precocious puberty secondary to ectopic hormone secretion should be treated by locating and removing source of hormone
8. **Complications** = short stature (bones fuse at early age); social and emotional adjustment issues

TABLE 11-1	Gynecologic Development by Age	
Age	**Hormone Levels**	**Characteristics**
Fetal–4 yrs old	High intrauterine FSH and LH that peaks at 20 wks gestation and decreases until birth FSH and LH increase again from birth until 6 months age then gradually decrease to low levels by 4 yr old	All oocytes formed and partially matured by 20 wks gestation Tanner stage 1 characteristics[a]
4–8 yrs old	Low FSH, LH, and androgen levels due to GnRH suppression	Tanner stage 1 characteristics Any sexual development considered precocious
8–11 yrs old	LH, FSH, and androgen levels begin to increase	Initial pubertal changes including early breast development and pubic and axillary hair growth
11–17 yrs old	Further increase of LH, FSH, and androgens to baseline mature levels Hormones secreted in pulsatile fashion (higher at night) due to sleep-associated increase in GnRH secretion	Puberty Progression through Tanner stages Development of secondary sexual characteristics and growth spurt Menarche in females (beginning of menstrual cycles) and further oocyte development
17–50 yrs old (females)	LH and FSH follow menstrual cycle Gradual increase in FSH and LH with ovarian insensitivity	Menstrual cycles Mature sexual characteristics
≥50 yrs old (females)	LH and FSH levels increase with onset of ovarian failure	Perimenopause: menstrual cycles become inconsistent (oligomenorrhea) Menopause: menstrual cycles cease (amenorrhea)

[a] See Table 11-2 for descriptions of Tanner stages.
FSH, follicle stimulating hormone; GnRH, gonadotropin-releasing hormone; LH, luteinizing hormone.

C. **Normal menstrual cycle (see Figure 11-2)**
   1. LH, FSH, estrogen, progesterone, and human chorionic gonadotropin (hCG) all play roles in the menstrual cycle
   2. **Follicular phase**
      a. Begins at first day of menses (menstruation)
      b. **FSH** stimulates **growth** of **ovarian follicle** (granulosa cells), which in turn secretes estradiol
      c. **Estradiol** induces **endometrial proliferation** and further increases FSH and LH secretion due to positive feedback of pituitary
   3. **Luteal phase**
      a. **LH surge** induces **ovulation**
      b. Residual follicle **(corpus luteum)** secretes estradiol and progesterone to **maintain endometrium** and induce development of secretory ducts
      c. High estradiol levels inhibit FSH and LH
      d. If egg is **not** fertilized, corpus luteum degrades, progesterone and estradiol levels decrease, and the **endometrial lining degrades** (menses)
   4. **Fertilization**
      a. If the egg is fertilized, it will implant in the endometrium
      b. Endometrial tissue secretes **hCG** to **maintain the corpus luteum**

FIGURE 11-1 Changes in hormone and oogonia (egg) levels with gestation and age. DHEA, dehydroepiandrosterone; FSH, follicle-stimulating hormone; hCG, human chorionic gonadotropin; LH, luteinizing hormone.

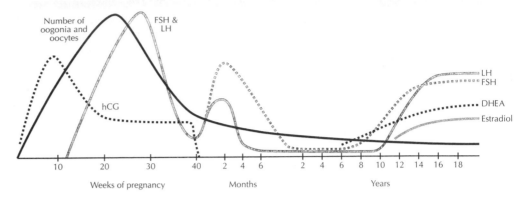

(Used with permission from Speroff L, Glass RH, Kase NG. *Clinical Gynecologic Endocrinology and Infertility.* 7th Ed. Baltimore: Williams & Wilkins, 1991.)

    c. Corpus luteum continues to secrete progesterone until sufficient production is achieved by a developing placenta (approximately 8–12 weeks)

D. **Menopause**

    1. **Permanent** end of menstruation due to **ceasing of ovarian function** in later middle age (~50 years old)

    2. Premature menopause is defined as ovarian failure before 40 years old (more likely with history of tobacco use, radiation therapy, chemotherapy, autoimmune disorders, or abdominal/pelvic surgery)

    3. During evolution of menopause (**perimenopausal** period) ovarian response to FSH and LH decreases while FSH and LH levels increase and estrogen levels fluctuate

    4. **H/P = hot flashes** (secondary to vasomotor instability), sweating, **menstrual irregularity** with eventual **amenorrhea,** fatigue, anxiety, irritability, depression, **dyspareunia** (due to vaginal wall atrophy and decreased lubrication), urinary frequency, dysuria, change in bowel habits; exam detects vaginal atrophy

    5. **Labs** = increased FSH, increased LH, decreased estradiol

    6. **Treatment =**

       a. Treatment focuses on **prevention of complications**

       b. Hormone replacement therapy was mainstay of therapy for many years, but its benefits have more recently been shown to be less than

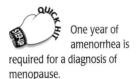

One year of amenorrhea is required for a diagnosis of menopause.

(vertical side tab) GYNECOLOGIC AND BREAST DISORDERS

TABLE 11-2	Tanner Stages for Female Breast and Hair Development	
Tanner Stage	**Breast Development**	**Pubic Hair Development**
1	Prepubertal—raised papilla (nipple) only	Prepubertal—no hair growth
2	Breast budding, areolar enlargement	Slight growth of fine labial hair
3	Further breast and areolar enlargement	Further growth of hair
4	Further breast enlargement—areola and papilla form secondary growth above level of breast	Hair becomes coarser and spreads over much of pubic region
5	Mature breast—areola recedes to level of breast while papilla remains extended	Coarse hair extends form pubic region to medial thighs

FIGURE 11-2 Hormone levels during the menstrual cycle with appropriate ovarian, endometrial, and basal body temperature responses. FSH, follicle-stimulating hormone; LH, luteinizing hormone.

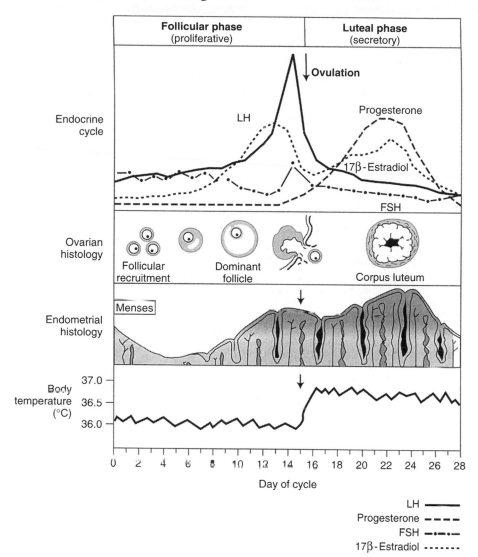

(Used with permission from Mehta S, Milder EA, Mirachi AJ, Milder E. *Step-Up: A High-Yield, Systems-Based Review for the USMLE Step 1*. 2nd Ed. Philadelphia: Lippincott Williams & Wilkins, 2003.)

previously believed, and it has been linked to increased risk for breast cancer and deep vein thrombosis

c. Unopposed estrogen therapy may decrease breast cancer risk but increases endometrial cancer risk; estrogen-progestin therapy may increase breast cancer risk but decreases endometrial risk

d. Calcium, vitamin D, bisphosphonates, and exercise to prevent osteoporosis

e. Lubricating agents to treat dyspareunia (painful intercourse)

f. Good cardiovascular follow up

g. Selective estrogen receptor modulators, such as raloxifene and tamoxifen, may serve a role in reducing osteoporosis and cardiovascular risks

h. Selective serotonin reuptake inhibitors (SSRIs) may reduce severity of hot flashes

7. **Complications** = osteoporosis, coronary artery disease

Increased risk of **osteoporosis** in menopausal women is due to **decreased estrogen** production by the ovaries.

TABLE 11-3	Roles of Hormones Involved in the Menstrual Cycle

Hormone	Effects
Luteinizing hormone (LH)	Mid-cycle **surge** induces **ovulation** Regulates cholesterol conversion to pregnenolone in ovarian theca cells as initial step in estrogen synthesis
Follicle-stimulating hormone (FSH)	Stimulates **development** of **ovarian follicle** Regulates ovarian granulosa cell activity to control estrogen synthesis
Estrogens (estradiol, estriol)	Stimulates **endometrial proliferation** Aids in follicle growth Induces LH surge High levels inhibit FSH secretion **Decrease** in levels leads to **menstruation** Principal role in sexual development
Progesterone	Stimulates **endometrial gland development** Inhibits uterine contraction Increases thickness of cervical mucus **Increases basal body temperature** Inhibits LH and FSH secretion; maintains pregnancy **Decrease** in levels leads to **menstruation**
Human chorionic gonadotropin (hCG)	Acts like LH after implantation of fertilized egg **Maintains corpus luteum viability** and progesterone secretion

II. Contraception (see Table 11-4)

A. Methods of contraception attempt to prevent pregnancy

B. The various forms of contraception are each associated with certain side effects

C. Method choice
1. Should consider likelihood of patient compliance
2. Side effects must be tolerated by patient
3. Certain methods may be contraindicated for comorbid medical conditions

III. Menstrual disorders and issues

A. **Amenorrhea**
1. Absence of menstruation
   a. **Primary**—absence of menses **(never** has happened) with normal secondary sexual characteristics by 16 years old or absence of both menses and secondary sexual characteristics by 14 years old
   b. **Secondary**—absence of menses for 6 months in patient with **prior history of menses**
2. Causes include **pregnancy, ovarian failure,** anatomical abnormality (mullerian duct dysgenesis, imperforate hymen, vaginal septum), hypothalamic-pituitary failure, congenital androgen insensitivity syndrome (XY genotype with female phenotype), thyroid dysfunction, polycystic ovary syndrome (PCOS), gonadal dysgenesis (Turner's syndrome), anorexia nervosa, excess prolactin secretion, severe malnutrition, menopause
3. **H/P =**
   a. History should address occurrence of any previous menstruation periods (i.e., primary or secondary amenorrhea), exercise and eating habits (substantial exercise or inadequate eating), family history, and medications
   b. Exam should note Tanner stages (see Table 11-2) and should check for normal sexual anatomy

TABLE 11-4 Methods of Contraception

Method	Description	Effectiveness		Side Effects
		Ideal (%)	Typical (%)	
Abstinence	• Not engaging in intercourse	100	100	• None
Rhythm method	• Recording occurrence of menses, daily basal body temperature, and cervical mucus to determine timing of cycle, occurrence of ovulation, and period of fertility	97	80	• May be useful in diagnosing infertility
Withdrawal method	• Withdrawal of penis from vagina immediately before ejaculation	96	81	• Decreased pleasure • Difficult to conduct in effective manner
Spermicide alone	• Insertion of anti-spermal jelly or cream into vagina immediately before intercourse	94	74	• Correct usage and quantity difficult to achieve consistently
Diaphragm / cervical cap	• Barrier inserted into vagina before intercourse to cover cervix • Used with spermicide and left in place for several hours after intercourse	94	80	• Inconvenient • Frequent poor compliance
Condom	• Barrier (most frequently latex) placed over penis and left in place until withdrawal following ejaculation • Frequently used with spermicide • Polyurethane condoms are currently being studied as an alternative to latex	97	86	• Risk of condom breakage • Latex significantly more effective than other materials (with possible exception of polyurethane) • Risk of latex allergy
Contraceptive sponge	• Polyurethane sponge implanted with spermicide that releases spermicide over 24 hours after insertion to inhibit fertilization	94	74	• Possible increased risk of toxic shock syndrome
Intrauterine device (IUD)	• Object inserted into uterus by physician and left in place for several years to incite an inflammatory response in the endometrium and prevent fertilization or successful implantation of a fertilized egg	99	98	• Risk of spontaneous abortion, ectopic pregnancy, and uterine perforation
Intravaginal ring	• Ring inserted intravaginally that releases ethinyl estradiol over 3 weeks to prevent ovulation • Replaced each month	99	98	• Withdrawal bleeding, device-related discomfort, headache
Oral contraceptive pills (OCPs)	• Either estrogen-progesterone combination or progesterone-alone pills that inhibit follicle development and ovulation (combination pill only), change endometrial quality, and increase cervical mucus viscosity to prevent fertilization to implantation	99	95	• Possible nausea, headache, weight gain • Increased risk of DVT • Milder effects for progesterone-only pills but slightly lower effectiveness
Medroxy-progesterone acetate (Depo-Provera)	• Progestin analogue injected by healthcare provider every 3 months that inhibits endometrial development	99	99	• Nausea, headache, weight gain

TABLE 11-4 (Continued)

Method	Description	Effectiveness Ideal (%)	Effectiveness Typical (%)	Side Effects
Medroxy-progesterone acetate/estradiol cypionate (Lunelle)	• Combination progestin analogue-estrogen injection administered by healthcare provider that prevents ovulation and inhibits endometrial development	99	99	• Weight gain, headaches, HTN, breakthrough bleeding • Less side effects than Depo-Provera • Currently not available in United States
Transdermal contraceptive patch	• Transdermal delivery of estradiol and progestin analogue to act in similar manner to OCPs • Patch must be changed weekly	99	95	• Risk of patch detachment • Nausea, headache, weight gain • Less effective in heavier women because of diffusion into adipose tissue
Morning-after pill	• Regimen of estradiol and progesterone taken within 72 hr of unprotected intercourse or intercourse with failed contraception method (e.g., poor withdrawal, broken condom) to prevent ovulation, inhibit fertilization, or interrupt new pregnancy	98	97	• Nausea, headache more severe than that seen with OCPs
Sterilization	• Cutting of vas deferens in men (vasectomy) or tubal ligation in women to prevent fertilization	~100	99	• May be difficult to reverse • Increased risk of ectopic pregnancy in cases of failure or after voluntary ligation reversal

DVT, deep venous thrombosis; HTN, hypertension.

4. **Labs** =
   a. β-**hCG test** used to rule out pregnancy
   b. TSH, T_4, and T_3-reuptake can diagnose thyroid dysfunction
   c. Increased **prolactin** suggests prolactin-secreting tumor
   d. FSH and LH levels measure hypothalamic-pituitary activity
   e. **Progestin challenge** (patient is observed for bleeding after 5-day administration of progesterone) and **estrogen-progesterone challenge** (patient is observed for bleeding after administration of estrogen and progesterone) can help detect anatomical abnormalities (bleeding indicates normal outflow tract), hormonal abnormalities, or hypothalamic-pituitary activity
5. **Treatment** =
   a. Modify behaviors (eating disorders, exercise) to allow menstruation
   b. Anatomical abnormalities require surgical correction
   c. Prolactinoma may be treated with bromocriptine or surgical excision
   d. Thyroid dysfunction treated according to specific pathology
6. **Complications** = patients with genetic disorders or ovarian failure may be **unable** to achieve normal menstrual cycles; in some untreatable patients with appropriate anatomy pregnancy may be accomplished through egg donation, in vitro fertilization, and hormone modulation
B. **Dysmenorrhea**
   1. Periodic pain associated with menses that may be primary (without pelvic pathology) or secondary (due to endometriosis, pelvic inflammatory disease [PID], uterine fibroids, ovarian cysts, or adenomyosis)

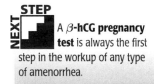
NEXT STEP A β-**hCG pregnancy test** is always the first step in the workup of any type of amenorrhea.

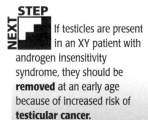
NEXT STEP If testicles are present in an XY patient with androgen insensitivity syndrome, they should be **removed** at an early age because of increased risk of **testicular cancer**.

GYNECOLOGIC AND BREAST DISORDERS

FIGURE 11-3 Approach to the patient with amenorrhea. GnRH, gonadotropin-releasing hormone; FSH, follicle-stimulating hormone; β-hCG, human chorionic gonadotropin; LH, luteinizing hormone. Neg, negative; PCOS, polycystic ovary syndrome; Pos, positive.

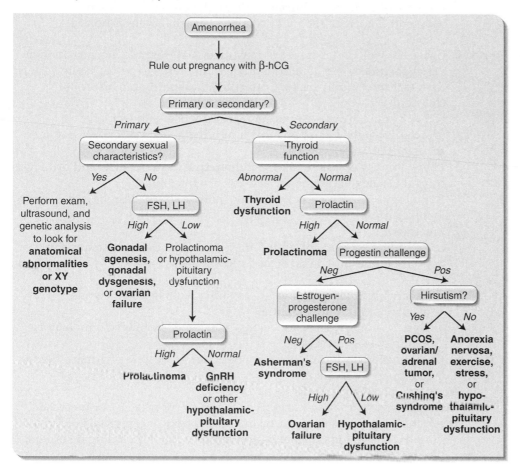

2. **H/P** = crampy lower abdominal pain associated with menstruation; nausea, vomiting, headache, diarrhea; mild abdominal tenderness

3. **Labs** = β-hCG and blood and vaginal cultures are helpful to rule out pregnancy and infection

4. **Radiology** = ultrasound (US) may be used to detect ovarian and uterine lesions; hysteroscopy or laparoscopy may be needed to detect intrauterine pathology, intra-abdominal pathology, or endometriosis

5. **Treatment** = nonsteroidal anti-inflammatory drugs (NSAIDs) or oral contraceptive pills (OCPs) for primary disorders; treat underlying disorder

C. **Premenstrual syndrome** (PMS)

1. Syndrome seen in women with normal functioning ovaries that **precedes menses** and is characterized by multiple pain, mood, and autonomic symptoms

2. Most women with menstrual cycles experience some symptoms, but **5–10% of women** have severe symptoms that **interfere with daily life**

3. **Risk factors** (for severe symptoms) = family history, depression

4. **H/P** =

   a. Weight gain, headache, abdominal or pelvic pain, abdominal bloating, change in bowel habits, depression, fatigue, irritability; breast tenderness, edema, abdominal tenderness

NEXT STEP Any woman of childbearing age with abdominal pain must be given a β-hCG pregnancy test to rule out **ectopic pregnancy.**

b. Findings precede menses and occur at similar time points in each cycle

5. **Treatment** = NSAIDs, OCPs, progestins; SSRIs may improve PMS accompanied by significant depression

D. **Endometriosis**

1. Presence of **endometrial tissue outside the uterus** (ovaries, broad ligament); ectopic tissue follows same menstrual cycle as normal tissue

2. Cause not well understood but may involve retrograde menstruation or vascular spread of endometrial tissue from uterus to pelvic cavity

3. **Risk factors** = family history, **infertility,** nulliparity (no history of childbirth)

4. **H/P** = dysmenorrhea, dyspareunia, painful bowel movements (dyschezia), **pelvic pain,** possible infertility; pelvic tenderness, palpable adhesions on uterus or ovaries

5. **Labs** = biopsy of lesions shows **endometrial tissue;** β-hCG and urinalysis helpful to rule out pregnancy and urinary tract infection

6. **Radiology** = laparoscopy will show **"powder-burn"** lesions and cysts on involved areas

7. **Treatment** =
   a. Recording a journal of symptoms is useful for defining treatment
   b. OCPs, progestins, danazol, or GnRH agonists may supply symptomatic relief
   c. Laparoscopic ablation may successfully remove lesions while maintaining fertility potential
   d. Hysterectomy, lysis of adhesions, or salpingo-oopherectomy may be required in severe cases

8. **Complications** = fertility may not be achieved despite pharmacologic or laparoscopic intervention

E. **Abnormal uterine bleeding**

1. **Irregular** menstruation, **excessive** menses (menorrhagia), or **increased duration** of menses that may be due to a variety of causes (e.g., uterine fibroids, cancer, hypothalamic-pituitary dysfunction, clotting disorders, threatened abortion)

2. **H/P** =
   a. Uterine bleeding that does not follow usual menstrual cycle or occurs in postmenopausal women
   b. Menses with **<21-day** or **>35-day intervals, lasting >7 days,** or **blood loss >80 mL** are considered abnormal

3. **Labs** =
   a. β-hCG used to rule out pregnancy
   b. CBC, coagulation studies, TSH, FSH, and LH are used to rule out anemia, coagulopathy, and endocrine abnormalities
   c. Pap smear and endometrial biopsy (possibly obtained during dilation and curettage) used to rule out cancer

4. **Radiology** = US may detect uterine lesions; hysteroscopy frequently indicated to visualize lesions and perform dilation and curettage (D&C)

5. **Treatment** =
   a. Treat underlying disorder
   b. OCPs may be used for cycle irregularity
   c. Endometrial ablation may be performed for severe or recurrent bleeding

F. **Polycystic ovary syndrome** (PCOS)

1. Hypothalamic-pituitary disease with LH and androgen overproduction leading to **amenorrhea, infertility,** and **virilization**

2. **Excess LH secretion** induces overproduction of androgens by ovaries

3. Some cases of PCOS may have hyperinsulinemia, which induces androgen production and increases risk of insulin resistance

Endometriosis is the **most common** cause of **female infertility** and may be responsible for up to 50% of cases.

GYNECOLOGIC AND BREAST DISORDERS

4. **Excess androgens** produced by ovaries and adrenals are converted to estrogen, which induces further ovarian androgen production
5. Amenorrhea and infertility due to abnormal LH levels and FSH inhibition by high estrogen level; virilization due to increased androgens
6. **H/P** =
   a. **Obesity** (frequently initial sign)
   b. **Hirsutism**—excess growth of facial, chest, and abdominal hair
   c. **Virilization**—balding, increased muscle mass, voice deepening, clitoral enlargement
   d. Amenorrhea or oligomenorrhea (infrequent menses)
   e. **Infertility**
   f. Bilateral ovarian enlargement on bimanual exam
7. **Labs** = increased LH, **LH:FSH ratio >3,** increased dehydroepiandrosterone (DHEA), increased androstendione; positive progestin challenge
8. **Radiology** = US shows **enlarged ovaries** with **multiple cysts**
9. **Treatment** =
   a. Clomiphene (anti-estrogen) induces follicle stimulation and maturation to allow pregnancy
   b. OCPs or progestins may be used to regulate menstrual cycles and decrease endometrial cancer risk
10. **Complications** = infertility; increased risk for diabetes mellitus (DM), hypertension, ischemic heart disease, ovarian torsion, and endometrial cancer

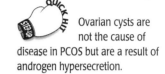

Patients with **PCOS** are at an increased risk for **endometrial cancer** secondary to chronically **high estrogen** levels.

Ovarian cysts are not the cause of disease in PCOS but are a result of androgen hypersecretion.

IV. Common gynecologic infections

A. **Vaginitis**
   1. Vaginal infection due to overgrowth of normal bacteria (*Gardnerella vaginalis*), protozoans (*Trichomonas*), or fungus (*Candida albicans*)
   2. **Risk factors** = OCP use, recent antibiotic use, pregnancy, DM, HIV, unprotected sex
   3. **H/P** = vaginal **irritation** or **pruritus,** vaginal discharge; exam detects vaginal inflammation with characteristic findings depending on cause (see Table 11-5 and Figure 11-4)

TABLE 11-5 Common Infectious Causes of Vaginitis

Characteristics	Gardnerella vaginalis	Trichomonas	Candida albicans
Physical exam	Mild vaginal inflammation	Vaginal and cervical inflammation, **cervical petechiae**	Significant vaginal inflammation
Discharge	Thin, white, fishy odor	Malodorous, frothy, **greenish**	Thick, white, **"cottage cheese-like"**
Wet mount (saline)	**Clue cells** (epithelial cells with multiple attached bacteria)	**Motile trichomonads**	Normal
Wet mount (KOH)	Fishy odor (positive whiff test)	Possible fishy odor	**Pseudohyphae**
Vaginal pH	>4.5	>4.5	**3.5–4.5**
Treatment	Metronidazole	Metronidazole (also **treat partner**)	Topical clotrimazole, miconazole, or nystatin, or oral fluconazole (single dose)

FIGURE 11-4 Vaginal Gram stain showing a true clue cell and abnormal bacteria characteristic of bacterial vaginosis.

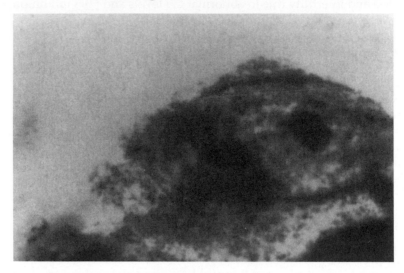

(Used with permission from Sweet RL, Gibbs RS. *Infectious Diseases of the Female Genital Tract.* 4th Ed. Philadelphia: Lippincott Williams & Wilkins, 2002.)

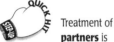

Lactobacilli are a common normal bacteria whose presence on a wet mount does **not** suggest infection.

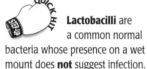

Treatment of **partners** is **unnecessary** for **G. vaginalis** or **C. albicans** but is **required** with **Trichomonas** infection (metronidazole).

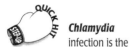

Chlamydia infection is the **most common STD** because it may be **asymptomatic** (especially in men) and frequently goes unrecognized.

N. gonorrhoeae is the most common cause of **septic arthritis** in young adults.

4. **Labs = wet mount** (smear of vaginal fluid examined under microscope) with saline or potassium hydroxide (KOH) and **vaginal pH** testing useful to distinguish cause
5. **Treatment** = antibiotics or antifungals, depending upon agent

B. **Toxic shock syndrome**
1. Severe systemic reaction to *Staphylococcus aureus* endotoxin associated with **prolonged tampon use,** prolonged intravaginal contraception use, or postpartum/postabortion infection
2. **H/P** = vomiting, diarrhea, sore throat, headache; high fever, generalized rash; severe cases develop **hypotension,** shock, respiratory distress, and **desquamation of palms and soles**
3. **Labs** = vaginal fluid culture shows *S. aureus*
4. **Treatment** =
    a. Remove tampon or other intravaginal objects
    b. Penicillinase-resistant β-lactam antibiotics and IV hydration
    c. Pressors may be needed for significant hypotension

V. **Sexually transmitted diseases (STDs)**
A. **Cervicitis**
1. Infection of cervical columnar epithelium due to *Neisseria gonorrhoeae* or *Chlamydia trachomatis*
2. Urethra, oral cavity, or rectal area may also become infected through sexual contact
3. **H/P** =
    a. Possibly asymptomatic (more likely in chlamydial infection)
    b. Dyspareunia, bleeding after intercourse, **purulent vaginal discharge** (milder for *Chlamydia*)
    c. **Urethritis** associated with purulent discharge and dysuria
    d. Rectal and pharyngeal infection are frequently asymptomatic
    e. Exam detects inflammation of cervix with associated discharge
4. **Labs** =
    a. Gram stain of cervical scraping shows gram-negative diplococci with *N. gonorrhoeae* (usually nothing seen with *Chlamydia* infection)

b. Culture on Thayer-Martin agar detects *N. gonorrhoeae*

c. **Immunoassays** useful for detecting both pathogens

5. **Treatment** = ceftriaxone for *N. gonorrhoeae*, doxycycline for *Chlamydia*; both antibiotics often given together because of **frequent dual infection;** sexual partners should be treated to reduce risk of re-infection

6. **Complication** = PID, septic arthritis

B. **Pelvic inflammatory disease** (PID)

1. Progressive *N. gonorrhoeae* or *Chlamydia* infection resulting in involvement of ovaries, uterus, fallopian tubes, or peritoneal cavity

2. Less frequently due to *Bacteroides, Escherichia coli,* or streptococci

3. **Risk factors** = multiple sexual partners, unprotected intercourse, prior PID, intrauterine device (IUD) use, douching, young age at first intercourse

4. **H/P** = lower abdominal pain starting within days of menses, nausea, vomiting, dysuria; purulent cervical discharge, abdominal tenderness, fever, **cervical motion tenderness,** adnexal tenderness, possible abdominal guarding

5. **Labs** =

   a. Increased white blood cell count, increased erythrocyte sedimentation rate (ESR)

   b. Gram stain, culture, immunoassays useful for identifying agent

   c. **Culdocentesis** (aspiration of intraperitoneal fluid from cul de sac posterior to uterus) yields pus

6. **Radiology** = US may detect inflamed and enlarged uterus, abscess of fallopian tubes or ovaries, or free fluid (technique utilized for diagnosis less now than in the past); laparoscopy may visualize inflamed tissue

7. **Treatment** = empiric antibiotics until specific agent identified (doxycycline, ceftriaxone, cefoxitin); treat as inpatient if high fevers or young age; treat sexual partners

8. **Complications** = **infertility** due to adhesion formation, chronic pelvic pain, **tubo-ovarian abscess, increased risk of ectopic pregnancy**

C. **Syphilis**

1. Disease caused by the spirochete *Treponema pallidum*

2. **H/P** = varies according to stage of disease

   a. **Primary**

      (1) 1 to 8 wks after exposure

      (2) Solitary **chancre** (firm papule that evolves into **painless ulcer)** forms near area of contact and heals spontaneously within 9 weeks

   b. **Secondary**

      (1) Begins as chancre heals and may last up to 12 weeks

      (2) Headache, malaise; fever, **maculopapular rash** on palms and soles, lymphadenopathy, papules in moist areas of body (condyloma lata)

      (3) Symptoms and lesions resolve spontaneously

   c. **Latent**

      (1) Asymptomatic

      (2) May last years

   d. **Tertiary**

      (1) 1/3 of patients progress beyond latent stage

      (2) Granulomatous lesions (**gummas**) of skin, bone, and liver

      (3) Loss of 2-point discrimination and proprioception secondary to dorsal column degeneration (**tabes dorsalis**), Argyll-Robertson pupils

3. **Labs** =

   a. VDRL and rapid plasma regain (RPR) are 80% sensitive screening tests

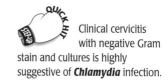
Clinical cervicitis with negative Gram stain and cultures is highly suggestive of **Chlamydia** infection.

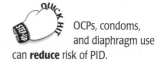
OCPs, condoms, and diaphragm use can **reduce** risk of PID.

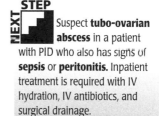
Suspect **tubo-ovarian abscess** in a patient with PID who also has signs of **sepsis** or **peritonitis.** Inpatient treatment is required with IV hydration, IV antibiotics, and surgical drainage.

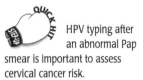

    b. Fluorescent treponemal antibody absorption (FTA-ABS) or microhemagglutination assay for antibodies to treponemes (MHA-TP) used to confirm diagnosis

    c. Spirochetes may be seen with dark-field microscopy

  4. **Treatment** = penicillin, doxycycline, or tetracycline; IV penicillin used in severe tertiary cases

  5. **Complications** = gummatous destruction of skin, bones, and liver; cardiovascular syphilis (aortic regurgitation, aortitis); neurosyphilis (cerebral atrophy, tabes dorsalis, meningitis)

D. **Genital herpes**—Disease caused by herpes simplex virus type 2 (most cases) or type 1 (less common) (see Chapter 10, Dermatology)

E. **Molluscum contagiosum** (see Chapter 10, Dermatology)

F. **Human papillomavirus** (HPV)

  1. Several types of papillomavirus that may be associated with **genital warts** (types 6 and 11) or **cervical cancer** (types 16, 18, 31, and 33)

  2. **H/P** = frequent small pink papules at site of contact; infection due to HPV types 6 or 11 may cause larger cauliflower-like warts on genital region

  3. **Labs** =

    a. An abnormal Pap smear should prompt HPV testing and colposcopy to look for lesions

    b. Biopsy of lesions may be used to confirm infection and determine virus type through HPV DNA analysis

  4. **Treatment** = cryotherapy, podophyllin, or laser therapy; **loop electrocautery excision procedure (LEEP);** cone biopsy allows a full biopsy and is curative for excised specimens with clear borders

  5. **Complications** = vaginal scarring for removal of large lesions, possible **increased risk** of **cervical cancer**

G. **Chancroid**

  1. Highly contagious disease caused by *Haemophilus ducreyi* seen most commonly in tropical or subtropical regions or in immunocompromised patients

  2. **H/P** = within 2 weeks of contact small papule forms in area of contact and transforms into **painful ulcer** with grayish base and foul odor; possible inguinal lymphadenopathy that may cause **significant inguinal swelling** (bubo formation)

  3. **Labs** = Gram stain of tissue at ulcer edge shows gram-positive rods

  4. **Treatment** = ceftriaxone, erythromycin, or azithromycin

H. **Lymphogranuloma venereum**

  1. Disease caused by L-1, L-2, or L-3 serotypes of *C. trachomatis* (differentiated from cervicitis); more common in developing nations

  2. **H/P** =

    a. Within 4 weeks of contact, malaise, headache, fever, and formation of papule at site of contact that becomes **painless ulcer**

    b. After 1 month **significant inguinal bubos** develop (more common in men than in women)

    c. May progress to bubo ulceration, elephantiasis (severe connective tissue swelling secondary to lymph vessel obstruction), fistula formation, and abscess formation

  3. **Labs** = immunoassays for *Chlamydia* may be helpful for diagnosis

  4. **Treatment** = tetracycline, erythromycin, or doxycycline

I. **Granuloma inguinale**

  1. Disease due to infection by *Donovania granulomatis*

  2. **H/P** =

    a. Papule on external genitalia forms several weeks after contact and rapidly becomes **painless ulcer** with **beefy red base** and **irregular borders**

    b. Mild lymphadenopathy may occur

c. Infection of ulcers may lead to significant scarring, vaginal stenosis, or elephantiasis

3. **Labs** = lesion biopsy on Giemsa stain shows **Donovan bodies** (red encapsulated intracellular bacteria)

4. **Treatment** = tetracycline for 3 weeks

VI. Gynecologic neoplasms

A. **Uterine fibroids** (uterine leiomyoma)

1. **Benign** uterine masses composed of smooth muscle; may vary in size with menstrual cycle and generally regress after menopause

2. **H/P** = possibly asymptomatic; possible heavy menses, abdominal pain, urinary frequency, or infertility; palpable mass on exam

3. **Radiology** = US or hysteroscopy used to locate or visualize mass

4. **Treatment** =
   a. Follow with US to detect **abnormal growth**
   b. Surgical resection indicated for highly symptomatic fibroids
   c. **Uterine artery embolization** following a pelvic MRI to rule out other soft tissue pathology may be performed to selectively infarct fibroids
   d. **Hysterectomy** may be performed for symptomatic fibroids in patients for whom fertility is not a concern

B. **Endometrial cancer**

1. Adenocarcinoma of uterine tissue related to **exposure to high estrogen levels;** most common in postmenopausal women

2. **Risk factors** = unopposed exogenous estrogen, PCOS, obesity, nulliparity, DM, hypertension, family history

3. **H/P** = heavy menses, mid-cycle bleeding, or **postmenopausal bleeding** with possible abdominal pain; ovaries or uterus may feel fixed in position if tumor has local extension

4. **Labs** = **increased CA-125** tumor marker (not specific for endometrial cancer and not always increased); endometrial biopsy shows hyperplastic abnormal glands with vascular invasion

5. **Radiology** = chest x-ray (CXR) and CT may be used to detect metastases

6. **Treatment** =
   a. Total abdominal hysterectomy, frequently with bilateral salpingo-oophorectomy (TAH/BSO) and radiation
   b. Hormone therapy (progesterone, tamoxifen) for tumors not cured by surgery and radiation
   c. Chemotherapy for advanced cases

7. **Complications** =
   a. Local extension to fallopian tubes, ovaries, and cervix
   b. Metastases to peritoneum, aortic and pelvic lymph nodes, lungs, and vagina
   c. 89% five-year survival rate with early detection; 17% five-year survival rate with metastases

C. **Cervical cancer**

1. Squamous cell cancer (85% cases) or adenocarcinoma (15% cases) of the cervix that results from progression of **cervical dysplasia**

2. **Risk factors** = early first intercourse, tobacco, **HPV** (types 16, 18, 31, or 33), multiple sexual partners

3. Cervical dysplasia
   a. Precancerous lesions of the cervix that progress to cervical cancer in 15% of cases
   b. Usually detected by Pap smear (abnormal cells seen on cytology)
   c. Graded by cell quality and depth of involvement on cone biopsy, best to worst:
      (1) Atypical squamous cells of undetermined significance (ASCUS)

Uterine fibroids do **not** continue to grow after menopause (because of estrogen sensitivity and decreased postmenopausal estrogen levels).

STEP
NEXT While **atrophic vaginitis** and **uterine fibroids** are the **most common causes** of vaginal **bleeding** in postmenopausal women, endometrial cancer must be ruled out for any postmenopausal woman presenting with this complaint (perform **endometrial biopsy**).

All women should receive **annual Pap smears** beginning approximately 3 years after the onset of vaginal intercourse or no later than 21 years of age. In those who have never engaged in intercourse, Pap smears may be deferred because of the low risk of cervical cancer related to HPV.

(2) Low-grade squamous intraepithelial lesion

(3) High-grade squamous intraepithelial lesion

(4) Carcinoma in situ

(5) Carcinoma

d. Followed with Pap smear every 3 to 6 months

e. Higher grade lesions treated with electrocautery, laser ablation, or cryosurgery

4. **H/P** = usually asymptomatic; possible postcoital bleeding, pelvic pain, or cervical discharge; cervical mass may be palpated

5. **Labs** = detected by **Pap smear**; punch biopsy of visible lesions; cone biopsy determines invasion

6. **Treatment** =

a. Carcinoma in situ treated with electrocautery (LEEP or conization), laser ablation, or cryotherapy

b. Cone biopsy may be curative if clear margins

c. Early stages of invasive cancer treated with hysterectomy

d. Radiation used in advanced cases

e. HPV vaccines are in development to reduce the risk of cancer

D. **Benign ovarian tumors**

1. Benign ovarian lesions with either functional ovarian cell, epithelial cell, or germ cell origin

2. **H/P** =

a. Frequently asymptomatic

TABLE 11-6	Common Types of Benign Ovarian Masses			
Tumor	**Origin**	**Characteristics**	**H/P**	**Treatment**
Follicular cyst	Ovarian follicle	**Granulosa** cells, cystic (<8 cm diameter), **may regress** over menstrual period	Abdominal pain and fullness; palpable tender mass on bimanual exam Peritoneal signs if torsion or rupture occur	**Observation;** ovarian cystectomy if mass does not regress or for increased suspicion of cancer
Lutein cyst	Corpus luteum	**Theca** cells, cystic or hemorrhagic corpus luteum, usually larger and firmer than follicular cyst, **may regress** over menstrual period	Abdominal pain; palpable tender mass on bimanual exam Greater risk of torsion or rupture than follicular cyst	**Observation;** ovarian cystectomy if mass does not regress or for increased suspicion of cancer
Mucinous or serous cystadenoma	Epithelial tissue	May resemble endometrial or tubal histology, cystic with serous or mucinous contents, may form calcifications **(psammoma bodies), may become extremely large**	Frequently asymptomatic until significant growth has occurred Palpable mass on bimanual exam that may be palpable during abdominal exam if large	Unilateral salpingo-oophorectomy; TAH/BSO if postmenopausal
Stromal cell tumor	Granulosa, theca, or Sertoli-Leydig cells	Secrete hormones appropriate to cells of origin, malignant potential	**Precocious puberty** (granulosa-theca cell tumors) or **virilization** (Sertoli-Leydig cell tumors)	Unilateral salpingo-oophorectomy; TAH/BSO if postmenopausal
Benign cystic teratoma	Germ cells	Composed of **multiple dermal tissues** including hair, teeth, and sebaceous glands	Frequently asymptomatic Oily contents may cause peritoneal irritation	Unilateral salpingo-oophorectomy; bilateral if abnormal ovarian development

TAH/BSO, total abdominal hysterectomy with bilateral salpingo-oophorectomy.

    b. Lower abdominal pain (more common with functional tumors or tumor torsion), nausea, vomiting, abdominal fullness (only after significant growth)

    c. Palpable ovarian mass on bimanual exam, possible abdominal tenderness

    d. In cases of ruptured mass patient may have guarding, rebound tenderness, and abdominal rigidity

3. **Labs = normal CA-125**; biopsy of tumor used to determine benign or malignant nature

4. **Radiology = US** used to evaluate type of mass (cystic or solid) and quality of mass (irregular, multiple septa, smooth edges)

5. **Treatment** = surgical excision ranging from ovarian cystectomy to TAH/BSO depending on tumor type and extent of involvement

6. **Complications** = tumor torsion, tumor rupture with hemorrhage

E. **Ovarian cancer**

1. Cancer of ovaries that may have one of several histologic forms; most cases are only diagnosed after considerable growth

2. **Risk factors = family history,** infertility, nulliparity, **BRCA1** or **BRCA2** gene mutations

3. **H/P =**

    a. Usually **asymptomatic until late in disease course**

    b. Abdominal pain, fatigue, weight loss, change in bowel habits; ascites, mass may be palpated on bimanual exam

4. **Labs = increased CA-125** (80% of cases); biopsy following laparoscopy or laporotomy shows lesions which may resemble epithelial, germ, granulosa, or theca cells

5. **Radiology** = US, CT, or MRI used to detect mass and extent of involvement

6. **Treatment =**

    a. TAH/BSO, chemotherapy

    b. Germ cell tumors treated with radiation

    c. Single oophorectomy may be performed for tumors detected early in patients wanting to maintain fertility

7. **Complications = poor prognosis**; usually in advanced stages by time of detection

VII. Disorders of the breast

A. **Fibrocystic changes**

1. Common **benign** masses found in women of childbearing age that change in size with menstrual cycle

2. **H/P** = multiple bilateral small tender breast masses, possible mild breast pain preceding menses; breast exam detects **mobile** masses that **vary in size during menstrual cycle**

3. **Labs** = biopsy (performed when atypical lesions suspected) shows epithelial hyperplasia

4. **Radiology** = mammograms (yearly imaging starting by age 40) should be used to identify and follow lesions; US useful for detecting cystic lesions

5. **Treatment** = caffeine reduction, OCPs, progesterone, or tamoxifen may improve symptoms in confirmed benign lesions

B. **Breast abscess**

1. Local infection of breast tissue due to *S. aureus* or streptococcus (superficial infections) or anaerobic bacteria (subareolar infections)

2. Most are related to **breast feeding**

3. **H/P** = painful mass in breast; palpable red breast mass, breast tenderness

4. **Labs** = fine needle aspiration (FNA) of abscess confirms infection

● US findings of cystic mass, smooth lesion edges, and few septa are more consistent with **benign** ovarian tumors.
● Findings of irregularity, nodularity, multiple septa, and pelvic extension are more suggestive of **malignancy.**

Monthly **self-breast examinations** after each menstrual period are the best way to distinguish **developing lesions** from **monthly variations** in breast tissue make-up, but have not been shown to decrease mortality.

Suspicious lesions on mammogram are those with **hyperdense regions** or **calcifications.**

5. **Treatment** = agent-appropriate oral or IV antibiotics; incision and drainage of fluctuant masses; continue breast feeding
6. **Complications** = fistula formation with recurrent abscesses

C. **Fibroadenoma**
1. Most common **benign** breast tumor; more common in **women <30 years old**
2. **H/P** = **solitary,** solid, and **mobile** mass with **well-defined edges**
3. **Labs** = biopsy (FNA or open) confirms benign nature
4. **Treatment** = surgical excision
5. **Complications** = recurrence is common

D. **Intraductal papilloma**
1. Benign lesions of ductal tissue that may carry malignant potential
2. **H/P** = bloody discharge from nipple upon stimulation
3. **Labs** = excisional biopsy used to rule out cancer; ductal lavage by microcatheter may be used to test for abnormal intraductal cells and is more accurate than examination of aspirated nipple fluid
4. **Treatment** = surgical excision

E. **Breast cancer**
1. Malignant neoplasms of the breast arising from either ductal (90% of cases, more aggressive) or lobular (10% of cases, less aggressive, more difficult to detect) tissue
2. **Risk factors** = family history (first-degree relative), ovarian cancer, endometrial cancer, prior breast cancer, increased estrogen exposure, early menarche, late menopause, nulliparity, late first pregnancy (>35 years old), BRCA1 or BRCA2 gene mutations
3. **H/P** =
   a. Possibly asymptomatic and undetected
   b. Painless breast lump, possible nipple discharge
   c. Palpable **solid** and **immobile** breast lump (when of sufficient size), peau d'orange (lymphatic obstruction causing lymphedema and skin thickening that makes breast look like an orange peel), possible nipple retraction
   d. Axillary lymphadenopathy in progressive cases

Nonbloody nipple discharge is consistent with a **noncancerous** pathology and frequently does **not** require excision.

Hormone replacement therapy has been linked to an **increased** incidence of breast cancer due to exogenous estrogen administration.

The **upper outer quadrant** is the most common site of breast cancer.

GYNECOLOGIC AND BREAST DISORDERS

FIGURE 11-5 Approach to the patient with a breast mass. FNA, fine needle aspiration.

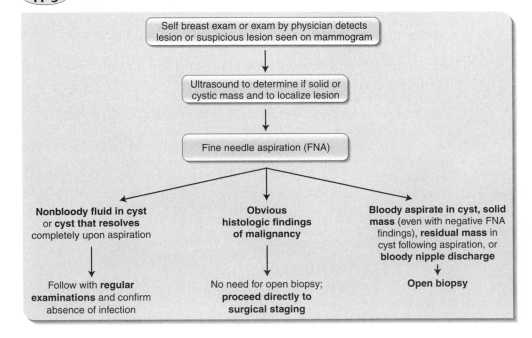

Self breast exam or exam by physician detects lesion or suspicious lesion seen on mammogram

↓

Ultrasound to determine if solid or cystic mass and to localize lesion

↓

Fine needle aspiration (FNA)

Nonbloody fluid in cyst or **cyst that resolves** completely upon aspiration

↓

Follow with **regular examinations** and confirm absence of infection

Obvious histologic findings of malignancy

↓

No need for open biopsy; **proceed directly to surgical staging**

Bloody aspirate in cyst, solid mass (even with negative FNA findings), **residual mass** in cyst following aspiration, or **bloody nipple discharge**

↓

Open biopsy

4. **Labs** =
   a. Biopsy confirms malignancy
   b. Testing for estrogen and progesterone receptors in tumor helps guide treatment
   c. Sentinel node biopsy helps determine extent of spread
5. **Radiology** = mammography is principal screening method; US may be used to differentiate cystic from solid lesions; CXR, bone scan, and CT may be used to identify metastases
6. **Treatment** =
   a. Carcinoma in situ or localized tumors treated with lumpectomy (partial mastectomy), axillary node dissection, and radiation
   b. More extensive tumors treated with radical mastectomy, lymph node dissection, and radiation
   c. Presence of positive nodes or metastases guides addition of chemotherapy
   d. Tumors with positive hormone receptors may be treated with tamoxifen
   e. Recurrent disease treated with chemotherapy
7. **Complications** =
   a. Tumors not responding to surgery and radiation will unlikely result in cure
   b. Metastases to bone, thoracic cavity, brain, and liver
   c. Tumors with positive hormone receptors and those seen in older patients carry better prognosis

FNA of a solid breast mass carries a **20%** chance of a **false negative**, so any negative FNA of a solid breast mass requires **open biopsy.**

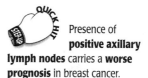
Presence of **positive axillary lymph nodes** carries a **worse prognosis** in breast cancer.

GYNECOLOGIC AND BREAST DISORDERS

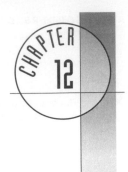

Obstetrics

QUICK HIT

Teratogens will either **kill** the fetus or will have **no effect** within the **initial 2 weeks** of gestation. They may cause **abnormal organ formation** between **2–12 weeks.**

QUICK HIT

Women at risk for poor nutrition during pregnancy include those who are teenagers, have a lower socioeconomic status, are underweight, or who smoke, are alcoholics, or drug abusers.

QUICK HIT

Daily caloric intake during pregnancy should be ~**2500** kcal.

QUICK HIT

Low-risk activity during pregnancy:

- **Exercise** is **encouraged** during pregnancy to improve maternal feelings of well-being, improve symptoms due to positional effects of the fetus, and to promote healthy blood sugar levels.
- Work and travel may be continued throughout pregnancy as long as fatigue and excessive stress are avoided (airline travel permitted up to 36 weeks' gestation).
- Sexual intercourse may be continued during pregnancy unless mother is considered high risk for spontaneous abortion, premature labor, or placenta previa.

I. Normal pregnancy physiology

A. Embryonic and fetal development begins with fertilization and takes approximately 38 weeks until fetal maturity occurs (see Figure 12-1)

B. Normal changes in maternal physiology during pregnancy
   1. Several physiologic changes occur in the mother in response to the maintenance of fetal viability (see Table 12-1)
   2. Normal changes in maternal physiology affect every organ system

II. Prenatal care

A. **Nutrition**
   1. Maternal nutritional demands alter during pregnancy in order to support both the mother and the developing fetus
   2. Some are specifically required to **reduce the risk of birth defects** (e.g., folate, iron) (see Table 12-2)
   3. Ideal weight gain
      a. 28–40 lbs. in women with a body mass index (BMI) <19.8
      b. 15–25 lbs. for BMI >26
      c. 25–35 lbs. for BMI 19.8–26 (~2 lbs in 1st trimester, 0.75–1 lb/week in 2nd and 3rd trimesters)

B. **Prenatal visits**
   1. **Good prenatal care** is vital to healthy fetal development; its goals are to prevent or manage conditions that may be harmful to the mother or fetus
   2. Maternal weight (to monitor weight gain), urinalysis (to detect urinary tract infection [UTI] and gestational diabetes mellitus [DM]), blood pressure, fundal height (to estimate fetal growth), and fetal heart sounds (confirms fetal viability) are evaluated at each visit
   3. Initial visit includes detailed history, physical and **risk assessment**
   4. Labs and ultrasound (US) are performed at certain time points during gestation to detect infection and fetal abnormalities (see Table 12-3)
   5. **Leopold maneuvers** (external abdominal examination) may be performed in 3rd trimester to determine fetal presentation
   6. Specialized tests are performed in women with increased risk for congenital abnormalities (>**35 years old,** history of spontaneous abortion, teratogen exposure, DM, history of fetal demise) (see Table 12-4)

III. Medical complications of pregnancy

A. **Gestational diabetes mellitus (DM)**
   1. **New onset** glucose intolerance that begins during pregnancy
   2. **Risk factors** = family history of DM, >25 years old, obesity, prior polyhydramnios, recurrent abortions, prior stillbirth, prior macrosomia, hypertension (HTN), African or Pacific Islander heritage

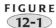

FIGURE
12-1 Timeline of fetal development during gestation.

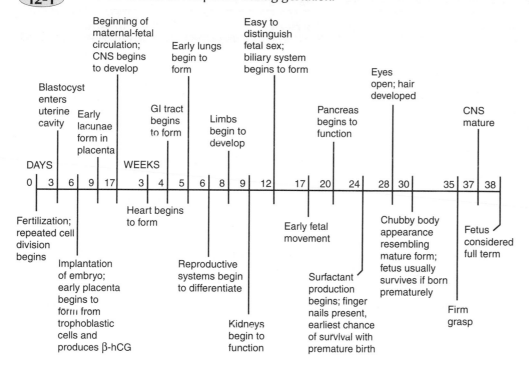

TABLE 12-1	**Normal Changes in Maternal Physiology during Pregnancy**
Anatomy/System	**Changes**
Cardiovascular	• Cardiac output increases 40% with associated increases in SV (10–30%) and HR (12–18 bpm) • Systolic murmur may be heard due to increased cardiac output • Myocardial O_2 demand increases • Systolic and diastolic blood pressures decrease slightly • Uterus displaces heart slightly superiorly
Respiratory	• Uterus displaces diaphragm superiorly and causes **decrease** of residual volume, **functional residual capacity,** and expiratory reserve volume • Total body O_2 consumption increases 20% • Tidal volume increases 40% with associated increase in minute ventilation due to stimulation by progesterone • P_{CO_2} decreases to ~30 mm Hg; dyspnea is frequent complaint despite increased minute ventilation and normal rate
Renal	• Renal plasma flow and glomerlular filtration rate increase 40% • Decrease in BUN and creatinine • Increased renal loss of bicarbonate to compensate for respiratory alkalosis • Blood and interstitial fluid volumes increase
Endocrine	• Non-diabetic hyperinsulinemia with associated mild glucose intolerance • Production of human placental lactogen contributes to glucose intolerance by interfering with insulin activity • Fasting triglycerides increase • Cortisol increases
Hematologic	• Increased RBC production • Hematocrit decreases due to increased blood volume • Hypercoagulable state
BUN, blood urea nitrogen; HR, heart rate; RBC, red blood cell; SV, stroke volume.	

TABLE 12-2 | **Important Increased Nutritional Demands during Pregnancy**

Substance	Increased Need	Reason for Need	Effects of Insufficiency
Calcium	1200 mg/day (50% increase)	Lactation reserves Increased utilization by fetus	Impaired maternal bone mineralization Hypertension Premature birth, low birth weight
Fluids	Adequate hydration important	Increased total maternal-fetal fluid volume	Relative dehydration
Folate	0.8–1 mg/day (should be started 4 wks before attempted conception)	Normal fetal neural tube development	Neural tube defects
Iron	30 mg/day (100% increase)	RBC production	Maternal anemia Premature birth, low birth weight, Maternal cardiac complications
Protein	60 g/day (30% increase)	Additional needs of maternal, fetal, and placental tissue	Impaired fetal and placental growth

RBC, red blood cell.

TABLE 12-3 | **Common Screening Tests Performed during Pregnancy**

Length of Gestation	Labs or Study Performed
Initial visit	CBC Blood antibody and Rh typing Pap smear Gonorrhea/chlamydia screening Urinalysis RPR or VDRL Rubella antibody titer PPD (selected populations) Hepatitis B surface antigen HIV screening (with maternal consent) Cystic fibrosis screening (selected populations)
16–18 wks	Quadruple screen[a] (maternal serum α-fetoprotein, hCG, unconjugated estradiol, maternal serum inhibin A) to look for trisomies 21 and 18 and neural tube defects
18–20 wks	US dating of pregnancy and assessment for gross fetal abnormalities
24–28 wks	1-hr glucose challenge to screen for gestational DM
32–36 wks	Cervical culture for *Neisseria gonorrhoeae* and *Chlamydia trachomatis* (selected populations) Group B streptococcus screening

[a] See Table 12-4 for description of quadruple screen.
CBC, complete blood count; DM, diabetes mellitus; hCG, human chorionic gonadotropin; PPD, purified protein derivative of tuberculin; Rh, rhesus factor; RPR, rapid plasma reagin; VDRL, Venereal Disease Research Laboratories.

TABLE 12-4 Prenatal Assessment in High-Risk Pregnancies

Test	Description	Indications
Quadruple screen	Maternal serum α-fetoprotein, estradiol, hCG, and maternal serum inhibin A levels measured to assess risk for neural tube defects and trisomies 18 and 21	• Performed in all pregnant women between 16–18 wks' gestation • Frequently initial marker for fetal complications
Amniocentesis	Transabdominal needle aspiration of amniotic fluid from amniotic sac after 16 wks' gestation to measure amniotic α-fetoprotein and determine karyotype (detects neural tube defects and chromosome disorders with greater sensitivity than triple screen alone)	• Abnormal quadruple screen, women >35 yr old, risk of Rh sensitization • Carries 1% risk of spontaneous abortion
Chorionic villi sampling	Transabdominal or transcervical aspiration of chorionic villus tissue between 9–12 wks' gestation to detect chromosomal abnormalities	• Early detection of chromosomal abnormalities in higher-risk patients (advanced age, history of children with genetic defects)
Percutaneous umbilical blood sampling	Blood collection from umbilical vein between 10–22 wks' gestation to identify chromosomal defects, fetal infection, Rh sensitization	• Late detection of genetic disorders, pregnancies with high risk for Rh sensitization
Lung maturity studies	Measurement of amniotic lecithin and sphingomyelin (collected by amniocentesis) to determine fetal lung maturity	• Imminent premature birth, need for premature delivery

hCG, human chorionic gonadotropin; Rh, rhesus factor.

3. **H/P** = usually asymptomatic
4. **Labs** = fasting glucose >105 mg/dL or **abnormal glucose tolerance test** performed at 24–28 weeks' gestation
5. **Treatment** =
   a. Strict glucose control through **diet** and **exercise**
   b. Glyburide or insulin may be used if indicated
   c. Periodic fetal US and nonstress tests (discussed later) performed to assess fetal well-being
   d. Cesarean section may be indicated for macrosomic babies
6. **Complications** =
   a. Maternal—hypoglycemia (secondary to therapy, may also occur after delivery), hypocalcemia, maternal polyhydramnios, preeclampsia, renal insufficiency, diabetic ketoacidosis, hyperosmolar hyperglycemic nonketotic coma, retinopathy
   b. Fetal—fetal macrosomia (baby of abnormally large size), intrauterine growth restriction (IUGR), neural tube defects, cardiac defects, intrauterine fetal demise
   c. Perinatal/postnatal—traumatic delivery, delayed neurologic maturity, fetal respiratory distress syndrome
B. **Pregestational diabetes mellitus (DM)**
   1. DM that exists **prior** to pregnancy; patient may or may not be aware of disease
   2. **H/P** = consistent with typical presentation of DM (see Chapter 5, Endocrine Disorders)
   3. **Labs** = increased serum glucose (prior to and during pregnancy), increased hemoglobin A_{1c} with poor control

 Maternal serum α-fetoprotein levels:
- This screening test is **only valid** if performed during the correct gestational window (**16–18 weeks' gestation**).
- **High** levels are associated with an increased risk of **neural tube defects** or multiple gestation.
- **Low** levels are associated with increased risk of **trisomies 21 and 18**.

 In **trisomy 18 all** quadruple-screen markers are **low** except inhibin A. In **trisomy 21** maternal serum α-fetoprotein and unconjugated estradiol are low, while **hCG** and **inhibin A** are **high**.

 Gestational DM occurs in ~1% of pregnancies.

 Gestational DM occurs most frequently in the **3rd trimester.** If mother presents with signs of DM earlier in pregnancy, suspect nongestational (type I or II) DM.

FIGURE
12-2 Screening for gestational diabetes mellitus performed at 24 to 28 weeks' gestation. GI, gastrointestinal.

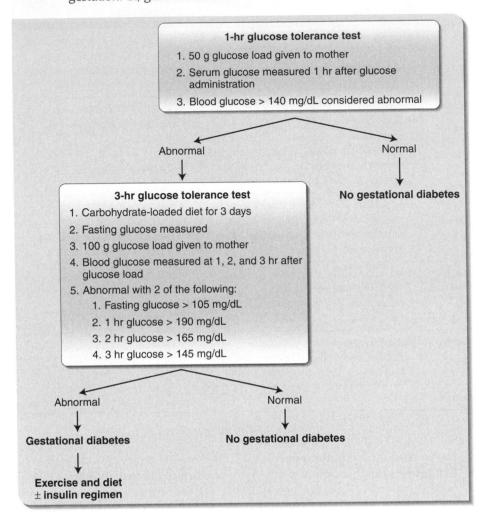

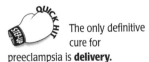

NEXT STEP Continue glucose assessment after birth because maternal glucose needs will change suddenly for patients with gestational DM and because the mother has a low risk of remaining diabetic after pregnancy.

The only definitive cure for preeclampsia is **delivery.**

4. **Treatment =**
   a. Try to control glucose with diet and exercise
   b. Insulin used for glucose control in type I and type II DM not adequately controlled with lifestyle modification
   c. US and echocardiogram (especially 3rd trimester) used to identify cardiac, neurologic, and growth abnormalities
   d. Early delivery after fetal lung assessment and corticosteroid administration recommended for poor glucose control or maternal complications

C. **Preeclampsia**
   1. Pregnancy-induced **HTN** with **proteinuria** and **edema** that develops after 20 weeks' gestation in 5% of pregnancies due to an unknown cause
   2. **Risk factors =** HTN, nulliparity, **prior history of preeclampsia,** <15 or >35 years old, multiple gestation (e.g., twins), vascular disease, African American ancestry
   3. **H/P =**
      a. Asymptomatic in mild cases
      b. **Edema** in **hands** and **face,** rapid weight gain, headache, epigastric abdominal pain, visual disturbances, hyperreflexia
      c. **Blood pressure >140/90** *or* **30 mmHg increase in systolic** *or* **15 mmHg increase in diastolic blood pressure** during pregnancy

4. **Labs** =
    a. Urinalysis shows 2+ proteinuria on dipstick or >4g protein/24 hours
    b. Complete blood count (CBC), electrolytes, blood urea nitrogen (BUN) and creatinine, liver function tests (LFTs), PT, PTT, and uric acid are useful to assess severity and rule out other pathology
    c. Fetal nonstress test and amniocentesis (less commonly) may be useful to assess fetal well-being

5. **Treatment** =
    a. If near term, **induce delivery**
    b. If mild and far from term, prescribe bed rest, frequent maternal examinations for worsening symptoms, daily protein assessment, and fetal nonstress tests
    c. If severe and far from term, closely monitor and maintain blood pressure <160/110 with diastolic blood pressure >90 using antihypertensive medications (hydralazine frequently used), give IV **MgSO$_4$ for seizure prophylaxis,** closely monitor maternal and fetal health, and induce delivery as soon as fetus is considered viable
    d. Continue antihypertensive medications and MgSO$_4$ for 24 hours postpartum and continue close observation for symptoms and lab abnormalities
    c. Mothers with preexistent HTN should continue their pregestational antihypertensive medications during pregnancy as long as they are not teratogenic (do not use β-blockers in the 1st trimesters, or angiotensin converting enzyme inhibitors [ACE-I] at any time during pregnancy)

6. **Complications** = eclampsia, seizures, stroke, IUGR, pulmonary edema, oligohydramnios; HELLP syndrome may also cause abruptio placenta, renal insufficiency, encephalopathy, and disseminated intravascular coagulation (DIC)

D. **Eclampsia**
1. Progression of preeclampsia leading to **maternal seizures** that may be severe and fatal if untreated
2. **H/P** = headaches, visual disturbances, and upper abdominal pain frequently precede onset of seizures
3. **Labs** = findings similar to preeclampsia
4. **Treatment** =
    a. Treatment is similar to that for preeclampsia with **delivery** being the definitive solution
    b. Use **MgSO$_4$** and **IV diazepam** to control seizures
    c. Stabilize patient with sufficient O$_2$ and blood pressure control
    d. Induce delivery as soon as mother stabilized
    e. **Continue** MgSO$_4$ and antihypertensive medications for **24 hours** following delivery because **25% of seizures** occur within 24 hours postpartum
5. **Complications** = significant risk of maternal and fetal death

E. **Maternal asthma** (preexisting)
1. Severe maternal asthma is associated with spontaneous abortion, intrauterine fetal demise, and IUGR
2. **H/P** = course of disease does not change during pregnancy from prior severity but exacerbations may be less tolerated by the mother due to normal physiologic changes of pregnancy
3. **Treatment** =
    a. **Activity limitation** and **avoidance of precipitating factors** is sufficient treatment in many cases
    b. Inhaled β-agonists may be used for mild exacerbations
    c. Inhaled cromolyn or corticosteroids may be added to regimen for poorly controlled asthma
    d. Oral corticosteroids are only used in severe cases, but are safe

QUICK HIT
Do not use **ACE-I** to stabilize blood pressure in pregnancy because of risk of **teratogenic** effects.

QUICK HIT
HELLP syndrome is a form of preeclampsia with poor fetal prognosis and 1% maternal mortality characterized by **H**emolysis, **E**levated **L**iver enzymes, and **L**ow **P**latelets.

NEXT STEP
Do not confuse **eclampsia** with **epilepsy.** Know the patient's history before making a diagnosis because induced delivery **will not** cure the **epileptic** patient.

QUICK HIT
Anticonvulsant use in pregnancy:
• **Phenobarbital** is the anticonvulsant of choice for treatment of **epilepsy** in early pregnancy because of lower risk of teratogenic effects.
• Clonazepam or carbamazepine may be used very carefully because of greater teratogenic risk.
• **Valproic acid** should **never** be used for epileptic seizure prophylaxis due to significant teratogenic risk.
• Diazepam may be used to break active seizures (80% effective).

4. **Complications** = increased risk of spontaneous abortion, intrauterine fetal death, and IUGR in untreated severe disease; oral corticosteroid use may be associated with IUGR and cleft palate (although unproven)

F. **Maternal nausea and vomiting**
1. Majority of pregnant women experience nausea and vomiting in the **1st trimester** of pregnancy (i.e., morning sickness); most cases improve by 2nd trimester
2. Most likely due to increases in chorionic gonadotropins or imbalance of progesterone and estrogen
3. **H/P** = nausea and vomiting that occurs frequently and may be daily; typically occurs in 1st trimester and improves after 12 weeks' gestation
4. **Treatment** = avoidance of large meals, elevating head in bed; antacids following meals may be helpful in worse cases

G. **Maternal deep venous thrombosis (DVT)**
1. Risk of DVT **increases** during pregnancy due to **venous stasis** and relative **increase** in **circulating clotting** factors
2. **H/P** = similar presentation to that in nonpregnant patients (see Chapter 1, Cardiovascular Disorders)
3. **Radiology** = US and Doppler studies are safe means of finding thrombosis
4. **Treatment** =
   a. IV heparin is used to treat active DVT (maintain PTT at 2 × normal) until delivery
   b. Low molecular weight heparin (enoxaparin) may be used in cases in which there is a significant amount of time until delivery but should be switched to unfractionated heparin ~2 weeks prior to delivery
   c. Anticoagulants should be continued following delivery for six weeks (warfarin may be used postpartum)
5. **Complications** = pulmonary embolus; heparin therapy may be complicated by hemorrhage or thrombocytopenia

H. **Maternal UTIs**
1. UTIs are **more common** during pregnancy due to decreased ureteral peristalsis (secondary to increased progesterone) and outflow obstruction
2. **H/P** = similar symptoms to nonpregnant patients (dysuria, urinary frequency, urgency) or asymptomatic
3. **Labs** = urinalysis shows white blood cells and nitrates; urine culture shows bacteria
4. **Treatment** = amoxicillin, nitrofurantoin, or cephalexin × 3–7 days; recurrent cases or pyelonephritis may require longer therapy

I. **Congenital infections**
1. Maternal infections during pregnancy that may have significant negative effects on fetal development or viability (see Table 12-7)
2. Prenatal screening is performed to detect certain infections that are of particular risk to the fetus

J. **Maternal drug use**
1. Several prescribed and illicit drugs can have a negative effect on pregnancy
2. **H/P** = a complete drug history should be collected to assess all potential fetal risks
3. **Treatment** =
   a. Appropriate counseling and education for drug abuse
   b. Stop teratogenic drugs during pregnancy (unless stopping drug is more harmful than use) and select alternative medications or therapies to treat medical conditions (see Table 12-6)
   c. Careful screening for related domestic abuse

Hyperemesis gravidum is severe nausea and vomiting that affects 1% of pregnant women. It may be complicated by electrolyte abnormalities and treated with avoidance of large meals, adequate hydration, and either H_2 antagonists or proton-pump inhibitors.

Warfarin has teratogenic effects and should **not** be used during pregnancy.

NEXT STEP Stop all anticoagulation during active labor until 6 hours after delivery to prevent severe hemorrhage.

Fluoroquinolones and trimethoprim-sulfamethoxazole (TMP-SMX, a sulfonamide) should not be used for treatment of UTI because of teratogenic effects.

Congenital infections are frequently referred to as the TORCHS infections: **T**oxoplasmosis, **O**ther (varicella-zoster, group B streptococcus, chlamydia, gonorrhea), **R**ubella/**R**ubeola, **C**ytomegalovirus, **H**erpes simplex/**H**epatitis B/**H**IV, **S**yphilis.

TABLE 12-5	Recreational Drug Use and Associated Risks to Mother and Fetus during Pregnancy	
Drug	**Maternal Risks**	**Fetal Risks**
Cocaine	**Arrhythmia,** myocardial infarction, subarachnoid hemorrhage, seizures, stroke, abruptio placenta	IUGR, prematurity, facial abnormalities, delayed intellectual development, **stroke**
Ethanol	Minimal	**Fetal alcohol syndrome** (mental retardation, IUGR, sensory and motor neuropathy, facial abnormalities), spontaneous abortion, intrauterine fetal demise
Hallucinogens	Personal endangerment (poor decision-making)	Possible developmental delays
Marijuana	Minimal	IUGR, prematurity
Opioids	**Infection** (from needles), narcotic withdrawal	Prematurity, IUGR, meconium aspiration, neonatal infections, **narcotic withdrawal** (may be fatal)
Stimulants	Lack of appetite and **malnutrition,** arrhythmia, withdrawal depression	IUGR
Tobacco	**Abruptio placenta, placenta previa**	Spontaneous abortion, prematurity, **IUGR,** intrauterine fetal demise, impaired intellectual development, higher risk of neonatal respiratory infections

IUGR, intrauterine growth restriction.

IV. Obstetric complications of pregnancy
  A. **Ectopic pregnancy**
   1. Implantation of zygote **outside of uterus**; most commonly occurs in **ampulla of fallopian tube** (95% of cases) but may also occur on ovary, cervix, or abdominal cavity
   2. **Risk factors = pelvic inflammatory disease,** sexually transmitted diseases, use of intrauterine device (IUD), gynecologic surgery, **prior ectopic pregnancy**, multiple sexual partners
   3. **H/P =**
   4. **Abdominal pain,** nausea, amenorrhea; scant vaginal bleeding, possible palpable pelvis mass
   5. In cases of rupture abdominal pain becomes severe and may be accompanied by hypotension, tachycardia, and peritoneal signs
   6. **Labs =** increased β-human chorionic gonadotropin (β-hCG) (urine or serum) indicates pregnancy; β-hCG in intrauterine pregnancy will double every 48 hours (β-hCG that is **low for time of gestation** should raise suspicion for ectopic pregnancy)
   7. **Radiology =**
     a. Transabdominal and transvaginal US should be able to visualize pregnancy once β-hCG reaches 6500 mIU/mL and 1500 mIU/mL, respectively
     b. **Absence of visible intrauterine pregnancy** should raise suspicion
     c. US may show free abdominal fluid if rupture has occurred
   8. **Treatment =** unruptured ectopic pregnancy of <6 weeks' gestation is treated with methotrexate to abort pregnancy; longer term or ruptured

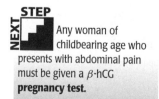
NEXT STEP Any woman of childbearing age who presents with abdominal pain must be given a β-hCG **pregnancy test.**

TABLE 12-6	Common Medications that Carry Teratogenic Risks
Medication	**Teratogenic Risks**
ACE-I	Renal abnormalities
Aminoglycosides	CN VIII damage, skeletal abnormalities
Carbamazepine	Facial abnormalities, IUGR, mental retardation, cardiovascular abnormalities, neural tube defects
Chemotherapeutics (all drug classes)	Intrauterine fetal demise (~30% pregnancies), severe IUGR, multiple anatomical abnormalities (palate, bones, limbs, genitals, etc.), mental retardation, spontaneous abortion
Diazepam	Cleft palate
DES	Vaginal and cervical cancer later in life (clear cell cancer)
Fluoroquinolones	Cartilage abnormalities
Heparin	Prematurity, intrauterine fetal demise; considered much safer than warfarin
Iodide	Goiter, hypothyroidism, mental retardation
OCPs	Intrauterine fetal demise, abnormal genitalia
Phenobarbital	Neonatal withdrawal
Phenytoin	Facial abnormalities, IUGR, mental retardation, cardiovascular abnormalities
Retinoids	CNS abnormalities, cardiovascular abnormalities, facial abnormalities, spontaneous abortion
Sulfonamides	Kernicterus (bile infiltration of brain)
Tetracycline	Skeletal abnormalities, limb abnormalities, teeth discoloration
Thalidomide	Limb abnormalities
Valproic acid	Neural tube defects (~1% pregnancies), facial abnormalities, cardiovascular abnormalities, skeletal abnormalities
Warfarin	Spontaneous abortion, IUGR, CNS abnormalities, facial abnormalities, mental retardation

ACE-I, angiotensin converting enzyme inhibitors; CN, cranial nerve; CNS, central nervous system; DES, diethylstilbestrol; IUGR, intrauterine growth restriction; OCPs, oral contraceptive pills.

ectopic pregnancy treated with IV hydration and **surgical excision** with attempt to preserve fallopian tube

9. **Complications** = unavoidable fetal death, severe maternal hemorrhage, increased risk of future ectopic pregnancy, infertility, Rh sensitization, **maternal death**

B. **Spontaneous abortion (miscarriage) (see Table 12-8)**
   1. **Non-elective** termination of pregnancy **prior to 20 weeks'** gestation
      a. 1st-trimester spontaneous abortions are usually due to **fetal chromosomal abnormalities**
      b. 2nd-trimester spontaneous abortions are usually due to infection, **cervical incompetence, uterine abnormalities,** hypercoagulable state, poor maternal health, or **drug use** (prescription or recreational)
   2. **Risk factors** = **increased maternal age,** multiple prior births, prior spontaneous abortion, uterine abnormalities

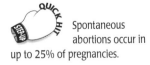

Spontaneous abortions occur in up to 25% of pregnancies.

TABLE 12-7 Congenital Infections and Effects upon the Fetus and Neonates

Maternal Infection	Possible Fetal/ Neonatal Effects	Diagnosis	Treatment
Toxoplasmosis	Hydrocephalus, intracranial calcifications, chorioretinitis	• Possible mononucleosis-like illness • Antibody screening may be helpful for diagnosis	• Pyrimethamine, sulfadiazine, and folinic acid • Mother should avoid gardening, raw meat, cat litter boxes, and unpasteurized milk
Varicella zoster	Prematurity, **encephalitis, pneumonia,** IUGR, **CNS abnormalities,** limb abnormalities High risk of neonatal death if birth occurs during active infection	• IgG titer screening in women with **no known history of disease**	• Varicella immune globulin given to nonimmune mother within 1 wk of exposure and to neonate if born during active infection • Vaccine is contraindicated during pregnancy (live attenuated virus carries risk of fetal infection)
Group B streptococcus	Respiratory distress, pneumonia, **meningitis**	• Antigen screening after 34 wks gestation	• IV β-lactams or clindamycin during labor
Gonorrhea/chlamydia	Increased risk of spontaneous abortion; neonatal sepsis, **conjunctivitis**	• Cervical culture and immunoassays	• Erythromycin given to mother
Rubella	Increased risk of spontaneous abortion, **congenital rubella syndrome** (IUGR, deafness, cardiovascular abnormalities, vision abnormalities, CNS abnormalities, hepatitis) if disease transmission occurs	• Early prenatal IgG screening	• Mother should be immunized before attempting to become pregnant • No treatment if infection develops during pregnancy • No proven benefit from rubella immune globulin
Rubeola (measles)	Increased risk of prematurity, IUGR, and spontaneous abortion; **high risk** (20% if term birth, 55% if preterm) **of neonatal death** if disease transmission occurs	• Clinical diagnosis in mother confirmed by IgM antibodies after rash develops	• Mother should be immunized before attempting to become pregnant • No treatment if infection develops during pregnancy • Vaccine is contraindicated during pregnancy (live attenuated virus carries risk of fetal infection)
Cytomegalovirus	IUGR, chorioretinitis, **CNS abnormalities,** mental retardation, vision abnormalities, deafness, hydrocephalus, hepatosplenomegaly	• Possible mononucleosis-like illness • Antibody screening may be helpful for diagnosis	• No treatment if infection develops during pregnancy • **Good hygiene** reduces risk of transmission
HIV	Viral transmission in utero (25% risk), **rapid progression** of disease to AIDS	• Early prenatal maternal blood screening • (consent required)	• **AZT** reduces risk of vertical transmission to ~8% • Use of combined therapies important
Hepatitis B	Increased risk of prematurity, IUGR; increased risk of neonatal death if acute disease develops	• Prenatal surface antigen screening	• Maternal **vaccination**; vaccination of neonate and administration of immune globulin shortly after birth
Herpes simplex	Increased risk of prematurity, IUGR, and spontaneous abortion; high risk of **neonatal death** or **CNS abnormalities** if disease transmission occurs	• Clinical diagnosis confirmed with viral culture or immunoassays	• Delivery by **caesarean section** to avoid disease transmission if active lesions present or if primary outbreak
Syphilis	Neonatal anemia, hepatosplenomegaly, skin lesions (**"blueberry muffin baby"**), pneumonia, hepatitis; 50% neonatal mortality	• Early prenatal RPR or VDRL	• Maternal penicillin

AZT, zidovudine; CNS, central nervous system; IUGR, intrauterine growth restriction; IV, intravenous; RPR, rapid plasma reagin; VDRL, Venereal Disease Research Laboratories.

OBSTETRICS

TABLE 12-8 Types of Spontaneous Abortions

Abortion Type	Threatened	Inevitable	Incomplete	Complete	Missed
Sign/Symptoms					
Uterine bleeding	In initial 20 wks of gestation	Initial 20 wks + pain	Initial 20 wks	Initial 20 wks	Present or with pain
Cervical os	Closed	Open	Open	Closed	Closed
Uterine contents expelled	None	None	Some	All	None
Diagnosis	US detects viable fetus	Possible detection of fetus by US	Based on history of expelled products of conception	Based on history of expelled products of conception	US detects unviable intrauterine fetus
Treatment	Bed rest, limited activity	D&C to remove uterine contents	D&C	None	D&C

D&C, dilation and curettage; US, ultrasound.

3. **H/P** = history should focus on prior abortions, birth history, prior gynecologic infections, and family history of congenital diseases; vaginal bleeding and possible open cervical os seen on examination
4. **Labs** = β-hCG used to assess gestational age and track progress of pregnancy
5. **Radiology** = US used to assess fetal viability
6. **Treatment** = dependent upon type of spontaneous abortion

C. **Intrauterine fetal demise**
   1. Intrauterine fetal death that occurs **after 20 weeks of gestation** and before the onset of labor
   2. Due to **placental** or **cord abnormalities** secondary to maternal cardiovascular or hematologic conditions, maternal HTN, **infection**, poor maternal health, or fetal congenital abnormalities
   3. **H/P** = pregnant patient notes no fetal activity; uterus small for length of gestation, no fetal movement, no fetal heart tones
   4. **Radiology** = US shows unviable intrauterine fetus with no heart activity
   5. **Treatment** = dilation and evacuation (D&E) used to remove fetus if before 24 weeks' gestation; induced labor used to deliver fetus if after 28 weeks
   6. **Complications** = DIC

D. **Intrauterine growth restriction (IUGR)**
   1. Fetal growth that lags behind gestational age
   2. Types
      a. **Symmetric**
         (1) 20% of cases
         (2) Overall decrease in fetal size
         (3) Early in pregnancy
         (4) Most commonly due to **congenital infection, chromosomal abnormalities,** or maternal drug use (illicit or recreational)
      b. **Asymmetric**
         (1) 80% of cases
         (2) Decreased abdominal size with preservation of head and extremities
         (3) Late in pregnancy
         (4) Due to multiple gestation, **poor maternal health,** or placental insufficiency

3. **H/P** = fundal height is **smaller** than expected for gestational age (beginning at 22 weeks' gestation, distance in centimeters from pubis to top of fundus should equal gestational age in weeks)

4. **Radiology** =
   a. US shows head circumference:abdominal circumference and femur length:abdominal circumference ratios **increased** in **asymmetric** IUGR and **normal** in **symmetric** IUGR
   b. US can be used to estimate fetal weight (<10th percentile in IUGR)
   c. US frequently detects oligohydramnios
   d. Doppler US studies may detect decreased fetal, umbilical, or maternal blood flow

5. **Treatment** =
   a. Fetal growth should be followed with US
   b. Nutritional supplementation, maternal O_2 therapy, and maternal bed rest may aid fetal growth
   c. Delivery should be induced if fetal growth slows further, maternal health worsens, or tests show fetal distress

E. **Oligohydramnios**

1. **Deficiency** of **amniotic fluid** in gestational sac
2. Associated with **IUGR**, fetal stress, fetal renal abnormalities, or poor fetal health
3. Significance of timing
   a. **1st trimester**—frequently results in **spontaneous abortion**
   b. **2nd trimester**—may be due to **fetal renal abnormalities**, maternal cause (preeclampsia, renal disease, HTN, collagen-vascular disease), placental thrombosis, or **amniocentesis**
   c. **3rd trimester**—associated with **premature rupture of membranes** (PROM), preeclampsia, abruptio placenta, or idiopathic causes
4. **H/P** = possibly asymptomatic; fundal height may be small for gestational age
5. **Radiology** = US used to determine amniotic volume and perform fetal assessment
6. **Treatment** = induce delivery of viable fetus if risk of fetal demise is significant (poor response of fetus to tests of well-being); hydration and bed rest may improve amniotic volume
7. **Complications** = spontaneous abortion, intrauterine fetal demise; abnormalities in limb, facial, and abdominal development due to **compression**

F. **Polyhydramnios**

1. **Excess** of amniotic fluid in gestational sac
2. May be due to insufficient swallowing of amniotic fluid (e.g., esophageal atresia) by fetus or increased fetal urination related to maternal DM, multiple gestation, fetal anemia, or chromosomal abnormalities
3. **H/P** = fundal height may be larger than expected for gestational age
4. **Radiology** = US used to assess amniotic fluid volume
5. **Treatment** = reduction of amniotic volume with amniocentesis, bed rest, **prevention of preterm labor with tocolytics**
6. **Complications** = preterm labor, PROM, fetal malpresentation, maternal respiratory compromise

G. **Premature rupture of membranes** (PROM)

1. Spontaneous **rupture of amniotic sac** with spillage of amniotic fluid **prior** to onset of labor
2. **Risk factors** = vaginal or cervical infection, cervical incompetence, poor maternal nutrition
3. **H/P** = loss of amniotic fluid from vagina; amniotic fluid may be seen on external vaginal examination

 The initial US finding for IUGR is frequently an **abdominal circumference** <**10th percentile** for gestational age.

 A fetal **nonstress test** and **biophysical profile** are easy ways to assess fetal well-being and risk of fetal demise due to a stressful environment.

 Excessive amniotic fluid frequently **re-accumulates** following percutaneous drainage.

 Internal manual examination should **not** be performed by the physician in cases of PROM because of an **increased risk of introducing infection** into the vaginal canal.

OBSTETRICS

4. **Labs** = **microscopic examination** of vaginal fluid will show **"ferning"** if amniotic fluid is present; vaginal fluid will turn **nitrazine paper blue** in presence of amniotic fluid; vaginal fluid should be cultured to detect infection

5. **Radiology** = US should be used to confirm oligohydramnios and to assess volume of residual amniotic fluid and fetal position

6. **Treatment** =
   a. Delivery should be induced if PROM occurs at **34 weeks' gestation or later**
   b. If amniotic fluid is infected (chorioamnionitis), delivery should be delayed until antibiotics are started
   c. If fetal lungs are **immature**, delivery should be delayed (tocolytics may be required) until lung maturity is reached; **corticosteroids** may be used to **speed lung maturity**

H. **Preterm labor**

1. Onset of labor **before 37 weeks** of gestation

2. **Risk factors** = **multiple gestation,** infection, **PROM,** previous preterm labor, polyhydramnios, cervical incompetence, poor nutrition, or lower socioeconomic status

3. **H/P** = signs of labor (8+ uterine contractions/hour, cervical dilation and effacement) **prior** to 37 weeks' gestation

4. **Labs** = vaginal and cervical cultures performed to detect infection

5. **Radiology** = US used to assess amniotic fluid volume, fetal well-being, and verify gestational age

6. **Treatment** =
   a. Hydration and bed rest stop preterm labor in 20% of patients
   b. **Tocolytic therapy** with **MgSO$_4$,** ritodrine, **terbutaline,** indomethacin, or nifedipine can be used to inhibit contractions
   c. Antibiotics given for prophylaxis against group B streptococcus or if evidence of active infection; corticosteroids may be given to hasten lung maturity

7. **Complications** = increased risk of neonatal complications and fetal respiratory distress syndrome

I. **Placenta previa**

1. **Implantation** of placenta **near cervical os** leading to antepartum hemorrhage

2. Types
   a. **Low implantation**—placenta implanted in lower uterus but does not infringe upon cervical os until dilation occurs
   b. **Partial** placenta previa—placenta partially covers os
   c. **Complete** placenta previa—placenta completely covers os

3. **Risk factors** = multiparity (prior pregnancy), increased maternal age, prior placenta previa, multiple gestation, uterine fibroids, history of abortion

4. **H/P** = **painless** vaginal bleeding in **3rd trimester** (30th week of gestation is most common time of onset)

5. **Radiology** = US determines location of placenta (transvaginal/translabial US more sensitive)

6. **Treatment** =
   a. Bed rest in cases of minor bleeding
   b. Once fetal lung maturity is achieved, perform delivery by **caesarean section**
   c. **Tocolytics** may be used to delay delivery and reduce maternal bleeding risk in cases of a preterm fetus with **immature lungs** and **mild maternal bleeding**
   d. Vaginal delivery may be performed with a low-lying placenta

7. **Complications** = severe hemorrhage, IUGR, malpresentation, PROM; **1%** of cases result in **maternal death**

Fetal lung maturity is determined by measuring lecithin (L) and sphingomyelin (S) levels in amniotic fluid and determining the **L:S ratio (L:S >2** with the presence of phosphatidylglycerol in amniotic fluid **suggests lung maturity).**

Manual or speculum vaginal examination should **not** be performed in cases of placenta previa to prevent inducing **greater hemorrhage.**

OBSTETRICS

FIGURE
12-3 Uterine profiles and cross-sections demonstrating normal placental implantation and examples of low-lying placenta, partial placenta previa, and complete placenta previa.

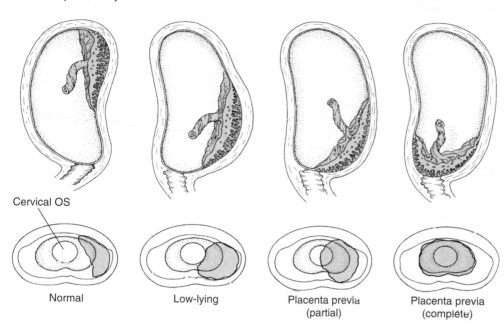

Cervical OS

| Normal | Low-lying | Placenta previa (partial) | Placenta previa (complete) |

(Taken from *OB-GYN Scenes and Procedures*. LifeART Nursing Collection.)

J. **Abruptio placenta**
   1. Premature separation of the placenta from uterine wall leading to **significant maternal hemorrhage**
   2. **Risk factors** = HTN, prior abruptio placenta, trauma, **tobacco use**, cocaine use, PROM, folate deficiency
   3. **H/P** = **painful** vaginal bleeding in **3rd trimester**, back pain, abdominal pain; pelvic and abdominal tenderness, **increased uterine tone**; hypotension occurs with severe hemorrhage
   4. **Radiology** = US **inconsistently** shows separation of placenta from uterus
   5. **Treatment** =
      a. Bed rest for very mild cases
      b. Delivery typically occurs rapidly secondary to uterine irritation, but **caesarean section** should be performed in cases of **hemodynamic instability**
      c. Transfusion is frequently required for significant hemorrhage
   6. **Complications** = DIC; **severe hemorrhage** that increases risk of maternal death; **fetal demise** occurs in 35% of cases; increased risk of abruption in future pregnancies

K. **Multiple gestation**
   1. Any pregnancy in which **more than one fetus** develops at the same time
   2. More likely to occur with fertility drug use
   3. Types
      a. **Monozygotic**—division of zygote resulting in development of identical fetuses; fetuses may or may not share amnion
      b. **Dizygotic**—fertilization of more than one egg by different sperm resulting in development of dissimilar (fraternal) fetuses and separate amnions
   4. Increased incidence of complications
      a. Maternal—HTN, DM, **preeclampsia, preterm labor**
      b. Fetal—**malpresentation,** placenta previa, abruptio placenta, PROM, **IUGR,** birth trauma, cerebral palsy, respiratory distress syndrome

Conjoined twins only occur in cases of **monozygotic** twinning.

If the umbilical cords for multiple fetuses are fused, **twin-twin transfusion syndrome** may result, in which one twin is **inadequately** perfused, leading to an increased risk of fetal complications.

5. **H/P** = fundal height large for gestational age; more than one fetal heart tone may be detected
6. **Radiology** = US detects 2+ gestational sacs
7. **Treatment** =
   a. Close maternal follow-up (weekly or biweekly) starting at 20 weeks' gestation
   b. Activity restriction, frequent assessment of fetal growth with US, and weekly nonstress tests starting at 36 weeks' gestation
   c. Preterm labor should be halted with tocolytic therapy
   d. Vertex-vertex (both heads downward) presentations may be delivered vaginally, but other presentations (e.g., vertex-transverse, vertex-breech) require caesarean section

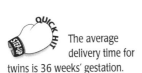

The average delivery time for twins is 36 weeks' gestation.

V. Labor and delivery

A. **Assessment of fetal well-being**

1. Tests of fetal activity, heart rate, and responses to stress used to confirm fetal well-being and to detect fetal distress

2. **Nonstress test**
   a. Used often during **prenatal assessment** and into labor
   b. Mother reclines in left lateral supine position
   c. Fetal heart rate monitored with external Doppler US; mother reports each fetal movement
   d. **Effects of fetal movement on heart rate** are noted
   e. Normal ("reactive") test is considered to be 2 or more 15-bpm accelerations of fetal heart rate lasting at least 15 seconds each within 20 minutes
   f. Nonreactive test prompts biophysical profile

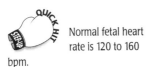

Normal fetal heart rate is 120 to 160 bpm.

3. **Biophysical profile**
   a. Performed in follow-up to nonreactive nonstress test
   b. **Nonstress test repeated** and US assessment performed
   c. US used to measure **Bishop Score—amniotic fluid index** (total linear measurement in centimeters of largest amniotic fluid pocket detected in each of four quadrants of amniotic sac), **fetal breathing rate, fetal movement, fetal tone** (extension of fetal spine or limb with return to flexion)
      (1) 2 points scored for each and for reactive nonstress test; 0 points in absence of criteria
      (2) Amniotic fluid index = 5–23 cm (2 points)
      (3) 1+ episode of rhythmic breathing lasting 20 seconds within a 30-minute period (2 points)
      (4) 2+ episodes of discrete fetal movement within a 30-minute period (2 points)
      (5) 1+ episodes of spine and limb extension with return to flexion (2 points)
   d. **Reassuring** profile is a score of **8 or 10; lower** score suggests **fetal distress**

4. **Contraction stress test**
   a. Used during labor to assess uteroplacental dysfunction
   b. Fetal heart rate recorded with external fetal monitor or fetal scalp electrode
   c. **Beat-to-beat variability** of ~5 bpm, **long-term heart rate variability,** and occasional **heart rate accelerations** (2+ accelerations of 15 bpm lasting at least 15 seconds within a 20−minute period) are **reassuring** signs
   d. **Decelerations** of heart rate from baseline may indicate fetal head compression, fetal hypoxia, or umbilical cord compression

TABLE 12-9 Types of Decelerations Seen on Fetal Heart Rate Tracings

Deceleration	Appearance	Cause	Treatment
Early	Decelerations begin and end **with** uterine contractions	Head compression	• None required • **Not a sign of fetal distress**
Late	Begin **after** initiation of uterine contraction and end **after** contraction has finished	**Uteroplacental insufficiency,** maternal venous compression, maternal hypotension, or abruption placenta; **may suggest fetal hypoxia**	• Test fetal blood from scalp sample to diagnose hypoxia or acidosis • Recurrent late decelerations or fetal hypoxia direct **prompt delivery**
Variable	**Inconsistent** onset, duration, and degree of decelerations	Umbilical cord compression	• Change mother's position

FIGURE 12-4 Examples of fetal heart and uterine tone tracings for early, late, and variable decelerations of fetal heart rate (FHR) following uterine contraction (UC).

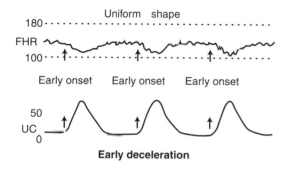

Early deceleration

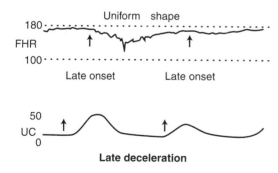

Late deceleration

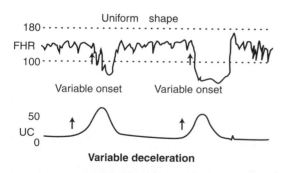

Variable deceleration

(Modified from Hon E. *An Introduction to Fetal Heart Rate Monitoring*. Los Angeles; University of Southern California, 1973. Also see Feibusch KC, Breaden RS, Badr, CD, Gomperts SN. *Prescription for the Boards: USMLE Step 2*. 3rd Ed. Philadelphia; Lippincott Williams & Wilkins, 2002.)

OBSTETRICS

5. **Fetal scalp blood sampling**
   a. Performed when a consistently abnormal fetal heart rate tracing seen or evidence of significant meconium in amniotic fluid detected
   b. Normal fetal blood pH is reassuring; **decreased pH** and **hypoxemia** indicate **fetal distress**

B. **Stages of labor**
   1. Labor (i.e., contractions and cervical effacement) typically begins 38–42 weeks' gestation and involves four stages of progression
   2. Nulliparous and multiparous women proceed through labor at different rates

C. **Induction of labor**
   1. Administration of **oxytocin** to initiate uterine contractions or speed progress of labor
   2. Indications
      a. Maternal—preeclampsia, DM, stalled stage of labor, chorioamnionitis
      b. Fetal—prolonged pregnancy (>40–42 weeks), IUGR, PROM, some congenital defects
   3. Contraindications to induction of labor are prior uterine surgery, fetal lung immaturity, malpresentation, and acute fetal distress

D. **Malpresentation**
   1. **Normal** fetal presentation (cephalic or vertex) is with fetal head down, chin tucked, and occiput directed towards birth canal
   2. **Face** (full hyperextension of neck) presentation occurs rarely and usually undergoes normal vaginal delivery if chin is anterior

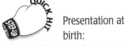

QUICK HIT

During the last few weeks of gestation a woman may experience multiple **false (Braxton-Hicks) contractions** not associated with true labor.

QUICK HIT

Presentation at birth:
- Normal presentation occurs in >95% of pregnancies.
- Prior to 28 weeks' gestation **25%** of pregnancies are in **breech** presentation, but the **majority** will assume **vertex** presentation by the time of birth.

TABLE 12-10 Stages of Labor

Stage	Beginning/End	Activity	Management	Duration Nulliparous	Multiparous
1	• Latent phase—start of uterine contractions until 4 cm cervical dilation • Active phase—4 cm cervical dilation until 10 cm cervical dilation with consistent progression	• Latent phase—cervical effacement and gradual dilation • Active phase—regular uterine contractions, quick progression of cervical dilation (1.5 cm/hr for nulliparous, 1 cm/hr for multiparous) and effacement, engagement of fetal head in pelvis	Monitor fetal heart rate and uterine contractions, assess progression of cervical changes periodically during active phase	6–18 hr (2/3 latent, 1/3 active)	2–10 hr
2	Full (10 cm) cervical dilation until delivery	Fetal descent through birth canal driven by uterine contractions	Monitor fetal heart rate and movement through birth canal	30 min–3 hr	5–30 min
3	Delivery of neonate until placental delivery	Placenta separates from uterine wall up to 30 min after delivery of neonate and emerges through birth canal, uterus contracts to expel placenta and prevent hemorrhage	Uterine massage, examination of placenta to confirm no intrauterine remnants	0–30 min	0–30 min
4	Initial postpartum hr	Hemodynamic stabilization of mother	Monitor maternal pulse and blood pressure, look for signs of hemorrhage	1 hr	1 hr

OBSTETRICS

FIGURE
12-5 Examples of frank (**A**), complete (**B**), and incomplete (**C**) variations of breech presentation.

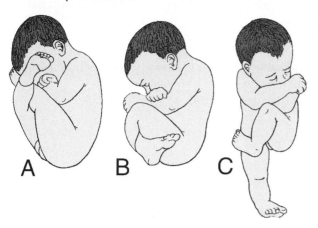

(Taken from LifeART *Obstetrics and Gynecology*. Philadelphia; Lippincott Williams & Wilkins.)

3. **Brow** (partial hyperextension of neck) presentation occurs very rarely and requires caesarean delivery if the head does not spontaneously correct to a normal presentation

4. **Breech presentation** is the most common **malpresentation**
   a. **Frank breech**—75% of cases; thighs flexed and knees extended
   b. **Complete breech**—thighs and knees flexed
   c. **Footling breech**—one or both legs extended
   d. **Risk factors** = prematurity, multiple gestation, polyhydramnios, uterine anomaly
   e. **H/P** = abdominal examination (i.e., Leopold maneuvers) detects fetal head in abdomen, vaginal exam may detect presenting part
   f. **Radiology** = US confirms fetal orientation
   g. **Treatment** = majority of cases will resolve prior to labor; **external cephalic version** may be applied to abdomen at 37 weeks' gestation to attempt repositioning of fetus (75% effective); vaginal delivery may be attempted for term fetuses in frank breech without other detected abnormalities; caesarean section performed in most cases (including frank breech) for delivery
   h. **Complications** = cord prolapse, head entrapment, fetal hypoxia, abruptio placenta, birth trauma

E. **Caesarean section**
   1. Delivery of fetus through incision in uterine wall
   2. Types
      a. **Classical**—vertical incision in anterior muscular portion of the uterus; chosen when fetus lies in transverse presentation, adhesions or fibroids prevent access to lower uterus, hysterectomy is scheduled to follow delivery, cervical cancer is present, or in postmortem delivery to remove living fetus from dead mother
      b. **Low transverse**—transverse incision in lower uterine segment; decreased risk of uterine rupture, bleeding, bowel adhesions, and infection (preferred to classical technique and performed more commonly)
   3. Indications
      a. Maternal—**eclampsia, prior uterine surgery, prior classic caesarean section,** cardiac disease, birth canal obstruction, maternal death, cervical cancer, active herpes simplex virus
      b. Fetal—**acute fetal distress, malpresentation,** cord prolapse, macrosomia

c. Combined maternal and fetal—failed induction of labor, placenta previa, abruptio placenta, cephalopelvic disproportion

4. In subsequent pregnancies, vaginal delivery may be attempted with use of **transverse** caesarean section

5. If **classical** incision utilized has been used previously, repeat caesarean delivery **must** be performed due to risk of uterine rupture

6. **Complications** = hemorrhage, infection and sepsis, thromboembolism, injury to surrounding structures

F. **Normal puerperium and postpartum activity**

1. **Care of the newborn**

   a. Immediate suction of mouth and nose to aid in breathing and to prevent aspiration

   b. Neonate is dried and wrapped in clothes to prevent heat loss

   c. Umbilical cord is clamped and cut; blood sample taken from cord to measure blood gases and blood type

   d. Onset of respiration within 30 seconds is confirmed; if spontaneous respiration does not begin, **resuscitation** must be initiated

   e. Tracheal injection of synthetic or exogenous surfactant may be given in cases of lung immaturity

   f. **Apgar score** performed at 1 and 5 minutes after birth; a score of **7+ at 1 minute** and **9+ at 5 minutes** is **reassuring**

2. **Maternal changes**

   a. Uterus decreases in size and cervix becomes firm over three weeks

   b. Uterine discharge (lochia) is red during initial days after birth but becomes paler and white by 10th day postpartum

   c. Vaginal wall gradually becomes firmer

   d. Total peripheral resistance increases rapidly due to elimination of uteroplacental circulation; diuresis causes significant weight loss in 1st week postpartum; cardiac output gradually returns to normal

   e. Mother may feel mild depression for few days after delivery ("postpartum blues"); most cases resolve without complications

   f. Menstruation returns 6–8 weeks postpartum in non-nursing mothers

   g. Ovulation and menstruation may not occur for several months in nursing mothers (93% effective in preventing pregnancy for 3 months after delivery if performed regularly)

G. **Postpartum bleeding**

1. Blood loss >500 mL/24 hours following vaginal delivery or >1000 mL/24 hours after caesarean section is abnormal

2. Due to **uterine atony** in most cases (more likely after multiple gestation, prolonged labor, and chorioamnionitis)

3. May also result from **birth canal trauma** or **retained placental tissue** (e.g., DIC)

4. **H/P** = excessive postpartum bleeding from genital tract; soft, boggy uterus palpable with uterine atony; vaginal examination may detect lacerations; examination of placenta after birth should detect any missing segments

 Risk of maternal mortality is 6× greater for caesarean section than vaginal delivery.

 Breast milk is considered the ideal infant nutrition because it contains important **IgA antibodies** for the newborn, is in **sufficient supply**, is **cost-free**, and enhances mother-infant bonding.

 Early breast milk (**colostrum**) is rich in proteins, fat, minerals, and contains IgA; after 1 week postpartum breast milk contains proteins, fat, water, and lactose.

 Uterine atony is more likely after multiple gestation, prolonged labor, and chorioamnionitis.

Retained placental tissue causes the most substantial volume of postpartum bleeding.

TABLE 12-11	Apgar Scoring System for Determining Neonatal Well-Being		
	Score		
Sign	**0**	**1**	**2**
Heart rate	None	<100 bpm	>100 bpm
Respirations	None	Poor, weak cry	Good, strong cry
Muscle tone	Poor	Some movement	Active movement
Response to stimulation	None	Grimace	Strong cry
Color	Blue, pale	Pink torso, blue extremities	Pink

5. **Radiology** = US may show retained placental tissue
6. **Treatment** =
   a. Uterine massage and oxytocin administration help increase uterine tone and decrease hemorrhage
   b. Surgical repair of lacerations should be performed
   c. Dilation and curettage (D&C) may successfully remove retained placental tissue
   d. Hysterectomy may need to be performed in severe or refractory cases

VI. Gestational trophoblastic neoplasms

A. Hydatidiform mole

1. **Benign** neoplasms of trophoblastic cells (cells that make up placenta) that infrequently become malignant; **benign** trophoblastic neoplasms make up **80%** of trophoblastic disease
2. Types
   a. Complete—46 XX genotype; completely derived from father (empty egg penetrated by sperm)
   b. Incomplete—69 XXY genotype; fertilization of egg by two sperm; associated with abnormal fetus
3. **Risk factors** = insufficient dietary folate or β-carotene, low socioeconomic status, very young (<20 years old) or older (>40 years old) at time of pregnancy, prior history of molar pregnancy, Asian heritage
4. **H/P** = heavy or irregular painless vaginal bleeding during **1st** or **2nd** trimester, excessive nausea, dizziness, anxiety; large fundal height for gestational age, expulsion of **"grape-like"** vesicles from vagina, no fetal movement or heart tones detected
5. **Labs** – β-hCG is **higher** than expected for gestational age
6. **Radiology** = US detects "**snow storm**" pattern in uterus without presence of gestational sac; use chest radiograph to rule out metastases to lung
7. **Treatment** = D&C to remove neoplasm; follow β-hCG for one year (levels should gradually decrease); avoid pregnancy for one year
8. **Complications** = malignant gestational trophoblastic neoplasm (10% of cases), choriocarcinoma (5% of cases, suggested by continued high β-hCG following D&C)

B. Choriocarcinoma

1. **Malignant** trophoblastic neoplasm that arises from hydatidiform moles (**50%** of cases) or following abortion, ectopic pregnancy, or normal pregnancy
2. **H/P** = vaginal bleeding, hemoptysis, dyspnea, headache, dizziness, rectal bleeding; enlarged uterus on examination with bleeding seen from cervical os
3. **Labs** = increased β-hCG
4. **Radiology** = US detects "**snow storm**" pattern in uterus; CT may detect metastases
5. **Treatment** = chemotherapy, radiation; follow β-hCG to track cure; perform hysterectomy for sustained high β-hCG
6. **Complications** = **metastases** to lungs, brain, liver, kidneys, or gastrointestinal tract; good prognosis unless presence of brain or liver metastases; frequently missed diagnosis if not due to progression from molar pregnancy

 NEXT STEP High β hCG is seen in both **hydatidiform mole** and **multiple gestation**; differentiate the conditions with US.

 NEXT STEP Highly suspect a molar pregnancy if **preeclampsia** occurs in the **first half** of pregnancy, and perform an US to confirm diagnosis.

Pediatrics

I. Development and health supervision

A. Physical growth

1. Characteristics of growth (weight, height, and head circumference) fall in a normal range; deviations from this range suggest abnormal growth, disease processes, or environmental concerns

2. Pediatrician should keep a record of growth on a chart

3. **Weight**
   a. Initial loss of weight in first few days after birth is normal; birth weight is regained by 2 weeks of age
   b. Birth **weight doubles** by ~4 months, triples at ~12 months, and **quadruples** at ~24 months
   c. From age 2 years to adolescence (age 13) annual weight gain is ~5 lb.
   d. Inadequate weight gain may be due to **poor food intake** (including poor feeding and abuse), chronic vomiting or diarrhea, **malabsorption,** neoplasm, or congenital heart disease
   e. Weight < 3rd percentile on growth charts or a consistently low weight for a given height suggests **failure to thrive** (see Chapter 3, Gastrointestinal Disorders)
   f. The prevalence of childhood obesity (body mass index >30) has steadily increased in the United States and is associated with rapid growth, sleep apnea, hypertension, slipped capital femoral epiphysis, precocious puberty, increased incidence of skin infections, social dysfunction, and earlier development of diabetes mellitus (DM)

4. **Height**
   a. **Height** (birth length) is increased by 50% at ~1 year of age, **doubles** at ~4 years old, and **triples** at ~13 years old
   b. Annual height gain from 2 years old to adolescence is ~2 inches/year
   c. Greater-than-normal height may be associated with familial tall stature, precocious puberty, acromegaly, hyperthyroidism, Klinefelter's syndrome, Marfan syndrome, or obesity
   d. Lower-than-normal height may be associated with familial short stature, Turner syndrome, constitutional growth delay, chronic renal failure, asthma, cystic fibrosis, immunologic disease, growth hormone deficiency, hypothyroidism, or cardiac disease

5. **Head circumference**
   a. Measured during first year of life
   b. ~5 cm growth during age 0–3 months, ~4 cm in 3–6 months, 2 cm in 6–9 months, and 1 cm in 9–12 months
   c. Macrocephaly may be associated with cerebral metabolic diseases (e.g., Tay-Sachs, maple syrup urine disease), hydrocephalus, increased intracranial pressure, skeletal dysplasia, acromegaly, or intracranial hemorrhage

    d. Microcephaly may be associated with fetal toxin exposure (e.g., fetal alcohol syndrome), chromosomal trisomies, congenital infection, or neural tube defects

6. Trend of growth abnormalities help suggest certain pathologies
    a. Normal growth rate that declines **after birth** suggests **postnatal** onset
    b. Growth that is **abnormal from the time of birth** suggests **prenatal** onset (genetic abnormalities, intrauterine pathology)
    c. Growth that is in low-normal range but eventually becomes closer to the mean suggests **constitutional growth delay**
    d. Growth that is **consistently** low-normal suggests genetic short stature (i.e., compare to parents)

7. **H/P** =
    a. Exam should look for other symptoms and signs that suggest a particular disease
        (1) Malabsorption—diarrhea
        (2) DM—hyperglycemia
        (3) Congenital heart disease—cyanosis, etc.
        (4) Signs of abuse—bruising, abnormal parent-child interaction
        (5) Psychosocial abnormalities—inattentiveness, apathy
    b. Growth should be assessed at **each health visit** to confirm normal patterns and catch abnormalities early

8. **Labs** = labs should be directed at diagnosis of a specific disease when clinical suspicion exists (for DM—blood glucose, for congenital heart disease—arterial blood gas, etc.)

9. **Treatment** =
    a. Treat underlying disorder
    b. Seek intervention for cases of abuse
    c. Provide parental education to help alleviate poor intake, poor-quality diets, or malnutrition and to help deal with psychosocial issues

B. **Developmental milestones**
1. **Social, physical,** and **intellectual** achievements are reached by children at characteristic ages (see Table 13-1)
2. Absence or delay of milestones may suggest developmental delays
3. Some delays are hereditary, but multiple or significant delays are a cause for concern
4. Multiple or persistent delays may be due to mental retardation, genetic disorders (e.g., fragile X syndrome, trisomy 21), language or hearing disorders, child abuse, or psychiatric conditions (e.g., attention deficit hyperactivity disorder [ADHD], autism)
5. Certain reflexes are prevalent during infancy but naturally disappear by **6 months** age; absence or persistence of infantile reflexes beyond 6 months (especially with a history of perinatal complications or suspected congenital malformation) may suggest central nervous system pathology (see Table 13-2)

C. **Childhood health maintenance**
1. Periodic physician visits are important during childhood to assess **growth,** detect growth and developmental **delays,** provide **vaccinations, screen** for certain disease processes, and provide **anticipatory guidance (see Table 13-3)**
    a. Visits ~1 week after birth and at 1 month old
    b. Visits at 2 months old then every 2 months (2, 4, 6 months) until 6 months old
    c. Visits every 3 months from 6–18 months old (6, 9, 12, 15, 18 months)
    d. Visits at 2 years old and annually thereafter
2. Screening during visits should address common medical concerns (vision, hearing, dentition, diseases in high-risk populations)
3. Anticipatory guidance should address **nutrition, development, daily care, accident prevention,** and **behavioral issues**

 It is **legally imperative** that **all suspected** cases of child abuse be **well documented** and be **reported** to the appropriate authorities.

 Ages for developmental milestones are **guidelines.** It is normal for milestones to occur at an appropriate **range of ages,** and parents should be reassured that milestones occur within such a range and not at concrete ages.

 STEP Be sure to collect a thorough **family history** while assessing growth or developmental delays in order to help distinguish a **hereditary** cause from an **organic** one.

 It is important to consider the **doctor-parent-child relationship** and the **ability** of the family **to understand** anticipatory advice when reviewing topics at each visit to ensure the greatest benefit to the child.

 Some teaching methods that maximize the communication of important information during a visit are **repetition, positive reinforcement,** limitation of number of topics discussed, and not focusing on minor points.

PEDIATRICS

TABLE 13-1 | Important Developmental Milestones During Childhood

Age	Social/Cognitive	Gross Motor	Fine Motor	Language
2 months	Social smile	Lifts head 45°	Eyes follow object to midline	Coos
4 months	Laughs Aware of caregiver Localizes sound	Lifts head 90°	Eyes follow object past midline	
6 months	Differentiates parents from others Separation anxiety	Rolls over Holds self up with hands Sits	Grasps/rakes Attempts to feed self	Babbles
9 months	Interactive games	Crawls	Grasps with thumb	First words
12 months	Parallel play	Pulls to stand Walks with help	Pincer grasp Makes tower of 2 blocks	~5–10-word vocabulary
18 months		Walks well Walks backwards	Makes tower of 4 blocks Uses cup or spoon	10–50-word vocabulary 2-word sentences
2 yrs	Dresses self with help	Runs Climbs stairs (initially 2 feet/step, then 1 foot/step)	Makes tower of 6 blocks	50–75-word vocabulary 3-word sentences
3 yrs	Magical thinking		Able to draw circle (○)	
4 yrs	Plays with others	Hops on 1 foot	Able to draw line image (+), later able to draw closed line drawing (△)	250+ word vocabulary 4-word sentences
6 yrs	Able to distinguish fantasy from reality	Skips	Draws a person	

TABLE 13-2 | Childhood Reflexes and Their Relation to Central Nervous System Pathology

Reflex	Description	Time of Disappearance	Area of CNS Associated with Abnormal Persistence or Disappearance
Moro	Extension of head causes extension and flexion of limbs; startle reflex	3 months	Medulla, vestibular nuclei
Grasp	Placing finger in palm causes grasping	3 months	Medulla, vestibular nuclei
Rooting	Rubbing cheek causes turning of mouth to stimuli	3 months	Medulla, trigeminal nuclei
Tonic neck	When head turned, arm on faced side extends and arm on opposite side flexes (fencer's position)	3 months	Medulla, vestibular nuclei
Placing	Rubbing foot dorsum causes foot to step up	2 months	Cortex

CNS, central nervous system.

TABLE 13-3	Screening Performed and Anticipatory Guidance Discussed during Regular Childhood Health Visits				
Visit	**Screening**	**Nutrition**	**Daily Care**	**Accident Prevention**	**Behavioral Issues**
Newborn/1 wk	Phenylketonuria, hypothyroidism, genetic metabolic disorders (maple syrup urine disease, cystic fibrosis, etc.) in high-risk patients; hearing; visual mobility and reflexes	Breast or bottle feeding	Crying, sleep position, bathing	Smoke detectors, baby furniture, car seats	Parent-child interaction
1 month	Visual mobility and reflexes	Breast or bottle feeding, fluoride supplements	Sleep, bowel and bladder habits	Sun exposure	Importance of close contact
2 months	Visual mobility and reflexes		Sleep, bowel habits	Close supervision, risks with ability to roll over	
4 months	Visual mobility and reflexes	Solid foods, fruits and vegetables	Teething	Keeping small objects out of reach	Vocal interaction
6 months	Visual mobility and reflexes	Cup training, daily caloric needs, finger foods, avoidance of milk or juice at bedtime	Shoes	Preparation for increased mobility ("child-proofing" the house), electrical socket covers, stair and door gates	Stranger anxiety, separation anxiety
9 months	Hgb/Hct; visual mobility and reflexes	Iron supplementation, self-feeding, spoon training	Tooth care, favorite toys	Aspiration risks	Communication, discipline
12 months	Visual mobility and reflexes; lead exposure; PPD in high-risk areas	Bottle weaning, eating at table, whole cow's milk		Poisoning risks, stair safety, burns	Speech, rules, positive reinforcement
15 months	Hgb/Hct; visual mobility and reflexes	Family meals			Toilet training, temper tantrums, punishment, listening to parent read
18 months	Visual mobility and reflexes	Reinforcement of utensil use	Nightmares, bedtime regimens	Supervised play, dangerous toys	Discipline, "terrible 2s", toilet training, games
2 yr	Lead exposure; visual mobility and reflexes	Avoiding unhealthy snacks, encouraging eating during meals	Transition from crib to bed, toothbrush training		Toddler independence, explanation of body parts, early play with other children
3 yr	Visual acuity; cholesterol (if family history of high cholesterol or CAD)	Healthy diet	Regular sleep schedule, television limitation	Water safety, animal safety	Day care or babysitters (earlier if both parents work), play with other children, reinforce consistent toileting, conversation

PEDIATRICS

TABLE 13-3 (*Continued*)

Visit	Screening	Nutrition	Daily Care	Accident Prevention	Behavioral Issues
4 yr	Hearing; lead exposure; visual acuity; PPD (every 2 yr if high-risk group)	Meals as time for family bonding	Self dental care	Pedestrian and bicycle safety, car seat or seat belt, dangers of strangers, guns, fires, poisons, teach phone number	Chores, interactions at day care or preschool, school preparation
6 yr	Lead exposure; visual acuity	Avoidance of excess weight	Exercise, hygiene, school activities	Swimming	Allowance, encourage learning and development, reading
10 yr	Hearing; visual acuity			Hazardous activities, drug use (including alcohol and tobacco)	Friends, sexual education, puberty, responsibility
12 yr	Hearing; visual acuity; PPD; Pap smear only if sexually active (girls)		Adequate sleep, school and extracurricular activities	Sexual responsibility	Body image, privacy issues
14 yr and older	Hearing; Hgb/Hct (girls); visual acuity; STD screening (if sexually active)	Weight maintenance	School and activities	Risk-taking behavior, driving, sexual responsibility	Dating, sexuality, goals, careers, independence issues

Note: anticipatory guidance from **prior** visits should be **reviewed** when appropriate.
CAD, coronary artery disease; Hgb/Hct, hemoglobin and hematocrit; PPD, purified protein derivative of tuberculin (TB test); STD, sexually transmitted disease.

The first dose of hepatitis B vaccine is typically administered shortly after birth before the infant leaves the hospital.

Haemophilus influenzae type b (Hib) vaccine is **unnecessary** in previously unvaccinated children **older than 5 years** because of the low risk of severe infection at this age and older. **Asplenic** children should **always** receive Hib and pneumococcal vaccines regardless of their age.

4. Vaccinations should be given at appropriate visits (see Table 13-4)
D. **Adolescence**
   1. Period of **rapid physical, psychosocial,** and **sexual growth** and maturity leading into adulthood
   2. Typically begins at 9–10 years old in girls and 9–11 years old in boys; development prior to these ages is considered precocious puberty
   3. Physical changes are classified by Tanner stages (also refer to Chapter 11, Gynecologic Disorders)
   4. Psychosocial issues
      a. Early adolescence (10–13 years old) is typified by concrete thinking and early independent behavior
      b. Middle adolescence (14–16 years old) is typified by emergence of **sexuality** (sexual identity, sexual activity), an increased **desire for independence** (conflict with parents, need for guidance, self-absorption), and abstract thought
      c. Late adolescence (17–21 years old) is typified by increased self-awareness, increased confidence in own abilities, a more open relationship with parents, and cognitive maturity
      d. Adolescents are at an increased risk for **risk-taking behaviors** (drug use, unprotected sexual activity, violence), **depression, suicidal ideation,** and **eating disorders**
   5. **H/P =**
      a. History during visits should **address risk factors**, physical changes, menstrual issues (girls), and **concerns of patient**

TABLE 13-4 Vaccination Schedule and Contraindications During Childhood Health Visits (2004 Recommendations)

Vaccine	Birth	1mo	2 mos	4 mos	6 mos	12 mos	15 mos	18 mos	24 mos	4–6 yr	11–12 yr	13–18 yr
DTaP[a]			DTaP	DTaP	DTaP		DTaP			DTaP		Td booster
Hib[b]			Hib	Hib	Hib	Hib						
Hep B[c]	Hep B		Hep B		Hep B							
IPV[d]			IPV	IPV		IPV				IPV		
MMR[e]						MMR			MMR			
VZV[f]						VZV						
PCV[g]			PCV	PCV	PCV							
Hep A[h]										Hep A		

[a] Diphtheria, tetanus, acellular pertussis (DTaP); contraindications = encephalopathy or anaphylaxis following prior dose.
[b] *Haemophilus influenzae* type b (Hib); no contraindications.
[c] Hepatitis B (Hep B); contraindications = allergy to yeast or anaphylaxis following prior dose.
[d] Inactivated polio vaccine (IPV); contraindications = pregnancy (or pregnant female at home) and anaphylaxis following prior dose.
[e] Measles, mumps, rubella (MMR); contraindications = pregnancy (or pregnant female at home), immunocompromise, HIV, blood transfusion with prior 1 year, allergy to neomycin, anaphylaxis following prior dose.
[f] Varicella zoster vaccine (VZV); contraindications = allergy to neomycin or gelatin, anaphylaxis following prior dose, tuberculosis infection, immunosuppression, HIV, transfusion recipient with prior 5 months, pregnancy (or pregnant female at home).
[g] Pneumococcal vaccine (PCV); no contraindications.
[h] Hepatitis A; recommended in southwest and western United States.

b. Examination should focus on sexual maturation, dermatological issues (e.g., acne, sun exposure, nevi), appropriate height and weight growth, and scrotal masses (detection of testicular cancer in boys)

6. **Treatment** =
   a. Majority of teenagers proceed through adolescence without serious incidents even though accidents are the #1 cause of death in this age group
   b. Risk-taking behavior may result in sexually transmitted diseases and drug addiction that need to be treated appropriately
   c. Emphasis should be placed on maintaining a good physician-patient relationship while addressing risk prevention

NEXT STEP Because of adolescents' want for independence and need for good self esteem, adolescent patients should be approached in a **nonjudgmental** fashion to perform an accurate history and physical exam.

Confidentiality between a physician and patient must be maintained during adolescence **unless life-threatening** concerns are involved (e.g., suicidal ideation, homicidal ideation, life-threatening disease), and this right may need to be stressed to parents.

TABLE 13-5 Tanner Stages for Male Genital and Pubic Hair Development

Tanner Stage	Penile/Testicular Development	Pubic Hair Development
1	Prepubertal; small genitals	Prepubertal; no hair growth
2	Testicular and scrotal enlargement with skin coarsening	Slight growth of fine genital and axillary hair
3	Penile enlargement and further testicular growth	Further growth of hair
4	Further penile glans enlargement and darkening of scrotal skin	Hair becomes coarser and spreads over much of pubic region
5	Adult genitalia	Coarse hair extends from pubic region to medial thighs

TABLE 13-6 Types of Congenital Immunodeficiency Disorders

Disease	Description	Diagnosis	Treatment
T cell disorders			
DiGeorge syndrome	Chromosomal deletion in 22q11 resulting in **thymic and parathyroid hypoplasia, congenital heart disease,** tetany, and abnormal facial structure; recurrent viral and fungal infections occur because of insufficient T cells	**Tetany** and **facial abnormalities** on exam should raise suspicion; decreased serum calcium; chest radiograph may show absence of thymic shadow; genetic screening can detect chromosomal abnormality	Calcium, vitamin D, thymic transplant, bone marrow transplant, surgical correction of heart abnormalities
Hyper-IgM disease	Defect in T cell CD40 ligand resulting in poor interaction with B cells, low IgG, and excessive IgM; infection by **encapsulated bacteria** and *Pneumocystis carinii*	Decreased IgG and IgA, **increased IgM;** possible decreased Hgb, Hct, platelets, and neutrophils	IVIG, TMP-SMX (*P. carinii* prophylaxis)
Chronic mucocutaneous candidiasis	Persistent infection of skin, mucous membranes, and nails by **Candida albicans** due to T cell deficiency; frequent associated adrenal pathology	Poor reaction to cutaneous *C. albicans* anergy test	Antifungal agents (e.g., fluconazole)
B cell disorders			
X-linked agammaglobulinemia	Abnormal B cell differentiation resulting in low B cell and antibody levels; X-linked disorder with **boys** experiencing recurrent bacterial infections after 6 months old	**No B cells in peripheral smear;** low total immunoglobulin levels	IVIG, appropriate antibiotics
IgA deficiency	Specific IgA deficiency due to abnormal immune globulin production by B cells; patients have increased incidence of respiratory and gastrointestinal infections	**Decreased IgA** with **normal** levels of **other immune globulins**	Treatment usually not needed; administration of **IVIG may worsen deficiency**
Common variable immunodeficiency	Autosomal disorder of B cell differentiation resulting in low immune globulin levels; patients experience increased respiratory and gastrointestinal infections beginning in 2nd decade of life; associated with increased risk of **malignant neoplasms** and **autoimmune disorders**	Low immune globulin levels; family history shows **both men and women affected**	IVIG, appropriate antibiotics
Combined B and T cell disorders			
Severe combined immunodeficiency syndrome (SCID)	Absent T cells and abnormal antibody function resulting in **severe immune compromise;** patients experience significant recurrent infections by all types of pathogens from an early age; **frequently fatal at an early age**	Significantly decreased WBCs, decreased immune globulins	IVIG, antibiotics, **bone marrow transplant; no live or attenuated vaccines** should be administered
Wiskott-Aldrich syndrome	X-linked disorder of immune development resulting in significant susceptibility to **encapsulated** bacteria and opportunistic pathogens; associated with **eczema** and **thrombocytopenia**	Recurrent infections in presence of **eczema** and **easy bleeding;** decreased platelets, decreased IgM with normal or high other immune globulins, abnormal T cell activity	**Splenectomy,** appropriate antibiotics, IVIG, bone marrow transplant
Ataxia-telangiectasia	Autosomal recessive disorder causing **cerebellar dysfunction, cutaneous telangiectasias,** impaired WBC development, and low IgA	**Telangiectasias** and **ataxia** develop after 3 yr old; recurrent infections begin a few years later; decreased WBCs, decreased IgA	IVIG may be helpful, but treatment usually unable to limit disease progression

TABLE 13-6 *(Continued)*

Disease	Description	Diagnosis	Treatment
Phagocytic cell disorders			
Chediak-Higashi syndrome	Autosomal recessive **dysfunction of neutrophils** resulting in recurrent *Staphylococcus aureus,* streptococcal, gram-negative bacteria, and fungal infections; associated with **abnormal platelets** and **albinism**	Large granules seen in granulocytes on peripheral smear	Appropriate antibiotics, bone marrow transplant
Chronic granulomatous disease	Defect in which neutrophils **cannot digest** engulfed bacteria resulting in recurrent bacterial and fungal infections	Cutaneous, pulmonary, and perirectal abscess formation; chronic lymphadenopathy	Appropriate antibiotics, prophylaxis with TMP-SMX, γ-interferon

Hct, hematocrit; Hgb, hemoglobin; IVIG, intravenous immune globulin; TMP-SMX, trimethoprim-sulfamethoxazole; WBC, white blood cell.

II. Immune disorders

A. Congenital immune deficiencies are uncommon and may be due to defects in T cells and/or B cells, or phagocytic cells (see Table 13-6)

B. **H/P** = frequent and **recurrent infections** beginning after three months of age including diseases caused by opportunistic pathogens; wound healing may be impaired

C. **Labs** = CBC detects general white blood cell (WBC) abnormalities; determination of specific WBCs affected (T cells, B cells, neutrophils, etc.) and peripheral blood smear can help determine precise cell type abnormality

D. **Treatment** — antibiotics (both prophylactic and therapeutic) are required to treat infections; severe immune deficiencies may require bone marrow transplant

E. **Complications** = recurrent infections, poor wound healing; death frequently occurs **prior to 3rd decade of life** (younger for severe deficiencies) because of body's inability to combat pathogens

III. Genetic disorders (chromosomal pathology)

A. **Sex chromosome disorders**

1. Diseases due to an abnormal number of **sex** chromosomes in the genetic karyotype

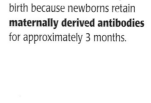

QUICK HIT
Presentation of immune disorders does not occur immediately after birth because newborns retain **maternally derived antibodies** for approximately 3 months.

QUICK HIT
Most pregnancies with a 45XO karyotype end in **spontaneous abortion.**

TABLE 13-7 **Common Sex Chromosome Disorders**

Condition	Karyotype	History and Physical
Turner syndrome	45XO or mosaicism	Female with **short stature, infertility,** abnormal genital formation, increased incidence for renal and cardiac defects **(coarctation of aorta),** craniofacial abnormalities (protruding ears, neck webbing, low occipital hairline)
Klinefelter's syndrome	47XXY	Male with **testicular atrophy,** tall and thin body, gynecomastia, infertility, mild mental retardation, and psychosocial adjustment abnormalities
XYY	47XYY	Male with tall body, significant acne, minimally increased risk for **violent and antisocial behavior**
XXX	47XXX	Female with increased incidence of mental retardation, menstrual abnormalities

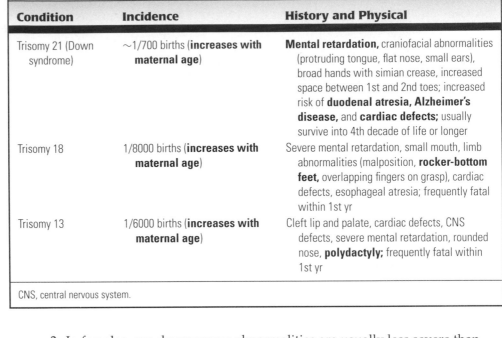

TABLE 13-8 Autosomal Trisomies		
Condition	**Incidence**	**History and Physical**
Trisomy 21 (Down syndrome)	~1/700 births (**increases with maternal age**)	**Mental retardation,** craniofacial abnormalities (protruding tongue, flat nose, small ears), broad hands with simian crease, increased space between 1st and 2nd toes; increased risk of **duodenal atresia, Alzheimer's disease,** and **cardiac defects;** usually survive into 4th decade of life or longer
Trisomy 18	1/8000 births (**increases with maternal age**)	Severe mental retardation, small mouth, limb abnormalities (malposition, **rocker-bottom feet,** overlapping fingers on grasp), cardiac defects, esophageal atresia; frequently fatal within 1st yr
Trisomy 13	1/6000 births (**increases with maternal age**)	Cleft lip and palate, cardiac defects, CNS defects, severe mental retardation, rounded nose, **polydactyly;** frequently fatal within 1st yr

CNS, central nervous system.

2. In females, sex chromosome abnormalities are usually less severe than autosomal disorders because **X chromosome inactivation** attempts to restore the normal number of active chromosomes and because Y chromosomes contain relatively **few** genes
3. **Labs** = karyotyping will reveal an abnormal number of sex chromosomes
4. **Treatment** =
   a. Growth hormone or androgen administration is used to treat short stature in Turner syndrome
   b. Special education or behavior counseling may be needed for mental impairments or antisocial behavior
   c. Generally, patients are able to live productive adult lives
B. **Trisomies**
   1. Syndromes that occur because of **autosomal nondisjunction** or **genetic translocation** during sex cell production that result in extra copies of autosomal genetic material

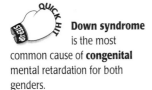

Down syndrome is the most common cause of **congenital** mental retardation for both genders.

TABLE 13-9 Common Deletion Syndromes		
Syndrome	**Deletion**	**History and Physical**
Cri du chat	Entire 5p chromosome arm	**High-pitched cat-like cry,** small head, low birth weight, mental retardation; early mortality may result from failure to thrive
Prader-Willi	15q11–15q13 (usually inherited from **father**)	**Overeating, obesity,** decreased muscular tone in infancy, mental retardation, small hands and feet; obesity-related complications may decrease lifespan
Angelman	15q11–15q13 (usually inherited from **mother**)	**Puppet-like movement, happy mood, unprovoked laughter,** mental retardation, seizures
Velocardiofacial	22q11	**Cleft palate,** cardiac defects, mild mental retardation, significant over-bite, association with DiGeorge syndrome; early mortality may result from associated cardiac complications or DiGeorge syndrome

PEDIATRICS

2. **Labs** =
   a. Karyotyping can detect extra chromosomes, and genetic screening can detect translocations
   b. Prenatal quadruple screen can help detect potentially affected fetuses, and amniocentesis may be used to confirm the diagnosis
3. **Treatment** =
   a. Supportive care
   b. Special education or selective environment used to handle mental retardation
   c. Surgical correction of anatomical defects when appropriate
   d. Genetic counseling and prenatal preparation recommended for parents

C. **Deletion syndromes**
   1. Diseases that result from deletion of all or part of an **autosomal** chromosome
   2. Usually severe disorders because of importance of missing genetic material
   3. **Labs** = high-resolution chromosome banding and fluorescence in situ hybridization techniques are useful for detecting small defects; karyotyping may detect substantial defects
   4. **Treatment** = supportive care; genetic counseling recommended for parents
   5. **Complications** = early mortality may result from associated abnormalities or diseases and not from deletions directly

D. **Fragile X syndrome**
   1. X-linked chromosomal disorder associated with mental retardation in **men;** women may be carriers and are unaffected
   2. End of X chromosome appears fragile and does not condense normally
   3. **H/P** = large face with **prominent jaw** and **large ears,** large testicles (macroorchidism), mental retardation, hyperactivity
   4. **Labs** = genetic screening detects hundreds of CGG repeats at end of X chromosome (number of repeats increases with each generation when inherited from a woman but not from a man); prenatal DNA analysis may be performed in mothers with a positive family history
   5. **Treatment** = appropriate genetic counseling for parents; special education and monitoring will likely be needed by affected males

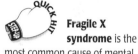

Fragile X syndrome is the most common cause of mental retardation in men.

TABLE 13-10 Important Pediatric Pathologies to Remember

Condition	Brief Description	Cross-Reference Chapter
Atrial/ventricular septal defect	Opening in septum of heart allowing shunting of blood	Chapter 1, Cardiovascular Disorders
Patent ductus arteriosus	Failure of ductus arteriosus to close after birth resulting in shunting of blood	Chapter 1, Cardiovascular Disorders
Tetralogy of Fallot	Ventricular septal defect, right ventricle hypertrophy, overriding aorta, and right ventricle outflow obstruction	Chapter 1, Cardiovascular Disorders
Croup	Inflammation of larynx	Chapter 2, Respiratory Disorders
Epiglottis	Infection of epiglottis leading to airway obstruction	Chapter 2, Respiratory Disorders
Respiratory distress of the newborn	Respiratory distress in premature infants due to surfactant deficiency	Chapter 2, Respiratory Disorders
Cystic fibrosis	Genetic exocrine gland disorder characterized by frequent respiratory infections and malabsorption	Chapter 2, Respiratory Disorders
Pyloric stenosis	Pyloric hypertrophy causing gastric obstruction	Chapter 3, Gastrointestinal Disorders
Intussusception	Telescoping of bowel into adjacent bowel resulting in obstruction	Chapter 3, Gastrointestinal Disorders
Wilm's tumor	Malignant renal tumor in children	Chapter 4, Genitourinary Disorders
Cretinism	Congenital hypothyroidism leading to poor physical and mental development	Chapter 5, Endocrine Disorders
Hemolytic disease of the newborn	Neonatal hemolysis due to Rh sensitization of the mother prior to birth	Chapter 6, Hematology/Oncology
Childhood leukemias	Malignant transformation of myeloid or lymphoid cells in bloodstream and bone marrow	Chapter 6, Hematology/Oncology
Neural tube disorders	Failure of neural tube to close during fetal development leading to spectrum of neurologic disorders	Chapter 8, Neurologic Disorders
Cerebral palsy	Neurologic injury during prenatal/perinatal insult leading to motor deficits	Chapter 8, Neurologic Disorders
Retinoblastoma	Malignant tumor of retina in children	Chapter 8, Neurologic Disorders
Developmental dysplasia of the hip	Poor development of acetabulum in fetus leading to congenital hip dislocation	Chapter 9, Musculoskeletal Disorders
Scoliosis	Non-correcting curvature of the spine	Chapter 9, Musculoskeletal Disorders
Acne vulgaris	Inflammation of hair follicles and sebaceous glands common in adolescence	Chapter 10, Dermatologic Disorders
Precocious puberty	Pubertal development beginning prior to anticipated age of sexual development	Chapter 11, Gynecologic Disorders
Primary amenorrhea	Absence of menses by time of anticipated initiation with normal secondary sexual characteristic development	Chapter 11, Gynecologic Disorders
Attention-deficit hyperactivity disorder	Problematic inattention and hyperactivity in school-age children	Chapter 14, Psychiatric Disorders

Rh, rhesus factor.

Psychiatric Disorders

I. Psychiatric evaluation

A. **History**

1. Patient's chief complaint (what he or she perceives as wrong) may **not** be the only issue that the physician needs to address

2. Review of systems (signs and symptoms), as well as past medical history should be performed to help detect if there are any **medical conditions** that may be causing a psychiatric disturbance

3. Family history should be explored to determine if certain psychiatric behaviors appear to be inherited

4. Social history should address **drug use,** employment history, legal issues, **relationships,** education, sexual history, and precipitating factors

B. **Examination and studies**

1. Physical examination should be used to detect contributory and comorbid medical conditions (frequently performed by other provider prior to psychiatric presentation)

2. Labs may be performed to aid in detection of any medical conditions or drug use

3. Head CT or MRI is useful for detecting cerebral lesions when suspected

C. **Mental status examination**

1. **Appearance, attitude, and behavior**

   a. Appearance and behavior help evaluate the patient's **ability to function** and **mental state** (e.g., depression, mania, psychosis, etc.)

   b. Attitude may suggest paranoia, personality disorders, or mood disorders

2. **Speech**

   a. Tone, rate, and volume should be noted

   b. Augmented qualities may suggest mania or aggressive behavior

   c. Reduced qualities may suggest depressed mood, social withdrawal, or impaired consciousness

3. **Mood and affect**

   a. **Mood** is the patient's **subjective** emotional state

   b. **Affect** is the way a patient **expresses** his or her state of mood

4. **Thought and language**

   a. **Production of thought** abnormalities include

      (1) **Impoverished** thought (decreased interaction with others or difficulty reasoning)

      (2) **Blocked** thoughts (sudden stops in thought processes)

      (3) **"Flight of ideas"** (rapid transitions from one incomplete thought to another)

   b. **Form of thought** abnormalities include

      (1) **Circumstantiality** (unnecessary details but arrival at a conclusion)

Ability to function generally refers to a patient's ability to live independently, perform normal activities of daily life, and function as a contributing member of society.

TABLE 14-1	**Multi-Axis Classification of Psychiatric Disorders**	
Axis	**Category**	**Examples**
I	Clinical psychiatric disorders	Mood disorders, anxiety disorders, substance abuse, delirium
II	Personality and development disorders	Borderline personality disorder, mental retardation
III	Medical conditions	Encephalopathy, neoplasm, HIV
IV	Psychosocial stresses	Support structures, social environment, occupational factors
V	Global assessment of functioning	(100-point scale that describes how well the patient has functioned in society)

     (2) **Tangentiality** (deviations from original topic to another one)
     (3) **Loose associations** (illogical jumps from one subject to another)
     (4) **"Word salad"** (using individual words without logical sense or sentence form)
     (5) **Neologisms** (using made-up words)
  c. **Thought content** may feature
     (1) **Abnormal fears** (phobias)
     (2) **Persistent thoughts** (obsessions)
     (3) **Urges** to perform a task (compulsions)
     (4) **False** beliefs **without** a realistic basis (delusions)
5. **Perception**
  a. Processing of sensory information
  b. **Hallucinations** and paranoid delusions are examples of abnormalities
6. **Cognition**
  a. **Level of consciousness** is capacity to interact with the environment
  b. **Orientation** is awareness of time, place, and identity
  c. **Concentration** is the ability to maintain attention to task
  d. **Memory** is the ability to retrieve mentally stored information
  e. **Intelligence** is the ability to learn, process, and retain new information
D. Psychiatric disorders may be described according to the multi-axis system

II. Mood disorders

A. **Major depressive disorder**
  1. Experience of significant depression that:
    a. Is not attributable to drug use, medical conditions, or bereavement
    b. Impacts the patient's ability to function
    c. Lasts >2 weeks
  2. Following resolution, these depressive episodes have a 50% chance of recurring
  3. Infrequently, patients may show signs of psychosis
  4. **H/P =**
    a. Diagnosis requires presence of **five symptoms** as listed below including either depressed mood or anhedonia (loss of interest in previously pleasurable activity) **lasting >2 weeks**
     (1) **Depressed mood or anhedonia**
     (2) Change in sleep patterns (insomnia, hypersomnia)
     (3) Feelings of guilt
     (4) Fatigue
     (5) Inability to concentrate
     (6) Changes in appetite (usually reduction)

Bereavement is **grief** following the death of a loved one and is characterized by sadness, difficulty concentrating, decreased appetite, insomnia, and recurrent thoughts or dreams of the deceased person. Symptoms appear periodically, may last >1 year, **self-resolve,** and **do not** affect ability to function.

The characteristics of major depressive disorder may be remembered with the mnemonic **SIGECAPS:** **S**adness (depressed mood), **I**nsomnia, **G**uilt, **E**nergy reduction (fatigue), **C**oncentration impairment, **A**ppetite changes, **P**sychomotor disturbances, **S**uicidal ideation.

(7) Psychomotor disturbances (impaired motor ability related to mental state)

(8) **Suicidal ideation**

5. **Treatment =**

a. Psychotherapy (cognitive or behavioral counseling and instruction designed to provide insight into condition and modify behavior) and pharmacological therapy are initial treatments (combined or alone) (see Table 14-2)

b. Electroconvulsive therapy (ECT) may be used for refractory or severe cases to decrease frequency of major depressive episodes

B. **Dysthymic disorder**

1. Feelings of **depression on more days than not** for >2 years with **no history of major depressive episodes**

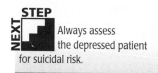

NEXT STEP Always assess the depressed patient for suicidal risk.

QUICK HIT Risks for **successful** suicide attempts include age >45 years, violent behavior, **drug use**, prior suicidal attempts, male gender, recent loss, **depression**, unemployment, or being single/widowed/divorced.

TABLE 14-2	Antidepressant Medications		
Drug/Class	**Mechanism**	**Indications**	**Adverse Effects**
Selective serotonin-reuptake inhibitors (SSRIs) (e.g., fluoxetine, sertraline, paroxetine)	Block presynaptic serotonin reuptake to increase synaptic free-serotonin concentration and postsynaptic serotonin receptor occupancy	First-line treatment for depression	Require 3-4 weeks of administration before they take effect; sexual dysfunction, increased risk of GI bleeding, may increase risk of suicidal ideation in adolescents
Tricyclic antidepressants (TCAs) (e.g., imipramine, amitriptyline, desipramine)	Block norepinephrine and serotonin reuptake to potentiate postsynaptic receptor activity	Second-line treatment for depression; may be useful in patients with comorbid neurologic pain	Easy to overdose and may be fatal at only 5 times therapeutic dose (due to cardiac QT interval prolongation that causes arrhythmias), sedation, weight gain, sexual dysfunction, anticholinergic symptoms,
Monoamine oxidase inhibitors (MAOIs) (e.g., phenelzine, isocarboxazid, tranylcypromine)	Block monoamine oxidase activity to inhibit deamination of serotonin, norepinephrine, and dopamine and increase levels of these substances	Second-line treatment for depression; may be particularly useful in treatment of depression with neurologic symptoms or in refractory cases	Dry mouth, indigestion, fatigue, headache, dizziness; consumption of foods containing tyramine (cheese, aged meats, beer) may cause hypertensive crisis
Bupropion	Poorly understood; may be related to inhibition of dopamine reuptake and augmentation of norepinephrine activity	Depression with fatigue and difficulty concentrating or comorbid ADHD	Headache, insomnia, weight loss
Venlafaxine	Inhibits reuptake of serotonin, norepinephrine, and dopamine	Refractory depression	Nausea, dizziness, insomnia, sedation, constipation, possible risk of overdose
Trazodone	Poorly understood but related to serotonin activity	Depression with significant insomnia	Hypotension, nausea, sedation
Mirtazapine	Blocks α_2 receptors and serotonin receptors to increase adrenergic neurotransmission	Depression with insomnia	Dry mouth, weight gain, sedation

ADHD, attention-deficit hyperactivity disorder; GI, gastrointestinal.

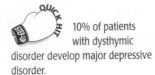

10% of patients with dysthymic disorder develop major depressive disorder.

On average, most bipolar patients experience four cycles of episodes in a 10-year period, but some may experience rapid cycles.

The characteristics of manic episodes may be remembered with the mnemonic **DIGFAST:** **D**istractibility, **I**nsomnia, **G**randiosity (feelings of), **F**light of ideas, **A**ctivity (increase in goal-oriented), **S**peech (pressured), **T**aking risks.

Adjustment disorder differs from **bereavement** in that the patient's ability to function normally is **impaired** in the **former** but **not** in the **latter.**

2. Milder but more chronic than major depressive disorder
3. **H/P** = Diagnosis requires depressed mood plus two or more of the symptoms below for a majority of days for >2 years and no history of major depressive episodes
   a. **Depressed mood**
   b. Change in sleep patterns
   c. Change in appetite
   d. Fatigue
   e. Inability to concentrate
4. **Treatment** = psychotherapy is initial treatment; pharmacologic agents may be used for continued depressive symptoms

C. **Bipolar disorder**
1. **Cyclic depression** and **mania** (or hypomania) that impairs patient's ability to function during episodes; patient is able to function normally between episodes
2. Types
   a. Bipolar I—depression alternates with manic episodes
   b. Bipolar II—depression occurs with occasional hypomanic episodes
3. **H/P** = depressive episodes are similar to those seen with major depressive disorder
   a. **Manic episodes** are characterized by **easy distractibility, insomnia,** feelings of grandiosity, flight of ideas, pressured speech, **increased goal-oriented activity,** increased risky pleasurable activity, and psychomotor agitation
   b. **Hypomanic episodes** are characterized by symptoms similar to those in mania but of a **milder degree** that **does not limit function**
   c. Diagnosis requires history of at least one manic or hypomanic episode (with three or more symptoms lasting >1 week) and recurrent major depressive episodes
4. **Treatment** =
   a. **Mood stabilizers** (lithium, carbamazepine, valproic acid, gabapentin, topiramate) are used to control and prevent manic and hypomanic episodes
   b. Lithium is frequently the first line drug for treatment of mania; its mechanism is unknown but likely involves inositol triphosphate activity
     (1) Adverse effects associated with lithium include hypothyroidism, polyuria, tremor, weight gain, renal insufficiency, teratogenesis, and confusion
     (2) Carbamazepine and valproic acid are more effective than lithium in patients with rapid cycling
   c. **Antidepressants** are used to treat depression
   d. Antipsychotic medications may be required for some patients with rapid cycling or refractory disease

D. **Cyclothymia**
1. Rapid cycling of hypomania and mild depression lasting >2 years without a period of normal mood >2 months
2. Mood level does not impair ability to function
3. **H/P** = symptoms of dysthymia that alternate with hypomanic episodes
4. **Treatment** = psychotherapy or mood stabilizers

E. **Adjustment disorder with depressed mood**
1. Behavioral and mood changes that occur within 3 months of a **stressful event** (e.g., death in family, assault, divorce) and cause significant impairment of ability to function
2. **H/P** =
   a. Sadness, inability to concentrate, **self-isolation,** change in sleep patterns, change in appetite

b. Symptoms begin within 3 months of stressful event and typically end 6 months after end of stressor

3. **Treatment** = psychotherapy; antidepressants may be used if psychotherapy alone is not able to permit normal daily functioning

III. Anxiety disorders

A. Panic disorder

1. Experience of recurrent, spontaneous panic attacks with associated fear that these episodes will occur; typically begins in late adolescence
2. **H/P** =
   a. **Recurrent panic attacks** (extreme anxiety and feeling of impending danger with chest pain, shortness of breath, palpitations, diaphoresis, nausea, dizziness, feeling of losing control, or chills or hot flashes) that occur without warning and last up to 30 minutes
   b. Diagnosis requires a history of recurrent episodes plus a **persistent fear that attacks will happen again**
3. **Treatment** =
   a. Psychotherapy may help alleviate fear between attacks and decrease panic attack occurrence
   b. Benzodiazepines (especially **alprazolam**) may be used to break attacks once they have started
   c. Selective serotonin reuptake inhibitors (SSRIs) may be useful for long-term therapy in patients with frequent attacks

Panic disorder:
- Increased incidence in patients with **mitral valve prolapse.**
- Occasionally associated with **agoraphobia** (fear of public places).

B. Specific phobia

1. Fear of a **particular object, activity,** or **situation** that causes patient to avoid feared subject; typically begins in childhood
2. **H/P** = encountering feared subject incites panic attack, and patient makes great effort to avoid feared subject; some patients may experience vasovagal response (fainting) during episodes
3. **Treatment** = psychotherapy involving desensitization through repeated exposure, relaxation techniques, hypnosis, or insight modification

C. Social phobia

1. Excessive fear of **social situations** and anxiety that results when the patient encounters such situations; typically begins in adolescence
2. **H/P** = social situations (e.g., performances, conversations) cause anxiety that may be mild or severe (i.e., panic attacks); patients avoid these situations and carry persistent fear of being embarrassed
3. **Treatment** =
   a. Psychotherapy
   b. β-Blockers may be used in mild cases to prevent tachycardia and diaphoresis
   c. Benzodiazepines may be useful in more symptomatic cases
   d. Monoamine oxidase inhibitors (MAOIs) may be used in refractory cases

D. Obsessive-compulsive disorder (OCD)

1. Significant, recurrent **obsessions** (e.g., feeling unclean, need for organization, recurrent images) and **compulsions** (e.g., counting, frequent or repetitive hand washing, placing items in a certain order) that **affect daily life** and function; typically begins in adolescence
2. **H/P** =
   a. Defined recurrent obsessions and compulsions that significantly affect ability to function and may take up considerable time in daily activity
   b. Patients are aware of behaviors but feel unable to control them
   c. Stressful events may exacerbate behaviors
   d. Diagnosis requires presence of obsessions and compulsions that significantly affect daily life

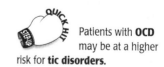

Patients with **OCD** may be at a higher risk for **tic disorders.**

TABLE 14-3	Anxiolytic Medications		
Drug	**Mechanism**	**Indications**	**Adverse Effects**
Benzodiazepines (e.g., alprazolam, clonazepam, diazepam)	Increase GABA inhibition of neuronal firing	Alprazolam has a rapid onset and short half-life and is particularly useful for treatment of panic disorder; clonazepam and diazepam are more useful for prolonged therapy	Sedation, confusion; stopping alprazolam usage is associated with withdrawal symptoms of restlessness, confusion, and insomnia (especially with frequent use)
Buspirone	Unclear, but related to serotonin and dopamine receptors	Anxiety disorders in which abuse or sedation is a concern	Headaches, dizziness

GABA, gamma aminobutyric acid.

3. **Treatment** = psychotherapy and pharmacologic therapy (SSRIs or clomipramine) help limit and control behavior

E. **Post-traumatic stress disorder (PTSD)**
1. Syndrome of anxiety symptoms that occur following **exposure to** a **significantly stressful event;** symptoms typically begin within three months of event
2. **H/P** =
   a. **Vivid dreams** or **recurrent intrusive thoughts** of traumatic event
   b. Avoidance of activity or settings associated with event, anhedonia, feelings of **detachment**, increased state of arousal, survivor guilt, social withdrawal
   c. Diagnosis requires patient to have been exposed to a traumatic event that caused significant distress, symptoms of reliving event through dreams or intrusive thoughts, avoidance of associations with event, and increased arousal lasting >1 month in acute cases and >3 months in chronic cases
3. **Treatment** = SSRIs, MAOIs, or mood stabilizers; psychotherapy may also be helpful in eliminating intrusive thoughts

F. **Generalized anxiety disorder**
1. Excessive, **persistent** anxiety that impairs ability to function and occurs more days than not for >6 months; typically begins in early adulthood
2. **Risk factors** = women two-times more likely than men
3. **H/P** =
   a. Anxiety about daily activities, inability to concentrate, restlessness, insomnia, irritability, muscle tension
   b. Diagnosis requires anxiety for majority of days plus three of above symptoms for >6 months
4. **Treatment** = psychotherapy and anxiolytics improve symptoms (see Table 14-3); SSRIs may be helpful in refractory cases

IV. **Psychotic disorders**
A. **Schizophrenia**
1. Severe psychotic disorder that causes significant limitations in ability to function; typically begins in late adolescence
2. **Risk factors** = family history; significantly higher rate in homeless and indigent patients likely secondary to their inability to function in society
3. **H/P** = periodic psychotic exacerbations with increased severity of symptoms; baseline function is generally impaired and worsens over time

It is **very difficult** to commit suicide using an overdose of benzodiazepines because their lethal dose is >1000 times the therapeutic dose. **Flumazenil** is a benzodiazepine antagonist that can reverse the effects of an overdose.

PSYCHIATRIC DISORDERS

TABLE 14-4 **Subtypes of Schizophrenia**

Subtype	Description
Paranoid	Excessive paranoia; hallucinations and ideas of reference may be particularly severe
Catatonic	Rigid posturing, poor response to stimuli
Disorganized	Flat affect, disorganized speech, inappropriate and disorganized behavior
Undifferentiated	Does not fit into other subtype descriptions

a. **Positive** symptoms—**delusions, hallucinations** (usually auditory), **disorganized thoughts and behavior,** thought broadcasting (belief that others can read the patient's thoughts or that thoughts are being transmitted to others), ideas of reference (belief that hidden meanings are found in common items)

b. **Negative** symptoms—**social withdrawal, flat affect** (displaying little emotional response to stimuli), apathy, anhedonia, inattentiveness

c. Patterns of certain symptoms may classify disease into subtypes (see Table 14-4)

d. Diagnosis requires presence of two or more symptoms plus impaired social function for >6 months

4. **Treatment =**

a. **Antipsychotics** (also known as neuroleptics) are the mainstay of therapy (see Table 14-5)

TABLE 14-5 **Antipsychotic Medications**

Drug Type	Mechanism	Indications	Adverse Effects
Atypical antipsychotics (clozapine, risperidone, olanzapine, sertindole, quetiapine)	Block **dopamine** and **serotonin** receptors	• **1st-line** drugs for maintenance therapy for psychotic disorders • Clozapine is most effective neuroleptic but is reserved for refractory psychosis due to risk of agranulocytosis	Anticholinergic effects, weight gain, arrhythmias, seizures; **clozapine** carries risk of **agranulocytosis;** frequency and severity of side effects is significantly **less** than seen with traditional neuroleptics
Traditional high-potency (haloperidol, droperidol, fluphenazine, thiothixene)	Block **dopamine** receptors	• Strong positive symptoms • Frequently 2nd-line drugs for maintenance therapy • **Fewer anticholinergic** side effects than other traditional drugs	**Extrapyramidal effects** (dystonia, parkinsonism), **tardive dyskinesia, anticholinergic effects** (sedation, constipation, urinary retention, hypotension), confusion, sexual dysfunction, **neuroleptic malignant syndrome,** seizures, arrhythmias
Traditional medium-potency (trifluoperazine, perphenazine)	Block dopamine receptors	• Strong positive symptoms • Frequently 2nd-line drugs for maintenance therapy • May be used in patients exhibiting significant extrapyramidal **and** anticholinergic side effects with other traditional neuroleptics	Similar to other traditional drugs
Traditional low-potency (thioridazine, chlorpromazine)	Block dopamine receptors	• Strong positive symptoms • Frequently 2nd-line drugs for maintenance therapy • **Fewer extrapyramidal** side effects than other traditional drugs	Similar to other traditional drugs

High-potency antipsychotics have **more extrapyramidal** side effects and **fewer anticholinergic** side effects. **Low**-potency antipsychotics have **fewer extrapyramidal** side effects and **more anticholinergic** side effects.

Tardive dyskinesia is a complication of antipsychotic medications that begins **after several months** of therapy and is characterized by **repetitive facial movements** (e.g., chewing, lip smacking). It should be treated by stopping the offending drug if the patient's condition allows, but may be **irreversible.**

Neuroleptic malignant syndrome is:

- An uncommon complication of antipsychotic medications that starts within **days** of usage and carries a high mortality rate.
- Characterized by **high fever, muscle rigidity,** decreased consciousness, and increased blood pressure and heart rate.
- Treated by immediately **stopping** use of the drug and administering **dantrolene.**

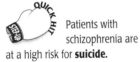

Patients with schizophrenia are at a high risk for **suicide.**

PSYCHIATRIC DISORDERS

b. Psychotic exacerbations may require hospitalization
c. Psychotherapy may be helpful to teach patient how to recognize symptoms

5. **Complications** =
   a. Generally poor prognosis with gradual deterioration over several years in ability to function in society
   b. Good prognostic factors include a history of mood disorder, mostly positive symptoms, and good support systems
   c. Prognostic factors for a worse outcome include mostly negative symptoms, motor or sensory neurologic signs, and poor support systems

B. **Other psychotic disorders**
   1. Psychotic disorders that are less common than schizophrenia but may demonstrate several similarities (see Table 14-6)
   2. Not due to organic causes
   3. May differ from schizophrenia by being of shorter duration (schizophreniform or brief psychotic disorder), accompanied by mood disorder (schizoaffective disorder), defined by the presence of delusions only (delusional disorder), or involving multiple persons (shared psychotic disorder)

V. Personality disorders

A. Persistent behavior that **deviates significantly from cultural norms**
   1. Manifested through perception of others, affect, interpersonal relationships, and impulse control

TABLE 14-6 Psychotic Disorders Not Classified as Schizophrenia

Disorder	Description	Treatment
Schizophreniform	Symptoms similar to schizophrenia but **last < 6 months;** patients return to normal function following resolution of psychotic episode; increased risk of true schizophrenia developing in future	Antipsychotics
Schizoaffective	Presence of **mood disorder with psychotic symptoms;** diagnosis requires presence of psychotic symptoms during normal mood for >2 weeks	Mood stabilizers, antidepressants; antipsychotics used for acute exacerbations
Delusional	Presence of 1 or more distinct **realistic delusions** lasting >1 month without any other psychotic symptoms; patient is able to function normally; **unrealistic delusions** are classified as **schizophreniform disorder or schizophrenia**	Antipsychotics
Brief psychotic	**Sudden** onset of psychotic symptoms (possibly stress-related) that last **<1 month**	Psychotherapy or low-dose antipsychotics; hospitalization necessary if symptoms affect ability to function
Shared psychotic (Folie à deux)	**Second patient** accepts and becomes involved in delusions of a psychotic patient	Group psychotherapy, antipsychotics; second patient's acceptance of delusions will wane if separated from primary patient

2. Behavior is **persistent** and **inflexible** despite situation
3. Behavior leads to impaired ability to function
4. Behavior begins in late adolescence
5. Behavior is not attributable to drug use, medical condition, or other psychiatric disorder

B. Clusters (see Table 14-7)
1. Classification system of personality disorders
2. Cluster A—odd or eccentric ("weird")
3. Cluster B—dramatic or emotional ("wild")
4. Cluster C—anxious or fearful ("wimpy")

VI. Substance abuse

A. Chronic use of a substance (e.g., drug) that impairs daily life and is notable for the development of tolerance (increasing doses are required for desired effect), withdrawal (symptoms that occur if use is stopped), desire to decrease use, feelings of loss of control over use, and significant amount of time devoted to procuring and using substance (see Table 14-8)

B. Intoxication is the reversible central nervous system (CNS) effect of a substance following usage

C. Dependence may be physical (causing withdrawal if not used) or compulsive (persistent use despite awareness of overuse)

VII. Eating disorders

A. **Anorexia nervosa**
1. Eating disorder in which patients **refuse to maintain normal body weight** through fasting, excessive exercise, or purging
2. Patients have distorted body image and believe that they are overweight
3. **Risk factors** — adolescence, high socioeconomic status; 90% of cases are women
4. **H/P** = body weight <85% ideal body weight, **fixation upon prevention of weight gain,** amenorrhea, cold intolerance, hypothermia, dry skin, lanugo hair growth (fine, short hair similar to that in the newborn), bradycardia
5. **Treatment** =
   a. Inpatient treatment is frequently required to aid in weight gain
   b. Psychotherapy involving family which focuses on body image, weight gain, sufficient caloric intake is needed to maintain long-term control
6. **Complications** = electrolyte abnormalities, arrhythmias (especially ventricular types)

B. **Bulimia**
1. Eating disorder in which patients **feel lack of control over eating behavior** and engage in binge eating but maintain **normal** body weight through purging, excessive exercise, or laxative use
2. **H/P** =
   a. Patients feel ashamed of condition and body weight drives self-image
   b. Dental enamel erosion (due to repeated vomiting), scars on hands (from inducing vomiting), parotid enlargement, oligomenorrhea
   c. Diagnosis requires history of binge eating followed by some form of compensatory behavior at least two times per week for >3 months
3. **Treatment** = psychotherapy directed at body image and reduction of binging-compensation cycles; SSRIs or MAOIs help in behavior modification

A patient who exhibits mild signs of a personality disorder but is able to function normally in society is said to have a **personality trait** and may not require treatment.

NEXT STEP Use the **CAGE** questionnaire to screen for drug abuse (especially alcohol). More than 1 "yes" response to any of these conditions should raise suspicion for excessive use:
Desire to **Cut down** on usage
Annoyance over others' suggestions to stop usage
Guilt over usage
Drug use upon waking (i.e., **Eye-opener**)

NEXT STEP Patients with anorexia nervosa should be screened for **depression**, and SSRIs should be included in treatment if depression is diagnosed.

Anorexia nervosa requiring hospitalization has >5% mortality.

PSYCHIATRIC DISORDERS

TABLE 14-7 Personality Disorders

Disorder	Characteristics	Treatment
Cluster A		
Paranoid	Persistent distrust of others, others' actions consistently interpreted as harmful or deceptive, reluctant to share information, frequent misinterpretation of comments, frequent angry reactions, common substance abuse	Supportive, nonjudgmental psychotherapy, low-dose antipsychotics
Schizoid	Inability to form close relationships, social detachment, emotionally restricted	Antipsychotics to initially resolve behavior, supportive psychotherapy focusing on achieving comfortable interactions with others
Schizotypal	Paranoia, ideas of reference, eccentric and inappropriate behavior, social anxiety, disorganized speech	Supportive psychotherapy focusing on recognition of reality, low dose antipsychotics or anxiolytics
Cluster B		
Antisocial	Aggressive behavior towards people and animals, destruction of property, illegal activity, pathological lying, irritability, risk-taking behavior, lack of responsibility, lack of remorse for actions; more common in men	Structured environment, psychotherapy with defined limit-setting may be helpful in controlling behavior
Borderline	Unstable relationships, need for attention, poor self-esteem, impulsivity, mood lability, suicidal ideation, sudden irritability, paranoia; much more common in women	Extensive psychotherapy employing multiple techniques combined with low-dose antipsychotics, SSRIs, or mood stabilizers
Histrionic	Dire need for attention, seductive behavior, emotional lability, shallow relationships, dramatic speech	Long-term psychotherapy focusing on relationship development and limit-setting
Narcissistic	Grandiosity, fantasies of success, manipulation of others, expectation of admiration, arrogance	Psychotherapy focusing on acceptance of shortcomings
Cluster C		
Avoidant	Fear or criticism and embarrassment, social withdrawal, fear of intimacy, poor self-esteem, reluctance to try new activities	Psychotherapy (initially individualized then group therapy later) focusing on self-confidence combined with antidepressants or anxiolytics
Dependent	Difficulty making decisions, fear of responsibility, need for supportive figure, lack of autonomy	Psychotherapy focusing on developing social skills and development of decisive behavior
Obsessive-compulsive	Preoccupied with details, perfectionistic, inflexible in beliefs, miserly, difficulty working with others, hoarding of worthless objects	Psychotherapy focusing on accepting alternative ideas and working with others
Not Fitting into Any Cluster		
Passive-aggressive	Passive resistance to rules, procrastinating, deliberately inefficient, sulking when not getting one's way	Supportive psychotherapy
Self-defeating	Self-sacrificing to maintain relationships, frequent complaints about status, frequent grudges, sabotages others efforts to help, refuses to admit to happiness	Psychotherapy focusing on insight of self-defeating behavior

TABLE 14-8	Characteristics of Substance Abuse			
Substance	Intoxication	Withdrawal	Complications of Chronic Use	Treatment
Alcohol	**Decreased inhibition,** slurred speech, **impaired coordination,** inattentiveness, decreased consciousness, retrograde amnesia	Diaphoresis, tachycardia, nausea, vomiting, tremor, **delirium tremens** (seizures, delirium)	**Malnutrition** (vitamin B$_{12}$, thiamine), encephalopathy (Wernicke-Korsakoff), **accidents,** suicide, **cirrhosis,** GI bleeding; higher incidence of abuse in patients with other psychiatric disorders	Supplemental nutrition, supportive psychotherapy or **group counseling** (Alcoholics Anonymous, etc.), disulfiram causes unpleasant nausea and vomiting if taken before alcohol consumption, benzodiazepines prevent delirium tremens during withdrawal
Amphetamines	**Hyperactivity,** psychomotor agitation, **pupillary dilation,** tachycardia, hypertension, psychosis	Anxiety, depression, increased appetite, fatigue	Psychosis	Rehabilitative counseling, antipsychotics, benzodiazepines
Benzodiazepines	Sedation, amnesia	Anxiety, insomnia, **seizures**	Minimal	Rehabilitative counseling, anticonvulsants
Caffeine	**Insomnia,** restlessness, tremor, anxiety, tachycardia	Headaches, fatigue	GI irritation	Gradual reduction in usage
Cocaine	**Euphoria,** tachycardia, psychomotor agitation, pupillary dilation, hypertension, paranoia, **grandiosity**	Sedation, depression, psychomotor retardation	Arrhythmias, **sudden cardiac death,** stroke	Reduction of hypertension, antipsychotics, benzodiazepines, rehabilitative counseling
Lysergic acid diethylamide (LSD)	**Hallucinations,** delusions, anxiety, paranoia, tachycardia, pupillary dilation, tremors	Minimal	Psychosis	Remove patient from dangerous environment until intoxication resolves, antipsychotics
Marijuana	**Euphoria,** paranoia, psychomotor retardation, impaired judgment, increased appetite, **conjunctival injection,** dry mouth	Minimal	**Amotivational syndrome,** infertility	Rehabilitative counseling
Nicotine (and other substances found in tobacco and cigarettes)	Restlessness	Insomnia, weight gain, irritability, inability to concentrate	**Cancer** (many different forms), **COPD,** increased respiratory infections, ischemic heart disease	Rehabilitative counseling, cutaneous (patch) or mucosal (gum) **nicotine** administration to reduce cravings for cigarettes, hypnosis, **bupropion**
Opioids	**Euphoria,** slurred speech, **pupillary constriction,** inattentiveness, decreased consciousness, **respiratory depression**	Depression, anxiety, **stomach cramps, nausea, vomiting,** diarrhea	Constipation, increased risk of **blood-borne infection** with IV drug use	**Methadone therapy,** inpatient rehabilitative counseling, naltrexone may prevent euphoria with use, naloxone is opioid antagonist used for acute overdose with significant respiratory depression
Phencyclidine (PCP) ("Angel dust")	Euphoria, impulsiveness, **aggressive behavior, nystagmus** (vertical and horizontal), hyperreflexia	**Sudden violent behavior**	Psychosis	Isolated containment until after resolution of intoxication, benzodiazepines, antipsychotics

COPD, chronic obstructive pulmonary disease; GI, gastrointestinal; IV, intravenous.

VIII. **Somatoform and factitious disorders**
  A. **Somatization disorder**
    1. **Multiple** recurrent **physical symptoms** that are **unintentional** and **cannot be explained by any medical condition;** typically begins in young adulthood
    2. **Risk factors** = women five times more likely than men
    3. **H/P** = diagnosis requires pain in four unrelated regions:
      a. Two gastrointestinal (GI) symptoms: nausea, vomiting, diarrhea, indigestion
      b. One sexual symptom: decreased libido, erectile dysfunction, menorrhagia
      c. One pseudo-neurologic symptom: ataxia, weakness, urinary retention, paresthesias, hallucinations
      d. Symptoms cannot be explained by medical conditions and are unintentional
    4. **Treatment** = psychotherapy may help alleviate symptoms; patients may be resistant to psychiatric treatment
  B. **Conversion disorder**
    1. Development of **sensory** or **motor deficits following stress** without associated medical conditions or intention
    2. **H/P** = onset of sensory (paresthesias, blindness, deafness) or motor (paralysis, loss of voice) deficits or pseudo-seizures that generally follow stressful situations; symptoms cannot be linked to any findings on examination
    3. **Treatment** = psychotherapy helps identify stressors with reactions and encourages normal responses to stressful situations
  C. **Hypochondriasis**
    1. Excessive fear that a minor symptom represents a serious illness that limits daily function; typically begins in middle age
    2. **H/P** =
      a. **Preoccupation with fear of having a serious illness** that persists despite a healthy medical evaluation, minor symptoms are frequently perceived as representative of severe disease, fear impairs ability to function
      b. Diagnosis requires above symptoms lasting >6 months
    3. **Treatment** =
      a. Regular physician visits help to alleviate fears
      b. Patient frequently resistant to psychiatric treatment
      c. Primary care physician should work with psychiatrist to review therapies
  D. **Body dysmorphic disorder**
    1. **Preoccupation with an imagined defect in appearance** that limits ability to function; typically begins in adolescence
    2. **H/P** = patient imagines physical defect in distinct body region, frequently presents to dermatologist or plastic surgeon to "improve" defect, and continues to imagine defect following surgery
    3. **Treatment** =
      a. Psychotherapy addressing self-perception
      b. Antidepressants may help in refractory cases
      c. Avoid performing needless surgery
  E. **Munchausen syndrome** (factitious disorder)
    1. **Intentional induction** of disease symptoms or signs by a patient that carries **no clear benefit** to patient
    2. May involve any organ system
    3. **H/P** =

NEXT **STEP** Conversion disorder in which the symptoms are **pain at multiple body sites** is called **pain disorder** and should be treated with psychotherapy and antidepressants. It may be distinguished from fibromyalgia by its relation to stressful events.

NEXT **STEP** Munchausen's syndrome *by proxy* is a disorder in which **parents** try to make their **children** appear to have a certain disease. It is considered **child abuse** and must be reported to the appropriate authorities.

a. Patient reports symptoms or signs of a given disease and attempts to induce disease process (self-injections of insulin or excrement, attempts to become infected by a pathogen, induction of GI illness, etc.)

b. Diagnosis requires **intentional production of symptoms or signs** by patient, **denial** of intention, **wandering** of patient from one physician to another, and **no clear incentive** for patient's actions

4. **Treatment =**
   a. Patient denial makes treatment difficult
   b. No unnecessary therapies should be administered
   c. If patient is willing, psychotherapy involving family may be beneficial

F. **Malingering**

1. **Intentional induction** of disease or reporting of symptoms by a **patient who will benefit** from appearing ill

2. **H/P =** patient reports symptoms for a certain disease in order to realize a personal gain (time off from work, financial compensation, particular therapy, etc.); patients will frequently leave site of care if they are confronted or realize that a goal is unattainable

3. **Treatment =** avoid necessary treatment; report suspicious activity to higher authority (psychiatrist, hospital patient data base, ethics committee)

IX. Delirium and dementia

A. **Delirium**

1. **Altered state of consciousness**
   a. Secondary to:
      (1) **Drugs** (e.g., alcohol, corticosteroids, benzodiazepines, oral contraceptive pills, antipsychotics, NSAIDs, chemotherapeutics, isoniazid, anticholinergics, antihistamines, antiarrhythmics)
      (2) Infection, **hypoxia,** or CNS abnormalities
   b. It is frequently quickly **reversible** once the underlying cause is identified and treated

2. **H/P =**
   a. Altered awareness of environment and level of consciousness that fluctuates
   b. Confusion, inattentiveness, impaired concentration, psychosis (delusions, paranoia, hallucinations), emotional lability, irritability
   c. Symptoms frequently worsen at night (i.e., "sun-downing")
   d. Mini-mental state examination (MMSE) may be used to test cognitive function (a score <25 indicates dysfunction)

3. **Labs =** should address potential metabolic or pharmacologic causes

4. **Radiology =** CT can be used to assess CNS insult

5. **Treatment = treat underlying cause;** antipsychotics and benzodiazepines may be used to decrease agitation

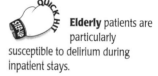
Elderly patients are particularly susceptible to delirium during inpatient stays.

B. **Dementia**

1. **Chronic progressive** cognitive impairment without changes in consciousness that may significantly limit ability to function (see Table 14-9)

2. Etiologies
   a. **Alzheimer's disease**—most common cause (>70% of cases) (see Chapter 8, Neurologic Disorders)
   b. **Vascular dementia**—dementia due to multiple cerebral infarcts (10% of cases); features **neurologic symptoms** in addition to dementia
   c. **Alcohol-induced**—due to chronic alcoholism; typically associated with aphasias

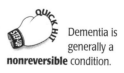
Dementia is generally a **nonreversible** condition.

FIGURE
14-1 Mini-mental state examination.

Score

1. Orientation to time—ask patient to identify year, season, date
   day, and month (1 point each, 5 total)
2. Orientation to place—ask patient to name country, state, town,
   hospital, floor (1 point each, 5 total)
3. Registration—name 3 words and ask patient to repeat them
   (1 point for each correct repeat, 3 total)
4. Attention and calculation—ask patient to spell "world" backwards
   or to count backward from 100 by 7s (5 points total)
5. Language (9 points total)
   a. point at a pen and a watch and ask patient to name
      them (1 point each)
   b. ask patient to repeat phrase "No ifs, ands, or buts"
      (1 point)
   c. give patient a sheet of paper and ask to hold it in the
      right hand, fold it in half, and put it on the floor
      (1 point for each activity)
   d. ask patient to close eyes (1 point)
   e. ask patient to write a sentence (1 point)
   f. ask patient to copy design below (1 point):

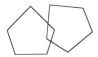

6. Recall—ask patient to repeat 3 objects recited earlier (1 point
   for each correct repeat, 3 total)

TOTAL SCORE

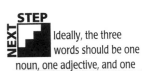

NEXT STEP Ideally, the three words should be one noun, one adjective, and one verb to avoid ease of recall due to patterns among words.

   d. Less common causes—Parkinson's disease, Huntington's disease,
      normal pressure hydrocephalus, endocrine diseases, metabolic
      diseases, neoplasms, infection
3. **H/P =**
   a. Impaired short and long-term memory, impaired abstract thought,
      poor judgment, personality changes, aphasia, fine motor impairment

TABLE 14-9 **Comparison of Delirium and Dementia**

Characteristic	Delirium	Dementia
Onset	Acute	Gradual
Daily course	Fluctuates between levels of consciousness; sun-downing	Generally consistent; sun-downing
Level of consciousness	Decreased	Normal
Orientation	Aware of self; impaired for time and place	Generally impaired
Thought production	Disorganized, flight of ideas	Impoverished
Psychotic features	Delusions, hallucinations	Minimal
Memory	Short-term impairment	Short and long-term impairment
Prognosis	Reversible	Usually nonreversible

b. Symptoms are initially mild and progress gradually (weeks to months)

c. MMSE shows impaired cognitive function

4. **Labs** = should be used to rule out endocrine or metabolic causes (glucose, vitamin B_{12}, thyroid hormones, electrolytes)

5. **Radiology** = CT or MRI of head may be useful for detecting cortical infarcts

6. **Treatment** =

a. Treat underlying cause if possible (metabolic, endocrine, infectious causes may be reversible)

b. **Occupational therapy** is helpful for extending independence and preventing accidents

c. Patient frequently will eventually require supervised care

d. Antipsychotics may be used to treat exacerbations of agitation

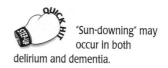

"Sun-downing" may occur in both delirium and dementia.

X. Pediatric psychiatric disorders

A. **Attention-deficit hyperactivity disorder (ADHD)**

1. Disorder of **inattention** and **hyperactivity** in school-age children that causes problems both at home and at school

2. **Risk factors** = four-times more common in males than females

3. **H/P** =

a. Inattention—**decreased attention span, difficulty following instructions,** carelessness in tasks, easily losing items, forgetful, poor listening, easy distractibility

b. Hyperactivity—fidgetiness, **impulsivity, inappropriate activity,** excessive talking, unable to remain quiet, impatience, interrupting of others

c. Children exhibit behaviors in **multiple settings**

d. Diagnosis requires child to have six inattention symptoms and six hyperactivity symptoms before turning 7 years old that limit ability to function

4. **Treatment** =

a. Psychostimulants (methylphenidate, pemoline) improve ability to focus and control behavior

b. Psychotherapy used to address child's self-esteem and help modify behavior

c. Bupropion, α-agonists, and tricyclic antidepressants (TCAs) are used in refractory cases

d. Limit consumption of food high in caffeine

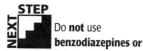

STEP **NEXT** Do **not** use **benzodiazepines or anticholinergics** in the treatment of delirium- or dementia-related agitation because they may **worsen** symptoms.

B. **Conduct disorder**

1. Repetitive disruptive and antisocial behavior that violates others' rights and social norms

2. **H/P** = **aggressive behavior** (violence, property destruction, illegal activity); diagnosis requires behavior lasting >1 year

3. **Treatment** = psychotherapy involving family; mood stabilizers may be used in severe cases

4. **Complications** = increased risk of substance abuse, **antisocial personality disorder**

C. **Tourette's syndrome**

1. Chronic tic disorder beginning in childhood; associated with ADHD and OCD

2. **H/P** = **multiple motor** (blinking, twitching, etc.) and **vocal** (sounds, words) **tics** that worsen with stress; diagnosis requires presence of tics for >1 year and beginning before patient is 18 years old

3. **Treatment** = psychotherapy with family addressing nature of tics; low-dose haloperidol, pimozide, or clonidine may reduce tic occurrence

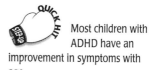

Most children with ADHD have an improvement in symptoms with age.

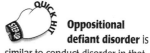

Oppositional defiant disorder is similar to conduct disorder in that patients exhibit aggressive behavior, but illegal and destructive activity does not occur.

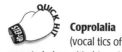

Coprolalia (vocal tics of repeated obscenities) is only seen in a **minority** of cases of Tourette's syndrome.

PSYCHIATRIC DISORDERS

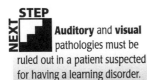

Tics typically **diminish** during sleep and focused activity.

STEP NEXT **Auditory** and **visual** pathologies must be ruled out in a patient suspected for having a learning disorder.

D. **Learning disorders**
  1. **Impairment in educational development** in a **healthy** child with **no** other psychiatric diagnosis or cognitive pathology (e.g., Down's syndrome, Fragile X syndrome)
  2. Disorder may be specific to ability to read, perform mathematics, or express thoughts
  3. **H/P =**
     a. Child demonstrating otherwise **normal intelligence** with **delays in certain academic goals**
     b. Children frequently have poor self-esteem
     c. Language delays or poor coordination may be evident
  4. **Labs** = scores on standardized tests are consistently lower than normal range
  5. **Treatment** = special education focusing on the specific learning disorder can help the child to improve his or her ability to learn

E. **Autism**
  1. Severe persistent impairment in **interpersonal interactions,** communication, and social activities; may be associated with mental retardation and schizophrenia
  2. **H/P =**
     a. Poor language development, **difficulty communicating with others,** impaired ability to interact with others
     b. Patient frequently demonstrates poor eye contact, unawareness of others, insistence on routine behavior (deviations from routine may cause inappropriate emotional responses)
  3. **Treatment =**
     a. Psychotherapy with peers and family may help improve social interaction
     b. Aggressive behavior may be treated with antipsychotics
     c. Supervised environment is usually required long term

Epidemiology and Ethics

I. Research studies

A. **Study requirements**

1. Subjects in a study must be **representative of the population** that the study seeks to examine
2. The study must contain a **sufficient number of subjects** to make it statistically significant
3. Subjects must give **informed consent**, except under special circumstances approved by an institutional review board (IRB) (e.g., trauma patients)
4. Proper **controls** should be included in studies that examine the efficacy of a given treatment
5. The interests of the patient must take priority over the interests of the study (study must be approved by IRB)

B. **Study designs** (see Table 15-1)

C. **Bias** (see Table 15-2)

II. Biostatistics

A. **Rates of disease**

1. **Incidence** = (# of new cases of a disease in a given time) / (total population)
2. **Prevalence** = (# of existing cases of a disease) / (total population)
3. **Disease frequency** = (# of people with a disease) / (at-risk population)
4. **Case fatality rate** = (people who die from a disease in a given time) / (# of cases of disease during given time)

B. **Risk of disease** (see Table 15-3)

1. **Relative risk (RR)**
   a. Risk of disease in people exposed to a given factor
   b. RR = (disease in exposed population) / (disease in unexposed population) = [A / (A + B)] / [C / (C + D)]
   c. **RR value**
      (1) **>1** suggests a **positive** relationship between exposure and disease
      (2) **<1** suggests a **negative** relationship between exposure and disease
      (3) **=1** suggests **no** relationship between exposure and disease
2. **Odds ratio (OR)**
   a. Odds of exposure among patients with a disease compared to odds of exposure among patients without a disease
   b. Estimate of relative risk
   c. OR = (A / C) / (B / D) = **(A × D) / (B × C)** (see Table 15-3)
3. **Attributable risk** (AR)
   a. Difference in rates of disease between exposed and unexposed populations
   b. AR = (rate of disease in exposed population) − (rate of disease in unexposed population)

 Investigator and observational bias may be avoided by **double-blinding** a study.

 Confounding variables are factors that affect **both** the experimental and control groups to interfere with the relationship **between** these groups.

 Relative risk is determined through **cohort** studies.

 Odds ratio is determined through **case-control** studies.

 The odds ratio is most accurate as an estimate of relative risk in cases of **rare diseases.**

EPIDEMIOLOGY AND ETHICS

TABLE 15-1 Study Designs Used in Clinical Research

Study Type	Description	Conclusions	Advantages	Disadvantages
Randomized clinical trial	• **Prospective comparison** of **experimental** treatment to **placebo** controls and **existing** therapies • **Double-blinded** to avoid bias • Patients **randomized** into study groups	Effectiveness of experimental treatment compared to controls and existing therapies	• **Gold standard** for testing therapies • May be controlled for several confounders	Often **costly** and **time consuming**
Case series	• Report of characteristics of a disease by examining multiple cases	Hypothesis for risk factors	• May be easy to complete • Provides insight into poorly understood conditions	Cannot be used to test hypotheses
Cohort study	• Examines a group of subjects **exposed** to a given situation or factor • May be **prospective** (exposed group identified and followed over time) or **retrospective** (examines exposed group in whom disease has already occurred)	**Relative risk**	• Able to examine **rare exposures** • Can study multiple effects of exposure	May be costly and time consuming; difficult to study rare diseases
Case-control study	• Retrospective comparison of patients with a **disease** to healthy controls; frequency of certain exposures in both groups is considered	**Odds ratio**	• Able to examine **rare diseases** • Can study multiple types of exposure • May examine small group size	Susceptible to **recall bias**; cannot determine disease incidence
Cross-sectional survey	• **Survey** of large number of people at one time to assess exposure and disease prevalence	Hypothesis for risk factors; disease prevalence	• Can be used as estimate for disease prevalence following exposure	Cannot be used to test hypotheses
Meta-analysis	• **Pooling** of multiple studies examining a given disease or exposure	Depends on original study type	• Larger study size • Can resolve conflicts in literature	Unable to eliminate limiting factors in original studies

Screening tests seek to **rule out** a disease in a patient.

Confirmatory tests are used to **validate** that a patient with a positive test truly has a disease.

C. **Statistics of diagnostic tests** (see Table 15-4)
   1. **Sensitivity**
      a. Probability that a screening test will be **positive** in **patients with a disease**
      b. Sensitivity = **A/(A + C)**
      c. Most acceptable screening tests are typically >80% sensitive
      d. **False negatives** occur in patients with a disease and a negative test; approximated by (1 − sensitivity)
   2. **Specificity**
      a. Probability that a test will be **negative** in **patients without a disease**
      b. Specificity = **D/(B + D)**
      c. Most acceptable confirmatory tests are typically >85% specific
      d. **False positives** occur in patients without a disease and a positive test; approximated by (1 − specificity)

TABLE 15-2 Types of Bias in Clinical Studies		
Type of Bias	**Description**	**Consequences**
Enrollment (selection)	**Nonrandom** assignment of subjects to study groups	Results of study not applicable to general population
Investigator	Subjective interpretation of data by **investigator** deviates towards **"desired"** conclusions	Results of study incorrectly resemble proposed hypothesis
Lead-time	Screening test provides **earlier diagnosis** in studied group compared to controls but has **no effect on time of survival**	Time from diagnosis to outcome increases to cause a false appearance of increased time of survival; time from disease occurrence to outcome actually remains the same regardless of screening
Length	Screening test **detects** several **slowly** progressive cases of a disease and **misses rapidly** progressive cases	Effectiveness of screening test is overstated
Observational	Subjects may respond to subjective questions in a different way than normal because **awareness** of the study changes their perception of the examined issue	Effectiveness of therapy is not accurately depicted by study group
Publication	Studies that show a difference between groups are **more likely to be published** than studies that do not show a difference	Data available for meta-analyses may not include studies that support the null hypothesis
Recall	Errors of memory within subjects due to **prior confounding experiences**	Patients with negative experiences are more likely to recall negative details
Self-selection	Patients with a certain **past medical history** may be more likely to participate in a study related to their condition	Subjects are not representative of the general population and introduce confounding variables

3. **Positive predictive value (PPV)**
   a. Probability that a patient with a positive test has a disease
   b. PPV = **A / (A + B)**
4. **Negative predictive value (NPV)**
   a. Probability that a patient with a negative test does not have a disease
   b. NPV = **D / (C + D)**

 A disease with a
- **high** prevalence will be associated with a high **positive** predictive value in a screening test.
- **low** prevalence will be associated with a high **negative** predictive value in a screening test.

TABLE 15-3 Calculation of Disease Risk			
		Disease	
		Yes	No
Exposure	Yes	**A**	**B**
	No	**C**	**D**
Relative risk (RR) = [A / (A + B)] / [C / (C + D)]; Odds ratio (OR) = (A / C) / (B / D) = **(A × D) / (B × C)**			

TABLE 15-4 **Analysis of Diagnostic Tests**		Disease	
		Yes	No
Test Positive		**A**	**B**
Negative		**C**	**D**

Sensitivity = A / (A + C); Specificity = D / (B + D); Positive predictive value (PPV) = A / (A + B); Negative predictive value (NPV) = D / (C + D)

D. **Types of error**
 1. **Null hypothesis**—states that there is no association between exposure and disease or treatment and response
 2. **Type I error**—null hypothesis is rejected even though it is true (**false positive**)
 3. **Type II error**—null hypothesis is not rejected even though it is false (**false negative**)
 4. Risk of these errors decreases with increasing sample size

E. **Significance**
 1. Statistically detectable difference between groups
 2. Probability value (**p-value**)
  a. Chance of a type I error occurring for a given result
  b. If **p <0.05,** the null hypothesis can be rejected (i.e., there is a significant relationship between groups)

III. Ethics
 A. **Rights of the patient**
  1. **Confidentiality**
   a. All information regarding the patient must be kept **private** between the **physician** and the **patient**
   b. The Health Insurance Portability and Accountability Act (HIPAA)
    (1) All patient account handling, billing, and medical records must be designed to maintain patient confidentiality
    (2) Exchange of patient information may only occur between care providers involved with the care of the patient in question
   c. Confidentiality is **not mandated** when the patient
    (1) Allows the physician to share information with designated others (family, etc.)
    (2) Carries a disease that is legally reportable (reported only to appropriate public officials)
    (3) Is considered to be **suicidal** or **homicidal**
    (4) Is an adolescent with a condition that is potentially harmful to self or others
  2. **Public reporting**
   a. Reporting of several diseases is required by law (including **HIV, STDs** hepatitis, Lyme disease, several food-borne illnesses, meningitis, rabies, and **tuberculosis**)
   b. Impaired ability to drive, **child abuse,** and **elder abuse** must be reported to authorities (exact legal requirements vary from state to state)
  3. **Informed consent**
   a. **Prior to any procedure or therapy,** the patient must be made aware of the indications, risks, and potential benefits of a proposed treatment;

The **null hypothesis** suggests that there is **no association** between exposure and disease or treatment and response. The **alternative hypothesis** suggests that there **is an association.**

Confidentiality should be maintained in **adolescents** seeking treatment for **STDs** or **pregnancy** (this point may need to be clarified with parents).

The patient should be made aware that certain diseases or conditions must be reported.

alternative treatments and their risks and the risks of refusing treatment must also be described

b. Informed consent or parental consent for minors is not required for emergent therapy (**implied consent**)

c. If a patient is not capable of making a decision, a designated surrogate decision maker is required for nonemergent care

4. **Disclosure**

a. Patients have the right to be made aware of their medical status, prognosis, treatment options, and medical errors in their care

b. If a family requests that a physician withhold information from the patient, physicians must deny the request unless it is determined that disclosing information would significantly harm the patient

B. **Patient decision making**

1. **Competency**

a. A competent patient is entitled to make all decisions regarding his or her medical care

b. To be judged competent, a patient must

(1) Not be diagnosed as presently psychotic

(2) Have an **understanding** of his or her **medical situation**

(3) Must be capable of making decisions that are in agreement with his or her history of values

c. Medical decisions for non-emancipated minors (i.e., <18 years old) are made by a minor's parents unless legally ruled to be not in the best interests of the child

2. **Durable power of attorney**

a. Legal documentation that designates a **second party** (e.g., family member) **as a surrogate decision maker** for medical issues

b. Designated individual should be able to make decisions **consistent with the patient's values**

c. Not valid in all U.S. states (e.g., NY)

3. **Living will**

a. Written document that details a patient's wishes in specific medical situations (resuscitation, ventilation, extraordinary maintenance of life)

b. May be less flexible than durable power of attorney

C. **End-of-life issues**

1. **Do-not-resuscitate order (DNR)**

a. A type of living will that details care in cases of coma, cardiac arrest, severe dementia, and terminal illness

b. DNR may refuse all nonpalliative therapies or may only restrict use of specific therapies (ventilation, cardiopulmonary resuscitation, feeding tubes, antibiotics, etc.)

2. **Life support**

a. Competent patients may request to have supportive measures withdrawn at any time

b. Wishes for life support (or withholding it) may be described in a living will or DNR

c. Physicians are able to remove respiratory care in cases in which there is **no living will** and the patient is **incapable** of voicing a decision **if the family and** the **physician** believe that removal of care is **consistent** with **what the patient would want**

3. **Physician-aided death**

a. Physician-assisted suicide occurs when a physician **supplies** a patient with a means of ending his or her life

b. Euthanasia is the **active administration by a physician** of a lethal agent to a patient in order to end suffering from a condition

c. Physician-assisted suicide is legal in few parts in the United States, and euthanasia is illegal in the entire United States

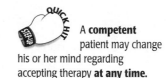 A **competent** patient may change his or her mind regarding accepting therapy **at any time.**

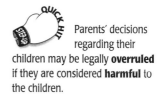 Parents' decisions regarding their children may be legally **overruled** if they are considered **harmful** to the children.

 Physicians are not required to supply therapies that are irrational for the current condition or when the maximum therapy has already failed.

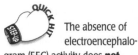

The absence of electroencephalo-gram (EEG) activity does **not** define brain death.

4. **Death**
   a. **Brain death** is defined as the irreversible **absence** of all brain activity (including the brainstem) in a patient lasting >6 hours
      (1) Absence of cephalic (i.e., cranial nerve) reflexes (e.g., gag, corneal, and caloric reflexes)
      (2) Apnea off of a ventilator for a duration sufficient to produce a normal hypercarbic drive
      (3) Absence of hypothermia or intoxication
      (4) Absent brain stem evoked responses, persistent isoelectric electroencephalogram (EEG), or absent cerebral circulation on radiologic testing
   b. **Heart death** is considered the inability to restore a spontaneous heartbeat in an asystolic patient
   c. **Hypothermic** patients must be warmed to normal body temperature before death can be declared
5. **Organ donation**
   a. Patients may declare themselves as organ donors prior to death (e.g., living will, driver's license)
   b. Hospitals receiving payments from Medicare are required to approach the family of the deceased regarding organ donation
   c. Patients and families may define exactly what organs may be donated
   d. Organs may be judged unsuitable for donation in cases of widespread or uncured **neoplasm, sepsis,** compromised organ function, organ-specific infection or disease, or **prolonged ischemia**

Index

Note: Page numbers followed by f indicate figure; those followed by t indicate table.